Teen Health Series

Part One

Understanding Stress and the Stress Response

Stress-Related Disorders

Disorders

SOURCEBOOK

Second Edition

Health Reference Series

Second Edition

Stress-Related Disorders
SOURCEBOOK

*Basic Consumer Health Information about Stress
and Stress-Related Disorders, Including Types of
Stress, Sources of Acute and Chronic Stress, the Im-
pact of Stress on the Body's Systems, and Mental and
Emotional Health Problems Associated with Stress,
Such as Depression, Anxiety Disorders, Substance
Abuse, Posttraumatic Stress Disorder, and Suicide;*

*Along with Advice about Getting Help for Stress-Related
Disorders, Information about Stress Management Techniques, a Glossary of Stress-Related Terms, and a Directory of Resources for Additional Help and Information*

Edited by
Amy L. Sutton

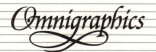

P.O. Box 13-1640 • Detroit, MI 48231

Bibliographic Note

Because this page cannot legibly accommodate all the copyright notices, the Bibliographic Note portion of the Preface constitutes an extension of the copyright notice.

Edited by Amy L. Sutton

Health Reference Series

Karen Bellenir, *Managing Editor*
David A. Cooke, M.D., *Medical Consultant*
Elizabeth Collins, *Permissions and Research Coordinator*
Cherry Stockdale, *Permissions Assistant*
EdIndex, Services for Publishers, *Indexers*

* * *

Omnigraphics, Inc.

Matthew P. Barbour, *Senior Vice President*
Kay Gill, *Vice President—Directories*
Kevin Hayes, *Operations Manager*

* * *

Peter E. Ruffner, *Publisher*

Copyright © 2007 Omnigraphics, Inc.

ISBN 978-0-7808-0996-3

Table of Contents

Visit www.healthreferenceseries.com to view *A Contents Guide to the Health Reference Series*, a listing of more than 13,000 topics and the volumes in which they are covered.

Part II: The Physical Effects of Stress

Part IV: Stress after Trauma, Loss, or Disaster

Part V: Controlling and Reducing Stress

Part VI: Additional Help and Information

Preface

About This Book

Nearly half of U.S. adults report concern about the stress in their lives, with work and money leading the list of major stressors. Stress is sometimes caused by traumatic events such as death, divorce, or mass disaster, but it often develops due to everyday frustrations with career, financial difficulties, technology, or caregiving. Stress impacts both physical and mental health by contributing to such problems as sleeplessness, reduced immunity, diabetes, depression, and anxiety. In severe cases, untreated or chronic stress may even lead to substance abuse, posttraumatic stress disorder, or suicide.

Stress-Related Disorders Sourcebook, Second Edition provides information about the origins and types of stress and describes physical and mental health disorders that may develop during and after stressful situations. Readers will learn about the link between stress and chronic pain, cardiovascular disease, and digestive disorders. The *Sourcebook* also discusses how stress contributes to mental health problems, including depression, anxiety disorders, posttraumatic stress disorder, and addiction to tobacco, alcohol, and drugs. Information about trauma, loss, and grief is presented, along with comprehensive facts about stress management techniques, such as relaxation training, meditation, exercise, and anger management. Tips on helping children and teens cope with stress are also offered, along with a glossary of related terms and a directory of resources.

How to Use This Book

This book is divided into parts and chapters. Parts focus on broad areas of interest. Chapters are devoted to single topics within a part.

Part I: Understanding Stress and the Stress Response provides an overview of the physical and mental symptoms of acute and chronic stress and identifies common causes of stress, including genes and personality traits, work, financial difficulties, caregiving responsibilities, and social isolation. It also offers insight into stress-related concerns in children, adolescents, men and women, and elderly adults.

Part II: The Physical Effects of Stress offers detailed information about how stress impacts the body's physical systems, including the brain and nerves, immune system, heart and blood vessels, hormones, and reproductive organs. This part also describes how stress alters weight, sleep, and chronic pain levels.

Part III: Stress and Mental Health Disorders discusses the link between stress and depression, panic disorder, obsessive-compulsive disorder, social phobia, specific phobias, and generalized anxiety disorder. Information about tobacco, alcohol, and drug addiction and their relationship to stress is also provided.

Part IV: Stress after Trauma, Loss, or Disaster explores typical stress reactions to trauma and loss and identifies severe stress reactions that may arise, such as posttraumatic stress disorder and suicide. This part also describes warning signs of suicide and offers suggestions for helping children and adolescents cope with devastating trauma.

Part V: Controlling and Reducing Stress identifies both traditional and alternative approaches to coping with stress. Tips on managing stress with nutrition and exercise, yoga and tai chi, massage therapy, meditation, and herbal remedies are included, as well as strategies for controlling anger, preventing road rage, reducing stress at work, and seeking social support.

Part VI: Additional Help and Information includes a glossary of important terms and a directory of government and private organizations that provide information to people with stress-related disorders.

Bibliographic Note

This volume contains documents and excerpts from publications issued by the following U.S. government agencies: Centers for Disease

Control and Prevention (CDC); National Cancer Institute (NCI); National Center for Complementary and Alternative Medicine (NCCAM); National Center for Posttraumatic Stress Disorder (NCPTSD); National Heart, Lung, and Blood Institute (NHLBI); National Highway Traffic Safety Administration (NHTSA); National Institute for Occupational Safety and Health (NIOSH); National Institute of Diabetes, Digestive, and Kidney Diseases (NIDDK); National Institute of Mental Health (NIMH); National Institute of Neurological Disorders and Stroke (NINDS); National Institute on Aging (NIA); National Institute on Alcohol Abuse and Alcoholism (NIAAA); National Institute on Drug Abuse (NIDA); National Institutes of Health (NIH); National Women's Health Information Center (NWHIC); Substance Abuse and Mental Health Services Administration (SAMHSA); U.S. Army Center for Health Promotion and Preventive Medicine; and the U.S. Food and Drug Administration (FDA).

In addition, this volume contains copyrighted documents from the following organizations and individuals: A.D.A.M., Inc.; Rachel Adelson; American Academy of Dermatology; American Academy of Periodontology; American Council for Headache Education; American Council on Consumer Interests; American Federation for Aging Research; American Heart Association; American Institute of Architects; American Psychological Association; Anorexia Nervosa and Related Eating Disorders, Inc.; Anxiety Disorders Association of America; Beth Azar; British Autogenic Society; Child Abuse Prevention Fund/Children's Hospital and Health System; Rebecca Clay; Cleveland Clinic Foundation; DePuy Orthopaedics, Inc.; Duke University Health System; Harris Interactive Inc.; HealthandAge Foundation; Helpguide.org; Hormone Foundation; International Society for Traumatic Stress Studies; Mount Sinai School of Medicine; National Center on Physical Activity and Disability; National Multiple Sclerosis Society; National Sleep Foundation; Nemours Center for Children's Health Media/TeensHealth.org; North Dakota State University Extension Service; Organization of Teratology Information Specialists; Regents of the University of California; Regents of the University of Michigan; University of Louisville Research Foundation; University of Minnesota Extension; and the Wisconsin Department of Health and Family Services, Division of Public Health.

Full citation information is provided on the first page of each chapter or section. Every effort has been made to secure all necessary rights to reprint the copyrighted material. If any omissions have been made, please contact Omnigraphics to make corrections for future editions.

Acknowledgements

Thanks go to the many organizations, agencies, and individuals who have contributed materials for this *Sourcebook* and to medical consultant Dr. David Cooke and document engineer Bruce Bellenir. Special thanks go to managing editor Karen Bellenir and permissions and research coordinator Liz Collins for their help and support.

About the Health Reference Series

The *Health Reference Series* is designed to provide basic medical information for patients, families, caregivers, and the general public. Each volume takes a particular topic and provides comprehensive coverage. This is especially important for people who may be dealing with a newly diagnosed disease or a chronic disorder in themselves or in a family member. People looking for preventive guidance, information about disease warning signs, medical statistics, and risk factors for health problems will also find answers to their questions in the *Health Reference Series*. The *Series*, however, is not intended to serve as a tool for diagnosing illness, in prescribing treatments, or as a substitute for the physician/patient relationship. All people concerned about medical symptoms or the possibility of disease are encouraged to seek professional care from an appropriate health care provider.

A Note about Spelling and Style

Health Reference Series editors use *Stedman's Medical Dictionary* as an authority for questions related to the spelling of medical terms and the *Chicago Manual of Style* for questions related to grammatical structures, punctuation, and other editorial concerns. Consistent adherence is not always possible, however, because the individual volumes within the *Series* include many documents from a wide variety of different producers and copyright holders, and the editor's primary goal is to present material from each source as accurately as is possible following the terms specified by each document's producer. This sometimes means that information in different chapters or sections may follow other guidelines and alternate spelling authorities. For example, occasionally a copyright holder may require that eponymous terms be shown in possessive forms (Crohn's disease *vs.* Crohn disease) or that British spelling norms be retained (leukaemia *vs.* leukemia).

Locating Information within the Health Reference Series

The *Health Reference Series* contains a wealth of information about a wide variety of medical topics. Ensuring easy access to all the fact sheets, research reports, in-depth discussions, and other material contained within the individual books of the *Series* remains one of our highest priorities. As the *Series* continues to grow in size and scope, however, locating the precise information needed by a reader may become more challenging.

A Contents Guide to the Health Reference Series was developed to direct readers to the specific volumes that address their concerns. It presents an extensive list of diseases, treatments, and other topics of general interest compiled from the Tables of Contents and major index headings. To access *A Contents Guide to the Health Reference Series*, visit www.healthreferenceseries.com.

Medical Consultant

Medical consultation services are provided to the *Health Reference Series* editors by David A. Cooke, M.D. Dr. Cooke is a graduate of Brandeis University, and he received his M.D. degree from the University of Michigan. He completed residency training at the University of Wisconsin Hospital and Clinics. He is board-certified in Internal Medicine. Dr. Cooke currently works as part of the University of Michigan Health System and practices in Ann Arbor, MI. In his free time, he enjoys writing, science fiction, and spending time with his family.

Our Advisory Board

We would like to thank the following board members for providing guidance to the development of this *Series*:

- Dr. Lynda Baker, Associate Professor of Library and Information Science, Wayne State University, Detroit, MI
- Nancy Bulgarelli, William Beaumont Hospital Library, Royal Oak, MI
- Karen Imarisio, Bloomfield Township Public Library, Bloomfield Township, MI
- Karen Morgan, Mardigian Library, University of Michigan-Dearborn, Dearborn, MI
- Rosemary Orlando, St. Clair Shores Public Library, St. Clair Shores, MI

Health Reference Series *Update Policy*

The inaugural book in the *Health Reference Series* was the first edition of *Cancer Sourcebook* published in 1989. Since then, the *Series* has been enthusiastically received by librarians and in the medical community. In order to maintain the standard of providing high-quality health information for the layperson the editorial staff at Omnigraphics felt it was necessary to implement a policy of updating volumes when warranted.

Medical researchers have been making tremendous strides, and it is the purpose of the *Health Reference Series* to stay current with the most recent advances. Each decision to update a volume is made on an individual basis. Some of the considerations include how much new information is available and the feedback we receive from people who use the books. If there is a topic you would like to see added to the update list, or an area of medical concern you feel has not been adequately addressed, please write to:

Editor
Health Reference Series
Omnigraphics, Inc.
P.O. Box 31-1640
Detroit, MI 48231
E-mail: editorial@omnigraphics.com

Chapter 1

Overview of Stress, Its Causes, and Stress-Related Disorders

Highlights

Stress affects most people to some degree. Acute (sudden, short-term) stress leads to rapid changes throughout the body. These changes could prove beneficial in a critical, life-or-death situation. Over time, however, repeated stressful situations put a strain on the body that may contribute to both physical and psychological problems. Chronic (long-term) stress can have real health consequences, and should be addressed like any other health concern.

Fortunately, research is showing that lifestyle changes and stress-reduction techniques can help people learn to manage their stress. In one study, people who received cognitive behavior training and were later exposed to stress had lower cortisol (stress hormone) levels as a result of the training. However, studies also show that many people must still learn these techniques and how to use them.

- The results of a national survey that were released in February 2006 show that: "Americans engage in unhealthy behaviors such as comfort eating, poor diet choices, smoking and inactivity to help deal with stress." The survey was conducted by American Psychological Association in partnership with the National Women's Health Resource Center and iVillage.com.

- A report issued in October 2006 by the American Academy of Pediatrics recommends more unstructured play time for children. The

"Stress," © 2007 A.D.A.M., Inc. Reprinted with permission.

report notes that today's over-scheduled, hurried lifestyle that many children experience is a source of stress and anxiety for some of them.

Introduction

The stress response of the body is somewhat like an airplane readying for take-off. Virtually all systems (the heart and blood vessels, the immune system, the lungs, the digestive system, the sensory organs, and brain) are modified to meet the perceived danger.

External and Internal Stressors

People can experience either external or internal stressors.

- External stressors include adverse physical conditions (such as pain or hot or cold temperatures) or stressful psychological environments (such as poor working conditions or abusive relationships). Humans, like animals, can experience external stressors.

- Internal stressors can also be physical (infections, inflammation) or psychological. An example of an internal psychological stressor is intense worry about a harmful event that may or may not occur. As far as anyone can tell, internal psychological stressors are rare or absent in most animals except humans.

Acute or Chronic Stress

Stressors can also be defined as short-term (acute) or long-term (chronic).

Acute stress: Acute stress is the reaction to an immediate threat, commonly known as the fight or flight response. The threat can be any situation that is experienced, even subconsciously or falsely, as a danger.

Common acute stressors include:

- noise (which can trigger a stress response even during sleep);
- crowding;
- isolation;
- hunger;
- danger;
- infection;

- high technology effects (playing video games, frequently ringing mobile phones); and
- imagining a threat or remembering a dangerous event.

Under most circumstances, once the acute threat has passed, the response becomes inactivated and levels of stress hormones return to normal, a condition called the relaxation response.

Chronic stress: Frequently, however, modern life poses ongoing stressful situations that are not short-lived. The urge to act (to fight or to flee) must therefore be controlled. Stress, then, becomes chronic. Common chronic stressors include:

- ongoing highly pressured work;
- long-term relationship problems;
- loneliness; and
- persistent financial worries.

The Body's Response

The best way to envision the effect of acute stress is to imagine yourself in a primitive situation, such as being chased by a bear.

The Brain's Response to Acute Stress

In response to seeing the bear, a part of the brain called the hypothalamic-pituitary-adrenal (HPA) system is activated.

Release of steroid hormones and the stress hormone cortisol: The HPA systems trigger the production and release of steroid hormones (glucocorticoids), including the primary stress hormone cortisol. Cortisol is very important in organizing systems throughout the body (including the heart, lungs, circulation, metabolism, immune systems, and skin) to deal quickly with the bear.

Release of catecholamines: The HPA system also releases certain neurotransmitters (chemical messengers) called catecholamines, particularly those known as dopamine, norepinephrine, and epinephrine (also called adrenaline).

Catecholamines activate an area inside the brain called the amygdala, which appears to trigger an emotional response to a stressful event. In the case of the bear, this emotion is most likely fear.

5

Effects on long- and short-term memory: During the stressful event, catecholamines also suppress activity in areas at the front of the brain concerned with short-term memory, concentration, inhibition, and rational thought. This sequence of mental events allows a person to react quickly, either to fight the bear or to flee from it. It also interferes with the ability to handle difficult social or intellectual tasks and behaviors during that time.

On the other hand, neurotransmitters at the same time signal the hippocampus (a nearby area in the brain) to store the emotionally loaded experience in long-term memory. In primitive times, this brain action would have been essential for survival, since long-lasting memories of dangerous stimuli (such as the large bear) would be critical for avoiding such threats in the future.

Response by the Heart, Lungs, and Circulation to Acute Stress

The stress response also affects the heart, lungs, and circulation:

- As the bear comes closer, the heart rate and blood pressure increase instantaneously.

- Breathing becomes rapid, and the lungs take in more oxygen.

- The spleen discharges red and white blood cells, allowing the blood to transport more oxygen throughout the body. Blood flow may actually increase 300–400%, priming the muscles, lungs, and brain for added demands.

The Immune System's Response to Acute Stress

The effect on the immune system from confrontation with the bear is similar to organizing a defensive line of soldiers to potentially critical areas. The steroid hormones reduce the activity in parts of the immune system, so that specific infection fighters (including important white blood cells) or other immune molecules can be repositioned. These immune-boosting troops are sent to the body's front lines where injury or infection is most likely to occur, such as the skin and the lymph nodes.

The Acute Response in the Mouth and Throat

As the bear gets closer, fluids are diverted from nonessential locations, including the mouth. This causes dryness and difficulty in talking. In addition, stress can cause spasms of the throat muscles, making it difficult to swallow.

The Skin's Response to Acute Stress

The stress effect moves blood flow away from the skin to support the heart and muscle tissues. This also reduces blood loss in the event that the bear causes a wound. The physical effect is a cool, clammy, sweaty skin. The scalp also tightens so that the hair seems to stand up.

Metabolic Response to Acute Stress

Stress shuts down digestive activity, a nonessential body function during short-term periods of hard physical work or crisis.

The Relaxation Response: The Resolution of Acute Stress

Once the threat has passed and the effect has not been harmful (for example, the bear has not wounded the human), the stress hormones return to normal. This is known as the relaxation response. In turn, the body's systems also return to normal.

Complications

In prehistoric times, the physical changes in response to stress were an essential adaptation for meeting natural threats. Even in the modern world, the stress response can be an asset for raising levels of performance during critical events such as a sports activity, an important meeting, or in situations of actual danger or crisis.

If stress becomes persistent and low-level, however, all parts of the body's stress apparatus (the brain, heart, lungs, vessels, and muscles) become chronically over- or under-activated. Such chronic stress may produce physical or psychological damage over time. Acute stress can also be harmful in certain situations, particularly in individuals with preexisting heart conditions.

Psychological Effects of Stress

Studies suggest that the inability to adapt to stress is associated with the onset of depression or anxiety. In one study, two thirds of subjects who experienced a stressful situation had nearly six times the risk of developing depression within that month.

Some evidence suggests that repeated release of stress hormone produces hyperactivity in the HPA system, and disrupts normal levels of serotonin, the nerve chemical that is critical for feelings of well-being. Certainly, on a more obvious level, stress reduces the quality of life by reducing feelings of pleasure and accomplishment. In addition, relationships are often threatened in times of stress.

Nevertheless, some stress may be beneficial. For example, some research has suggested that stress may be a risk factor for suicide. However, a 2003 study found a higher risk for suicide only in women reporting both low and very high stress. Those with moderate stress levels had the lowest risk.

Heart Disease

The effects of mental stress on heart disease are controversial. Stress can certainly influence the activity of the heart when it activates the automatic part of the nervous system that affects many organs, including the heart. Such actions and others could theoretically affect the heart badly in several ways:

- Sudden stress increases the pumping action and rate of the heart, while at the same time causing the arteries to constrict (narrow). This restricts blood flow to the heart. A 2002 study suggested that such actions may be responsible for some cases of acute stress that have been associated with a higher risk for serious heart problems. These problems include heart rhythm abnormalities and heart attacks, and even death in people with heart disease.

- Emotional effects of stress alter the heart rhythms, which could pose a risk for serious arrhythmias (rhythm abnormalities) in people with existing heart rhythm disturbances.

- Stress causes blood to become stickier (possibly in preparation of potential injury), increasing the likelihood of an artery-clogging blood clot.

- Stress appears to impair the clearance of fat molecules in the body, raising blood-cholesterol levels, at least temporarily.

- Chronic stress may lead to the production of immune factors called cytokines. Cytokines produce a damaging inflammatory response, which is now believed to be responsible for damage to the arteries. Such damage contributes to heart disease.

- Studies have reported an association between stress and hypertension (high blood pressure), which may be more pronounced in men than in women. According to some evidence, people who regularly experience sudden spikes in blood pressure (caused by mental stress) may, over time, develop injuries in the inner lining of their blood vessels. In one 20-year study, for example, men who periodically measured highest on the stress scale were twice as likely to have high blood pressure as those with normal stress.

Evidence is still needed to confirm any clear-cut relationship between stress and heart disease. For example, a 2002 study in Scotland found no greater risk for actual heart disease or heart events even in men who reported higher mental stress. In fact, higher stress was associated with fewer heart events. Men with high stress levels did tend to complain of chest pain and to go to the hospital for it more often than those with lower stress. They also went to the hospital more often.

Evidence has linked stress to heart disease in men, particularly in work situations where they lack control. The association between stress and heart problems in women is weaker, and there is some evidence that the ways women cope with stress may be more heart-protective. In one study, men were more apt than women to use alcohol or eat less healthily in response to stress than women, which might account for their higher heart risks from stress. Different stressors may affect genders differently. In one study, work stress was associated with a higher risk for heart disease in men, but marital stress—not work stress—was associated with more severe heart disease in women with existing heart problems.

Stress reduction and heart disease: Studies in 2001 and 2002 suggest that treatments that reduce psychological distress improve long-term outlook in people with heart disease, including after a heart attack. Some evidence indicates that stress management programs may reduce the risk of heart attacks by up to 75% in people with heart disease. Specific stress management techniques may help some problems but not others. For example, acupuncture in one study helped people with heart failure but had no effect on blood pressure. Relaxation methods, on the other hand, may help hypertensive individuals.

Stroke

One survey revealed that men who had a more intense response to stressful situations, such as waiting in line or problems at work, were more likely to have strokes than those who did not report such distress.

In some people, prolonged or frequent mental stress causes an exaggerated increase in blood pressure. In fact, a 2001 study has linked for the first time a higher risk for stroke in adult white men and elevated blood pressure during times of stress.

Effect on the Immune System

Chronic stress affects the immune system in complicated ways, and may produce various effects.

Susceptibility to infections: Chronic stress appears to blunt the immune system's response to infections, and may even impair a person's response to immunizations. Several studies have shown that people under chronic stress have low white blood cell counts and are vulnerable to colds. And once any person catches a cold or flu, stress can make symptoms worse. People who carry the herpes virus or HIV may be more susceptible to viral activation following exposure to stress. Even more serious, some research has found that HIV-infected men with high stress levels progress more rapidly to AIDS when compared to those with lower stress levels.

Inflammatory response: Some evidence suggests that chronic stress triggers an over-production of certain immune factors called cytokines, which in excess levels can have very damaging effects. In fact, such findings may partly explain the association between chronic stress and numerous diseases, including heart disease and asthma.

Cancer

Current evidence does not support the idea that stress causes cancer or recurrence in cancer survivors. For example, a 2002 study reported no association between stressful life events and recurrence in women who had been treated for breast cancer. Nevertheless, some animal studies suggest that lack of control over stress (not simply stress itself) had negative effects on immune function and contributed to tumor growth. Although stress reduction techniques have no effect on survival rates, studies show that they are very helpful in improving a cancer patient's quality of life.

Gastrointestinal Problems

The brain and intestines are strongly related, and are controlled by many of the same hormones and parts of the nervous system. Indeed, some research suggests that the gut itself has features of a primitive brain. It is not surprising then that prolonged stress can disrupt the digestive system, irritating the large intestine and causing diarrhea, constipation, cramping, and bloating. Excessive production of digestive acids in the stomach may cause a painful burning.

Irritable bowel syndrome: Irritable bowel syndrome (or spastic colon) is strongly related to stress. With this condition, the large intestine becomes irritated, and its muscular contractions are spastic rather than smooth and wave-like. The abdomen is bloated, and the patient experiences cramping and alternating periods of constipation and diarrhea. Sleep disturbances due to stress can make irritable bowel syndrome even worse.

Peptic ulcers: It is now well-established that most peptic ulcers are either caused by the *H. pylori* bacteria or the use of nonsteroidal anti-inflammatory (NSAID) medications (such as aspirin and ibuprofen). Nevertheless, studies still suggest that stress may predispose someone to ulcers, or sustain existing ulcers. Some experts estimate that social and psychological factors play some contributing role in 30–60% of peptic ulcer cases, whether they are caused by *H. pylori* or NSAIDs. In any case, some experts believe that the anecdotal relationship between stress and ulcers is so strong that attention to psychological factors is still warranted.

Inflammatory bowel disease: Although stress is not a cause of inflammatory bowel disease (Crohn disease or ulcerative colitis), there are reports of an association between stress and symptom flare-ups. One study, for example, found that while short-term (past month) stress did not significantly exacerbate ulcerative colitis symptoms, long-term perceived stress tripled the rate of flare-ups compared to patients who did not report feelings of stress.

Eating Problems

Stress can have varying effects on eating problems and weight.

Weight gain: Often stress is related to weight gain and obesity. Many people develop cravings for salt, fat, and sugar to counteract tension and, therefore, gain weight. Weight gain can occur even with a healthy diet, however, in some people exposed to stress. In addition, the weight gained is often abdominal fat, a predictor of diabetes and heart problems.

The release of cortisol, a major stress hormone, appears to promote abdominal fat and may be the primary connection between stress and weight gain. Cortisol is a glucocorticoid, and glucocorticoids, along with insulin, appear to be responsible for stress-related food cravings. A 2005 study showed that such hormonally induced cravings for "comfort foods" may have a biological benefit for managing stress. Ingestion of comfort foods appears to reduce the negative hormonal and behavioral changes associated with stress, which might lessen the impact of stress on an individual. However, the long-term health risks of carrying excess abdominal fat are significant.

Weight loss: Some people suffer a loss of appetite and lose weight during periods of stress. In rare cases, stress may trigger hyperactivity of the thyroid gland, stimulating appetite but causing the body to burn up calories at a faster than normal rate.

Eating disorders: Chronically elevated levels of stress chemicals have been observed in patients with anorexia and bulimia. Some studies, however, have not found any strong link between stress and eating disorders. More work is needed to determine if changes in stress hormones are a cause or result of eating disorders.

Diabetes

Chronic stress has been associated with the development of insulin resistance, a condition in which the body is unable to use insulin effectively to regulate glucose (blood sugar). Insulin resistance is a primary factor in diabetes. Stress can also exacerbate existing diabetes by impairing the patient's ability to manage the disease effectively.

Pain

Researchers are attempting to find the relationship between pain and emotion, but the area is complicated by many factors, including effects of personality types, fear of pain, and stress itself.

Muscular and joint pain: Chronic pain caused by arthritis and other conditions may be intensified by stress (according to a study on patients with rheumatoid arthritis, however, stress management techniques do not appear to have much effect on arthritic pain). Psychological distress also plays a significant role in the severity of back pain. Some studies have clearly associated job dissatisfaction and depression to back problems, although it is still unclear if stress is a direct cause of the back pain.

Headaches: Tension-type headache episodes are highly associated with stress and stressful events. Sometimes the headache doesn't even start until long after a stressful event is over. Some research suggests that tension-type headache sufferers may actually have some biological predisposition for translating stress into muscle contractions. Among the wide range of possible migraine triggers is emotional stress (although the headaches often erupt after the stress has eased). One study suggested that women with migraines tend to have personalities that over-respond to stressful situations.

Sleep Disturbances

The tensions of unresolved stress frequently cause insomnia, generally keeping the stressed person awake or causing awakening in the middle of the night or early morning. In fact, evidence suggests that stress hormones can increase during sleep in anticipation of a specific waking time.

Sexual and Reproductive Dysfunction

Sexual function: Stress can lead to diminished sexual desire and an inability to achieve orgasm in women. Stress response can also cause temporary impotence in men. Part of the stress response involves the release of brain chemicals that constrict the smooth muscles of the penis and its arteries. This constriction reduces the blood flow into and increases the blood flow out of the penis, which can prevent erection.

Premenstrual syndrome: Some studies indicate that the stress response in women with premenstrual syndrome may be more intense than in those without the syndrome.

Fertility: Stress may even affect fertility. Stress hormones have an impact on the hypothalamus gland, which produces reproductive hormones. Severely elevated cortisol levels can even shut down menstruation. One interesting small study reported a significantly higher incidence of pregnancy loss in women who experienced both high stress and prolonged menstrual cycles. Another reported that women with stressful jobs had shorter periods than women with low-stress jobs.

Effects on pregnancy: Old wives' tales about a pregnant woman's emotions affecting her baby may have some credence. Stress may cause physiologic alterations, such as increased adrenal hormone levels or resistance in the arteries, which may interfere with normal blood flow to the placenta. Maternal stress during pregnancy has been linked to a higher risk for miscarriage, lower birth weights, and increased incidence of premature births. Some evidence also suggests that stress experienced by expectant mothers can even influence the way in which the baby's brain and nervous system will react to stressful events. Indeed, one study found a higher rate of crying and low attention in infants of mothers who had been stressed during pregnancy.

Memory, Concentration, and Learning

Stress affects the brain, particularly memory, but the effects differ significantly depending on whether the stress is acute or chronic.

Effect of acute stress on memory and concentration: Studies indicate that the immediate effect of acute stress impairs short-term memory, particularly verbal memory. On the plus side, high levels of stress hormone during acute stress have been associated with enhanced memory storage and greater concentration on immediate events.

Effect of chronic stress on memory: If stress becomes chronic, sufferers often experience loss of concentration at work and at home, and they may become inefficient and accident-prone. In children, the physiologic responses to chronic stress can clearly inhibit learning. Chronic stress in older people may play an even more important role in memory loss than the aging process. In one study, for example, older adults with low stress hormone levels tested as well as younger adults in cognitive tests: those with higher stress levels tested 20–50% lower.

Studies have connected long-term exposure to excess amounts of cortisol (a major stress hormone) to shrinking of the hippocampus, the brain's memory center. For example, two studies reported that groups who suffered from posttraumatic stress disorder (Vietnam veterans and women who suffered from sexual abuse) displayed up to 8% shrinking of the hippocampus. It is not yet known if this shrinking is reversible.

Other Disorders

Allergies: Stress has been related to skin allergies. In fact, some research suggests that stress, not indoor pollutants, may actually be a cause of the so-called sick-building syndrome. Sick-building syndrome produces allergy-like symptoms, such as eczema, headaches, asthma, and sinus problems, in office workers.

Skin disorders: Stress plays a role in worsening numerous skin conditions, including hives, psoriasis, acne, rosacea, and eczema. Unexplained itching may also be caused by stress.

Unexplained hair loss (alopecia areata): Alopecia areata is hair loss that occurs in localized (individual) patches. The cause is unknown, but stress is suspected as a player in this condition. For example, hair loss often occurs during periods of intense stress, such as mourning.

Teeth and gums: Stress has now been implicated in increasing the risk for periodontal disease, which is disease in the gums that can cause tooth loss.

Substance Abuse

People under chronic stress often turn to alcohol abuse or tobacco use for relief. The damage these self-destructive habits cause under ordinary circumstances is compounded by the physiological effects of stress itself. Many people also resort to abnormal eating patterns or passive activities, such as watching television. The results of a national survey, released in February 2006, show that: "Americans engage in unhealthy behaviors such as comfort eating, poor diet choices, smoking, and inactivity to help deal with stress."

Alcohol affects receptors in the brain that reduce stress. Lack of nicotine increases stress in smokers, which creates a cycle of dependency on smoking. One study indicated that nicotine has calming effects in women but not in men. In fact, in the study, smoking increased aggression in men.

The cycle is self-perpetuating: a sedentary routine, an unhealthy diet, alcohol abuse, and smoking all promote heart disease. They also interfere with sleep patterns, and lead to increased rather than reduced tension levels. Drinking four or five cups of coffee, for example, can cause changes in blood pressure and stress hormone levels similar to those produced by chronic stress. Animal fats, simple sugars, and salt are known contributors to health problems.

Conditions with Similar Symptoms

The physical symptoms of anxiety disorders mirror many symptoms of stress, including:

- a fast heart rate;
- rapid, shallow breathing; and
- increased muscle tension.

Anxiety is an emotional disorder, however, and is characterized by feelings of apprehension, uncertainty, fear, or panic. Unlike stress, the triggers for anxiety are not necessarily or even usually associated with specific stressful or threatening conditions. Some individuals with anxiety disorders have numerous physical complaints, such as headaches, gastrointestinal disturbances, dizziness, and chest pain. Severe cases of anxiety disorders are debilitating, and interfere with career, family, and social spheres.

Depression

Depression can be a disabling condition, and, like anxiety disorders, may result from chronic stress. A 2005 study of Canadian workers found that individuals with a high level of work-related stress are more than twice as likely to experience a major depressive episode, compared with people under less stress. Evidence also suggests that certain people may be genetically susceptible to depression after stressful life events. Depression also mimics some of the symptoms of stress, including changes in appetite, sleep patterns, and concentration. Serious depression, however, is distinguished from stress by feelings of sadness, hopelessness, loss of interest in life, and, sometimes, thoughts of suicide. Acute depression is also accompanied by significant changes in the patient's functioning. Professional therapy may be needed in order to determine if depression is caused by stress, or if it is the primary problem.

Posttraumatic Stress Disorder Symptoms

Posttraumatic stress disorder (PTSD) is a reaction to a very traumatic event, and it is actually classified as an anxiety disorder. The event that brings on PTSD is usually outside the norm of human experience, such as intense combat or sexual assault. The patient struggles to forget the traumatic event and frequently develops emotional numbness and event-related amnesia. Often, however, there is a mental flashback, and the patient re-experiences the painful circumstance in the form of dreams and disturbing thoughts and memories. These thoughts and dreams resemble or recall the trauma. Other symptoms may include lack of pleasure in formerly enjoyed activities, hopelessness, irritability, mood swings, sleep problems, inability to concentrate, and an excessive startle-response to noise.

Treatment

Perhaps the best general approach for treating stress can be found in the elegant passage by Reinhold Niebuhr, "Grant me the courage to change the things I can change, the serenity to accept the things I can't change, and the wisdom to know the difference." The process of learning to control stress is life-long, and will not only contribute to better health, but a greater ability to succeed in one's own agenda.

When to Seek Professional Help for Stress

Stress can be a factor in a variety of physical and emotional illnesses, which should be professionally treated. Many stress symptoms are mild and can be managed by over-the-counter medications (for example, aspirin, acetaminophen, or ibuprofen for tension headaches; antacids, anti-diarrhea medications, or laxatives for mild stomach distress). A physician should be consulted, however, for physical symptoms that are out of the ordinary, particularly those that get worse or wake a person up at night. A mental health professional should be consulted for unmanageable acute stress or for severe anxiety or depression. Often short-term therapy can resolve stress-related emotional problems.

Considerations for Choosing a Strategy for Reducing Stress

In choosing specific strategies for treating stress, several factors should be considered.

- No single method is always successful: A combination of approaches is generally most effective.

- What works for one person does not necessarily work for someone else.

- Stress can be positive as well as negative. Appropriate and controllable stress provides interest and excitement and motivates the individual to greater achievement. A lack of stress may lead to boredom and depression.

Stress may play a part in making people vulnerable to illness. A physician or psychologist should be consulted if there are any indications of accompanying medical or psychological conditions, such as heart symptoms, significant pain, anxiety, or depression.

Overcoming Obstacles to Treatment

People often succeed in relieving stress for the short-term. However, they go back to previous ways of stressful thinking and behaving because of outside pressure, long-held beliefs, or habits.

The following are some obstacles to managing stress:

- The fight or flight urge: The very idea of relaxation can feel threatening, because it is perceived as letting down one's guard. For example, an over-demanding boss may put a subordinate into a psychological state of fighting-readiness, even though there is no safe opportunity for the subordinate to fight back or express anger. Stress builds up, but the worker has the illusion, even subconsciously, that the stress itself is providing safety or preparedness. For this reason, the employee does nothing to correct the condition.

- Many people are afraid of being perceived as selfish if they engage in stress-reducing activities that benefit only themselves. The truth is that self-sacrifice (in the form of not reducing one's stress) may be inappropriate and even damaging, if the person making the sacrifice is unhappy, angry, or physically unwell.

- Some people believe that certain emotional responses to stress, such as anger, are natural and unchangeable features of personality. Research has shown, however, that with cognitive behavioral therapy, individuals can be taught to change their emotional reactions to stressful events.

It is essential to remember that reducing stress and staying relaxed clears the mind, so it can begin appropriate actions to get rid of the stress-ridden conditions.

Stress Reduction and Effects on Health

Although treating stress cannot cure medical problems, stress management can be a very important part of medical treatment. Specific stress reduction approaches may benefit different medical problems. For example, acupuncture in one study helped reduce harmful heart muscle actions in people with heart failure, but it had no effect on blood pressure. Relaxation methods, on the other hand, may help people

18

with high blood pressure. Stress reduction may improve well-being and quality of life for many patients who are experiencing stress because of severe or chronic medical conditions.

Important Note: Stress reduction techniques should never be used as the only treatment, or in place of proven treatments, for any medical condition.

Risk Factors

At some point in their lives virtually everyone will experience stressful events or situations that overwhelm their natural coping mechanisms. In one poll, 89% of respondents indicated that they had experienced serious stress in their lives. Some people are simply biologically prone to stress. Many outside factors influence susceptibility as well.

Conditions Most Likely to Produce Stress-Related Health Problems

Conditions that are most likely to be associated with stress and negative physical effects include the following:

- An accumulation of persistent stressful situations, particularly those that a person cannot easily control (for example, high-pressured work plus an unhappy relationship).

- Persistent stress following a severe acute response to a traumatic event (such as an automobile accident).

- Acute stress accompanying serious illness, such as heart disease.

Factors That Influence the Response to Stress

People respond to stress differently, depending on different factors:

- **Early nurturing:** Abusive behavior towards children may cause long-term abnormalities in the hypothalamus-pituitary system, which regulates stress.

- **Personality traits:** Certain people have personality traits that cause them to over-respond to stressful events.

- **Genetic factors:** Some people have genetic factors that affect stress, such as having a more or less efficient relaxation response.

19

One 2001 study found a genetic abnormality in serotonin regulation that was connected with a heightened reaction of heart rates and blood pressure in response to stress. (Serotonin is a brain chemical involved with feelings of well-being.)

- **Immune regulated diseases:** Certain diseases that are associated with immune abnormalities (such as rheumatoid arthritis or eczema) may actually weaken a response to stress.

- **The length and quality of stressors:** Naturally, the longer the duration and more intense the stressors, the more harmful the effects.

Individuals at Higher Risk for Stress

Studies indicate that the following people are more vulnerable to the effects of stress than others:

- Older adults: As people age, achieving a relaxation response after a stressful event becomes more difficult. Aging may simply wear out the systems in the brain that respond to stress, so that they become inefficient. The elderly, too, are very often exposed to major stressors such as medical problems, the loss of a spouse and friends, a change in a living situation, and financial worries. No one is immune to stress, however, and it may simply go unnoticed in the very young and old.

- Women in general and working mothers specifically: Working mothers, regardless of whether they are married or single, face higher stress levels and possibly adverse health effects, most likely because they bear a greater and more diffuse work load than men or other women. This has been observed in women in the United States and in Europe. Such stress may also have a domino and harmful effect on their children. It is not clear, however, if stress has the same adverse effects on women's hearts as it does on men's.

- Less educated individuals

- Divorced or widowed individuals: Numerous studies indicate that unmarried people generally do not live as long as their married contemporaries.

- Anyone experiencing financial strain, particularly long-term unemployed and those without health insurance

- People who are isolated or lonely
- People who are targets of racial or sexual discrimination
- People who live in cities

Childhood Factors

Children are frequent victims of stress because they are often unable to communicate their feelings accurately. They also have trouble communicating their responses to events over which they have no control. Certain physical symptoms, notably repeated abdominal pain without a known cause, may be indicators of stress in children.

Various conditions can affect their susceptibility to stress.

Low birth weight: A 2002 study reported that low birth weight and slow growth up until age 7 was related to stress in adulthood. It appears that children who compensated for the low birth weight with higher weight gain after birth did not have as high risk for stress later on.

Parental stress: Parental stress, especially in mothers, is a particularly powerful source of stress in children, even more important than poverty or overcrowding. In a 2002 study, for example, young children of mothers who were highly stressed (particularly if they were depressed) tended to be at high risk for developing stress-related problems. This was especially true if the mothers were stressed during both the child's infancy and early years. Some evidence even supports the old idea that stress during pregnancy can have adverse effects on the infant's mood and behavior. Older children with stressed mothers may become aggressive and anti-social. One study suggested that stress-reduction techniques in parents may improve their children's behavior.

Gender differences in adolescent stress: Adolescent boys and girls experience equal amounts of stress, but the source and effects may differ. Girls tend to become stressed from interpersonal situations, and stress is more likely to lead to depression in girls than in boys. For boys, however, specific events, such as changing schools or getting poor grades, appear to be the major sources of stress.

A report issued in October 2006 by the American Academy of Pediatrics recommends more unstructured play time for children. The report notes that today's over-scheduled, hurried lifestyle that many

21

children experience is a source of stress and anxiety in some children.

Work and Stress

In a 1999 study of 46,000 workers, health care costs were 147% higher in workers who were stressed or depressed than in others who were not. Furthermore, according to one survey, 40% of American workers describe their jobs as very stressful, making job-related stress an important and preventable health hazard.

Several studies are now suggesting that job-related stress is as great a threat to health as smoking or not exercising. Stress impairs concentration, causes sleeplessness, and increases the risk for illness, back problems, accidents, and lost time from work. Work stress can lead to harassment or even violence while on the job. At its most extreme, chronic stress places a burden on the heart and circulation that in some cases may be fatal. The Japanese even have a word for sudden death due to overwork: *karoushi*.

Not all work stress is harmful. However, studies suggest the following job-related stressors may increase people's—particularly men's—health risks:

- having no say in decisions that affect one's responsibilities;

- unrelenting and unreasonable performance demands;

- lack of effective communication and conflict-resolution methods among workers and employers;

- lack of job security;

- night-shift work, long hours, or both;

- too much time spent away from home and family; and

- wages not matching levels of responsibility.

Reducing stress on the job: Many institutions within the current culture, while paying lip service to stress reduction, put intense pressure on individuals to behave in ways that increase tension. Yet, there are numerous effective management tools and techniques available to reduce stress. Furthermore, treatment for work-related stress has proven benefits for both the employee and employer. In one study, at the end of 2 years, a company that instituted a stress management program saved nearly $150,000 in workmen's compensations costs (the cost of the program was only $6,000). Other studies in 2002 and 2003 reported specific health benefits resulting from workplace stress-management programs. In one of the studies, workers with hypertension experienced reduced blood pressure after even a brief (16-hour) program that helped them manage stress behaviorally.

In general, however, few workplaces offer stress management programs, and it is usually up to the employee to find their own ways to reduce stress. Here are some suggestions:

- Seek out someone in the Human Resources department or a sympathetic manager and communicate concerns about job stress. Work with them in a non-confrontational way to improve working conditions, letting them know that productivity can be improved if some of the pressure is off.

- Establish or reinforce a network of friends at work and at home.

- Restructure priorities and eliminate unnecessary tasks.

- Learn to focus on positive outcomes.

- If the job is unendurable, plan and execute a career change. Send out resumes or work on transfers within the company.

- If this isn't possible, be sure to schedule daily pleasant activities and physical exercise during free time.

It may be helpful to keep in mind that bosses are also victimized by the same stressful conditions they are imposing. For example, in a 2001 study of male managers in three Swedish companies, those who worked in a bureaucracy had greater stress-related heart risks than those who worked in companies with social supports.

Caregiving

Caregivers of family members: Studies show that caregivers of physically or mentally disabled family members are at risk for chronic stress. Furthermore, a 1999 study reported that overall mortality rates were over 60% higher in caregivers who were under constant stress. Spouses caring for a disabled partner are particularly vulnerable to a range of stress-related health threats, including influenza, depression, heart disease, and even poorer survival rates. Caring for a spouse with even minor disabilities can induce severe stress.

Specific risk factors that put caregivers at higher risk for severe stress, or stress-related illnesses, include:

- Caregiving wives: Some studies suggest that wives experience significantly greater stress from caregiving than husbands do. In a 2000 study, caregiving wives tended to feel more negative about their husbands than caregiving husbands felt about their wives.

- Having a low income

- Being African-American: African-American people tend to be in poorer physical health, and have lower incomes than Caucasians. They therefore face greater stress as caregivers to their spouses than their white counterparts.

- Living alone with the patient

- Helping a highly dependent patient

- Having a difficult relationship with the patient

Intervention programs that are aimed at helping the caregiver approach the situation positively can reduce stress, and help the caregiver maintain a positive attitude. A 2002 program also demonstrated that moderate-intensity exercise was very helpful in reducing stress and improving sleep in caregivers.

Health professional caregivers: Caregiving among the health professionals is also a high risk factor for stress. One 2000 study, for example, found that registered nurses with low job control, high job demands, and low work-related social support experienced very dramatic health declines, both physically and emotionally.

Anxiety Disorders

People who are less emotionally stable or have high anxiety levels tend to experience specific events as more stressful than others. Some experts describe an exaggerated negative response to stress as "catastrophizing" the event (turning it into a catastrophe). Nevertheless, a 2003 study of patients with anxiety disorder did not find any differences in actual physical response to stress (heart rate, blood pressure, release of stress hormones) compared to people without anxiety.

Lacking a Social Network

The lack of an established network of family and friends predisposes one to stress disorders and stress-related health problems, including heart disease and infections. A 2000 study, meanwhile, reported that older people who maintain active relationships with their adult children are buffered against the adverse health effects of chronic stress-inducing situations, such as low income or lower social class. One study suggested this may be because people who live alone are unable to discuss negative feelings as a means to relieve their stress.

Studies of people who remain happy and healthy despite many life stresses conclude that most have very good networks of social support. One study indicated that support even from strangers reduced blood pressure surges in people undergoing a stressful event. Many studies suggest that having a pet helps reduce medical problems aggravated by stress, including heart disease and high blood pressure.

Lifestyle Changes

A healthy lifestyle is an essential companion to any stress-reduction program. General health and stress resistance can be enhanced by regular exercise, a diet rich in a variety of whole grains, vegetables, and fruits, and by avoiding excessive alcohol, caffeine, and tobacco.

Of interest, a 2003 study suggested that fish oil, which has been associated with a lower risk for heart disease and stroke, may blunt some of the harmful effects of mental stress on the heart.

In one 2002 study, high doses of vitamin C reduced stress levels and blood pressure. The doses given were higher than the recommended upper limit of 2,000 mg per day. High doses may cause headaches and diarrhea. Long-term use increases risk for kidney stones and has other adverse effects in specific individuals.

Exercise

Exercise in combination with stress management techniques is extremely important for many reasons:

- Exercise is an effective distraction from stressful events.

- Exercise may directly blunt the harmful effects of stress on blood pressure and the heart (exercise protects the heart in any case).

Usually, a varied exercise regime is more interesting, and thus easier to stick to. Start slowly. Strenuous exercise in people who are not used to it can be very dangerous and any exercise program should be discussed with a physician. In addition, half of all people who begin a vigorous training regime drop out within a year. The key is to find activities that are exciting, challenging, and satisfying. The following are some suggestions:

- Sign up for aerobics classes at a gym.

- Brisk walking is an excellent aerobic exercise that is free and available to nearly anyone. Even short brisk walks can relieve bouts of stress.

- Swimming is an ideal exercise for many stressed people including pregnant women, individuals with musculoskeletal problems, and those who suffer exercise-induced asthma.

- Yoga or tai chi can be very effective, combining many of the benefits of breathing, muscle relaxation, and meditation while toning and stretching the muscles. The benefits of yoga may be considerable. Numerous studies have found it beneficial for many conditions in which stress is an important factor, such as anxiety, headaches, high blood pressure, and asthma. It also elevates mood and improves concentration and the ability to focus.

As in other areas of stress management, making a plan and executing it successfully develops feelings of mastery and control, which are very beneficial in and of themselves. Start small. Just 10 minutes of exercise three times a week can build a good base for novices. Gradually build up the length of these every-other-day sessions to 30 minutes or more.

Cognitive-Behavioral Techniques

Cognitive-behavioral techniques (CBTs) are among the most effective ways of reducing stress. A 2005 study found that CBT training can have a long-term impact on one's ability to cope with stress. In the study, participants received CBT training and were exposed to a stressful situation 4 months later. The participants who had received CBT training had significantly less stress-induced cortisol responses compared with individuals who had received no stress management training. This effect was observed in both men and women, although the CBTs had a greater effect on men. CBT may be particularly helpful when the source of stress is chronic pain or a chronic disease. In fact, in a study of patients with HIV, CBT was more helpful than support groups for improving well-being and quality of life.

A typical CBT approach includes identifying sources of stress, restructuring priorities, changing one's response to stress, and finding methods for managing and reducing stress.

Identifying sources of stress: One key component in most CBT approaches is a diary that keeps an informal inventory of daily events and activities. While this exercise might itself seem stress producing (and yet one more chore), it need not be done in painstaking detail. A few words accompanying a time and date are usually enough to serve as reminders of significant events or activities.

The first step is to note activities that put a strain on energy and time, trigger anger or anxiety, or precipitate a negative physical response (such as a sour stomach or headache).

Also note positive experiences, such as those that are mentally or physically refreshing or produce a sense of accomplishment.

After a week or two, try to identify two or three events or activities that have been significantly upsetting or overwhelming.

Questioning the sources of stress: Individuals should then ask themselves the following questions:

- Do these stressful activities meet my goals or someone else's?

- Have I taken on tasks that I can reasonably accomplish?

- Which tasks are under my control and which ones aren't?

Restructuring priorities—Adding stress-reducing activities: The next step is to attempt to shift the balance from stress-producing to stress-reducing activities. Eliminating stress is rarely practical or feasible, but there are many ways to reduce its impact.

Consider as many relief options as possible. Examples include:

- Listen to music. Music is an effective stress reducer in both healthy individuals and people with health problems. In a 2001 study, for example, students who listened to a well-known gentle classical piece of music during a stressful task had reduced feelings of anxiety, heart rate, and blood pressure.

- Take long weekends or, ideally, vacations.

- If the source of stress is in the home, plan times away, even if it is only an hour or two a week.

- Replace unnecessary time-consuming chores with pleasurable or interesting activities.

- Make time for recreation. This is as essential as paying bills or shopping for groceries.

- Own a pet. In a 2001 study of people with high blood pressure, pet owners had much lower blood pressure increase in response to stress than non-owners. Note that owning a pet was beneficial only for people who like animals to begin with.

Discuss feelings: The concept of communication and letting your feelings out has been so excessively promoted and parodied that it has nearly lost its value as good psychological advice. Nevertheless, feelings of anger or frustration that are not expressed in an acceptable way may lead to hostility, a sense of helplessness, and depression.

Expressing feelings does not mean venting frustration on waiters and subordinates, boring friends with emotional minutia, or wallowing in self-pity. In fact, because blood pressure may spike when certain chronically hostile individuals become angry, some therapists strongly advise that just talking, not simply venting anger, is the best approach, especially for these people.

The primary goal is to explain and assert one's needs to a trusted individual in as positive a way as possible. Direct communication may not even be necessary. Writing in a journal, writing a poem, or composing a letter that is never mailed may be sufficient.

Expressing one's feelings solves only half of the communication puzzle. Learning to listen, empathize, and respond to others with understanding is just as important for maintaining the strong relationships necessary for emotional fulfillment and reduced stress.

Keep perspective and look for the positive: Reversing negative ideas and learning to focus on positive outcomes helps reduce tension and achieve goals. The following steps, using an example of a person who is alarmed at the prospect of giving a speech, may be useful:

- First, identify the worst possible outcomes (forgetting the speech, stumbling over words, humiliation, audience contempt).

- Rate the likelihood of these bad outcomes happening (probably very low or that speaker wouldn't have been selected in the first place).

- Envision a favorable result (a well-rounded, articulate presentation with rewarding applause).

- Develop a specific plan to achieve the positive outcome (preparing in front of a mirror, using a video camera or tape recorder, relaxation exercises).

- Try to recall previous situations that initially seemed negative but ended well.

Use humor: Research has shown that humor is a very effective mechanism for coping with acute stress. Keeping a sense of humor during difficult situations is a common recommendation from stress management experts. Laughter not only releases the tension of pent-up feelings and helps keep perspective, but it appears to have actual physical effects that reduce stress hormone levels. It is not uncommon for people to recall laughing intensely even during tragic events, such as the death of a loved one, and to remember this laughter as helping them to endure the emotional pain.

Relaxation and Other Alternative Techniques

Relaxation methods: Since stress is here to stay, everyone needs to develop methods to promote the relaxation response, the natural unwinding of the stress response. Relaxation lowers blood pressure, respiration, and pulse rates, releases muscle tension, and eases emotional strains. This response is highly individualized, but there are certain approaches that seem to work.

Combinations are probably best. For example, in a study of children and adolescents with adjustment disorder and depression, a combination of yoga, a brief massage, and progressive muscle relaxation effectively reduced both feelings of anxiety and stress hormone levels. A 2005 study of organ transplant recipients showed that training in meditation and gentle yoga led to significant improvements in quality of sleep and lessened anxiety and depression.

No one should expect a total resolution of stress from these approaches, but if done regularly, these programs can be very effective.

Acupuncture: Some evidence suggests that acupuncture may also be helpful. It might even improve some physical factors associated with stress and health problems. For example, in a study of heart failure patients, acupuncture improved stress-related heart muscle activity, which could be an important benefit in these patients. However, acupuncture had no effect on stress-related blood pressure or heart rate.

Hypnosis: Hypnosis may also benefit some people with severe stress. In one study of patients with irritable bowel, stress reduction by hypnosis correlated with improvement in many bowel symptoms.

Relaxation Methods

Deep breathing exercises: During stress, breathing becomes shallow and rapid. Taking a deep breath is an automatic and effective technique for winding down. Deep breathing exercises consciously intensify this natural physiologic reaction and can be very useful during a stressful situation, or for maintaining a relaxed state during the day.

- Inhale through the nose slowly and deeply to the count of 10.

- Make sure that the stomach and abdomen expand, but the chest does not rise.

- Exhale through the nose, slowly and completely, also to the count of 10.

- To help quiet the mind, concentrate fully on breathing and counting through each cycle.

- Repeat five to 10 times, and make a habit of doing the exercise several times each day, even when not feeling stressed.

Muscle relaxation: Muscle relaxation techniques, often combined with deep breathing, are simple to learn and very useful for getting to sleep. In the beginning it is useful to have a friend or partner check for tension by lifting an arm and dropping it. The arm should fall freely. Practice makes the exercise much more effective and produces relaxation much more rapidly. Small studies have reported beneficial effects on blood pressure in patients with high blood pressure who use this technique.

- After lying down in a comfortable position without crossing the limbs, concentrate on each part of the body.

- Maintain a slow, deep breathing pattern throughout this exercise.

- Tense each muscle as tightly as possible for a count of five to 10, and then release it completely.

- Experience the muscle as totally relaxed and lead-heavy.

- Begin with the top of the head and progress downward to focus on all the muscles in the body.

- Be sure to include the forehead, ears, eyes, mouth, neck, shoulders, arms and hands, fingers, chest, belly, thighs, calves, and feet.

- Once the external review is complete, imagine tensing and releasing internal muscles.

Meditation: Meditation, used for many years in Eastern cultures, is now widely accepted in this country as a relaxation technique. The goal of all meditative procedures, both religious and therapeutic, is to quiet the mind (essentially, to relax thought). Small studies have suggested that regular meditation can benefit the heart and help reduce blood pressure. Better research is needed, however, to confirm such claims.

Some recommend meditating for no longer than 20 minutes in the morning after awakening and then again in early evening before dinner. Even once a day is helpful. Note: Meditating before going to bed may cause some people to wake up in the middle of the night, alert and unable to return to sleep.

New practitioners should understand that it can be difficult to quiet the mind, and should not be discouraged by lack of immediate results. Several techniques are available. A few are discussed here.

The only potential risks from meditating are in people with psychosis, in whom meditating may trigger a psychotic event.

- **Mindfulness meditation:** Mindfulness is a common practice that focuses on breathing. It employs the basic technique used in other forms of meditation.

  - Sit upright with the spine straight, either cross-legged or sitting on a firm chair with both feet on the floor, uncrossed.

  - With the eyes closed or gently looking a few feet ahead, observe the exhalation of the breath.

  - As the mind wanders, simply note it as a fact and returns to the "out" breath. It may be helpful to imagine your thoughts as clouds dissipating away.

- **Transcendental meditation (TM):** TM uses a mantra (a word that has a specific chanting sound but no meaning). The meditator repeats the word silently, letting thoughts come and go. In one study, TM was as effective as exercise in elevating mood.

31

- **Mini-meditation:** The method involves heightening awareness of the immediate surrounding environment. Choose a routine activity when alone. For example:

  - While washing dishes, concentrate on the feel of the water and dishes.

  - Allow the mind to wander to any immediate sensory experience (sounds outside the window, smells from the stove, colors in the room).

  - If the mind begins to think about the past or future, or fills with unformed thoughts or worries, redirect it gently back.

  - This redirection of brain activity from your thoughts and worries to your senses disrupts the stress response and prompts relaxation. It also helps promote an emotional and sensual appreciation of simple pleasures already present in a person's life.

Biofeedback: Biofeedback is a technique that measures bodily functions, like breathing, heart rate, blood pressure, skin temperature, and muscle tension. By watching these measurements, you can learn how to alter these functions by relaxing or holding pleasant images in your mind.

- During biofeedback, electric leads are taped to a subject's head.

- The person is encouraged to relax using methods such as those described above.

- Brain waves are measured and an audible signal is emitted when alpha waves are detected, a frequency which coincides with a state of deep relaxation.

- By repeating the process, subjects associate the sound with the relaxed state and learn to achieve relaxation by themselves.

Massage therapy: A 2005 report that reviewed data from multiple studies showed that massage therapy decreases cortisol levels. Another 2005 study showed that massage from a stable romantic partner can reduce physiological responses to a subsequent stressful event. In the study, women who received instructed shoulder-neck-massage from their partners before being exposed to stress had lowered cortisol responses, and smaller heart rate increases after the stressful event. Interestingly, massage was more beneficial than receiving social support from the partner, indicating the power of physical touch in managing stress.

Several massage therapies are available and some are listed here. Many massage techniques are available, such as the following:

- Swedish massage is the standard massage technique. It uses long smooth strokes, and kneading and tapping of the muscles.

- Shiatsu applies intense pressure to the same points targeted in acupuncture. It can be painful, but people report deep relaxation afterward.

- Reflexology manipulates acupuncture points in the hands and feet.

Herbal and Natural Remedies

Some people who experience chronic stress seek herbal or natural remedies. It should be strongly noted, however, that just as with standard drugs, so-called natural remedies can cause problems, sometimes serious ones.

Probiotics: Probiotics are helpful bacterial strains that by themselves may provide a barrier against harmful bacteria. They do so through various mechanisms, such as excreting certain acids (for example, lactate, acetate) that inhibit harmful bacteria. They may also compete with them for nutrients. Stress reduces levels of these bacteria. Research even suggests that probiotics may help maintain remission in patients with IBD [inflammatory bowel disease]. In one small 2002 study, people suffering from stress and exhaustion significantly reduced their stress symptoms and gastrointestinal complaints when they took a probiotic supplement for 6 months. The specific bacteria that might be beneficial, however, are not fully known. The most well-known probiotics are the lactobacilli strains, such as acidophilus, which is found in yogurt and other fermented milk products. Others, however, may prove to be more important, such as *Bifidobacterium* and GG lactobacilli. Other probiotics include the lactobacilli *rhamnosus, casel, plantarium, bulgaricus,* and *salivarius,* and also *Enterococcus faecium* and *Streptococcus thermophilus.*

Aromatherapy: The smell of lavender has long been associated with a calming effect. In a Japanese study, 14 women who were put in a room with a lavender scent experienced reduced mental stress. Several aromatherapies are now used for relaxation. Use caution, however, as some of the exotic plant extracts in these formulas have been associated with a wide range of skin allergies.

Valerian: Valerian is an herb that has sedative qualities and may reduce stress and associated physical effects. This herb is on the U.S. Food and Drug Administration's [FDA] list of generally safe products. Of note, however, the herb's effects could be dangerously increased if it is used with standard sedatives. Other interactions and long-term side effects are unknown. Side effects include vivid dreams. High doses of valerian can cause blurred vision, excitability, and changes in heart rhythm.

Herbs and Supplements

Generally, manufacturers of herbal remedies and dietary supplements do not need FDA approval to sell their products. Just like a drug, however, herbs and supplements can affect the body's chemistry, and therefore have the potential to produce side effects that may be harmful. There have been numerous reported cases of serious and even lethal side effects from herbal products. Always check with your doctor before using any herbal remedies or dietary supplements.

Special warning on kava: Kava has been commonly used to reduce anxiety and stress. It is now highly associated with liver injury and even liver failure in a few cases. Experts now strongly warn against its use.

People seeking relief from stress should be wary of things that promise a quick cure, or plans that include the purchase of expensive treatments. These treatments may be useless and sometimes even dangerous.

References

Ginsburg KR and the Committee on Communications and Committee on Psychosocial Aspects of Child and Family Health. Clinical Report: The Importance of Play in Promoting Healthy Child Development and Maintaining Strong Parent-Child Bonds. Last accessed on 17 October, 2006.

Dallman MF, Pecoraro NC, la Fleur SE. Chronic stress and comfort foods: self-medication and abdominal obesity. *Brain Behav Immun.* 2005;19:275–280.

Wang J. Work stress as a risk factor for major depressive episode(s). *Psychol Med.* 2005;35:865–871.

Hammerfald K, Grau M, et al. Persistent effects of cognitive-behavioral stress management on cortisol responses to acute stress in healthy subjects-A randomized controlled trial. *Psychoneuroendocrinology.* 2005 Sep 22; epub ahead of print.

Kreitzer MJ, Gross CR, Ye X, et al. Longitudinal impact of mindfulness meditation on illness burden in solid-organ transplant recipients. *Prog Transplant.* 2005;15:166–172.

Field T, Hernandez-Reif M, Diego M, et al. Cortisol decreases and serotonin and dopamine increase following massage therapy. *Int J Neurosci.* 2005;115:1397–1413.

Ditzen B, Neumann I, Bodenmann G, et al. Romantic Partner Interaction Reduces Endocrine and Autonomic Stress Responses in Women. New Research Abstracts, Annual Meeting of the American Psychiatric Association. Washington, D.C. 2005. Abstract NR140.

Chapter 2

Stressed Out Nation: Many Americans Cope with Stress in Unhealthy Ways

More than half of working adults—and 47 percent of all Americans—say they are concerned with the amount of stress in their lives, according to a new telephone survey conducted Jan. 12–24 [2006] by APA's [American Psychological Association's] Practice Directorate in partnership with the National Women's Health Resource Center and iVillage.com.

Moreover, the survey finds that people experiencing stress are more likely to report hypertension, anxiety, depression, or obesity. The survey, which sampled 2,152 adults who are 18 years or older, is part of the Practice Directorate's "Mind/Body Health: For a Healthy Mind and Body, Talk to a Psychologist" campaign. The initiative aims to highlight psychology's role at the intersection between mental and physical well-being.

By focusing on the physical and mental toll of stress, the campaign is shining light on how many Americans react to both work- and family-related stress—by engaging in unhealthy behaviors, such as comfort eating, making poor diet choices, smoking, and being inactive, says Helen Mitternight, assistant executive director of public relations in the Practice Directorate.

"Americans are stressed out, and they are dealing with that stress in an unhealthy way," says Mitternight.

Stambor, Z. (2006). Stressed out nation. *Monitor on Psychology, 37* (4), 28–29. Copyright © 2006 by the American Psychological Association. Reprinted with permission.

However, on a positive note, she notes, nearly 20 percent of those most concerned about stress said that seeing a mental health professional could help them get back on track and relieve some of their stress.

Gender Differences

Stress is particularly prevalent for the primary decision-maker in the household for health issues, says Mitternight. Since 73 percent of women identify themselves as such, women feel the brunt of the health-care burden, she adds.

"Women are the health-care managers of their families," says Amber McCracken, director of communications for the National Women's Health Resource Center. "From taking care of their own health to serving as the caregivers for their children, partner, and parents, each aspect of care brings stress. Unfortunately, too often women do not take the necessary steps to alleviate that stress, and their own physical health suffers."

Moreover, men and women exhibit their stress differently, the survey found. Women are more likely than men to report feelings of nervousness, wanting to cry, or lacking energy. Men, 40 percent of whom consider themselves the primary health-care decision-maker, are prone to describing their stressed condition as sleepless, irritable, or angry.

Those gender differences are magnified in men and women's coping mechanisms, the survey found. For instance, nearly 31 percent of women say they are comfort eaters, while only 19 percent of men report eating to deal with their problems. The urge to comfort-eat can have complex consequences, as the survey found that comfort eaters are more likely to exhibit higher levels of the most common stress symptoms, including fatigue, lack of energy, nervousness, and sleeplessness.

The survey also found that 21 percent of participants who ate at a fast-food restaurant in the week prior to the survey reported being very concerned about stress, while only 13 percent of people who did not eat at a fast-food restaurant in the week prior to the survey were very concerned about stress. Not surprisingly, the fast-food-eaters were also more likely to experience more serious health problems like hypertension and high cholesterol.

Mind/Body Connection

The survey suggests that for most Americans, stress results from a conglomeration of concerns. For instance, an office worker stressing out over a project deadline may quickly down a hamburger and fries while he or she works to save time. In turn, that stress-fueled decision may next lead to health worries.

The office worker's stressors are not unique, as more than half the survey respondents included concerns about money, work, family-member health problems, or the state of the world today, as some of their leading sources of stress. More than 40 percent of participants also cited the health of immediate family members and caring for their children as common stressors.

An effective means of dealing with stress, suggests Russ Newman, Ph.D., J.D., executive director of APA's Practice Directorate, is learning how to cope.

"Everybody experiences stress," says Newman. "The key is how effectively people deal with and manage stress. People who turn to comfort food or smoking are starting a vicious cycle. Their attempts to reduce stress can actually lead to health problems that result in even more stress."

To help break the cycle, Newman suggests that stressed people pay attention to their behaviors and lifestyle choices. Additionally, he notes that although some behaviors can be particularly difficult to change, working with a psychologist can help modify those actions.

The survey sponsors released the results at February press event in New York City that garnered national media attention on TV news shows such as "Good Morning America" and in newspapers such as *USA Today*. In addition to the media campaign, the sponsors are pairing the results with additional tips on how to manage stress. iVillage is also posting a Stress Smarts Quiz on its website to help readers understand the seriousness of their stress.

Chapter 3

Signs and Symptoms of Stress

What is stress?

Life can be stressful. We all face different challenges and obstacles, and sometimes the pressure is hard to handle. When we feel over-whelmed, under the gun, or unsure of how to meet the demands placed on us, we experience stress. In small doses, stress can be a good thing. It can give you the push you need, motivating you to do your best and to stay focused and alert. Stress is what keeps you on your toes dur-ing a presentation at work or drives you to study for your midterm when you'd rather be watching TV. But when the going gets too tough and life's demands exceed your ability to cope, stress becomes a threat to both your physical and emotional well-being.

Stress is a psychological and physiological response to events that upset our personal balance in some way. These events or demands are known as stressors. We usually think of stressors as being negative, such as an exhausting work schedule or a rocky relationship. How-ever, anything that forces us to adjust can be a stressor. This includes

"Stress: Signs, Symptoms, Causes, and Effects," by Ellen Jaffe-Gill, M.A., Melinda Smith, M.A., Lisa Flores Dumke, M.A., Heather Larson, and Jeanne Segal, Ph.D., reprinted with permission from http://www.helpguide.org/mental/stress _signs.htm. © 2007 Helpguide.org. All rights reserved. Helpguide provides a detailed list of related references for this article, including links to informa-tion from other websites. For a complete list of Helpguide's current resources related to stress signs and symptoms, causes of stress, burnout, and stress re-lief and relaxation techniques, visit www.helpguide.org.

41

positive events such as getting married or receiving a promotion. Regardless of whether an event is good or bad, if the changes it brings strain our coping skills and adaptive resources, the end result is the subjective feeling of stress and the body's biological stress response.

According to the American Psychological Association, fifty-four percent of Americans are concerned about the level of stress in their everyday lives.

What causes stress and its symptoms?

The potential causes of stress are numerous. Your stress may be linked to outside factors such as the state of the world, the environment in which you live or work, or your family. Your stress can also come from your own irresponsible behavior, negative attitudes and feelings, or unrealistic expectations.

Furthermore, the causes of stress are highly individual. What you consider stressful depends on many factors, including your personality, general outlook on life, problem-solving abilities, and social support system. Something that's stressful to you may be neutral or even enjoyable to someone else. For example, your morning commute may make you anxious and tense because you worry that traffic will make you late. Others, however, may find the trip relaxing because they allow more than enough time and enjoy playing music or listening to books while they drive.

Stressors can be divided into three broad categories:

- **Frustrations:** Frustrations are obstacles that prevent you from meeting your needs or achieving personal goals. They can be external—such as discrimination, an unsatisfying job, divorce, or the death of a loved one—or internal. Examples of internal frustrations include physical handicaps, the lack of a desired ability or trait, and other real or perceived personal limitations.

- **Conflicts:** Stressors involving two or more incompatible needs or goals are known as conflicts. For example, a working mother might feel torn over a job offer that would advance her career, but take time away from her family. Sometimes the conflict involves a choice between two desirable options, such as deciding between two acceptance offers from equally appealing colleges. At other times, the decision involves disagreeable alternatives.

- **Pressures:** Stress can stem from the expectations of others or the demands you place on yourself. You may feel pressure to get good grades in order to please your parents or get into a good school. Or you may feel pressure to excel at work, make a difference in your community, or be the perfect mother.

Whether or not the source of stress causes significant emotional and physical symptoms depends in part on the nature of the stressor itself. Stressors that involve central aspects of your life or that persist for extended periods of time are more likely to result in severe distress and disruption of functioning. Furthermore, the more stressful situations or life changes you're dealing with at one time, the more intense the symptoms of stress.

What are the signs and symptoms of stress?

Stress affects the mind, body, and behavior in many ways. The specific signs and symptoms of stress vary from person to person, but all have the potential to harm your health, emotional well-being, and relationships with others. Below is a partial list of stress signs and symptoms that a person undergoing stress might experience.

- Intellectual symptoms: How stress can affect your mind
  - Memory problems
  - Difficulty making decisions
  - Inability to concentrate
  - Confusion
  - Seeing only the negative
  - Repetitive or racing thoughts
  - Poor judgment
  - Loss of objectivity
  - Desire to escape or run away
- Emotional symptoms: How stress can make you feel
  - Moody and hypersensitive
  - Restlessness and anxiety
  - Depression
  - Anger and resentment
  - Easily irritated and "on edge"
  - Sense of being overwhelmed

- Lack of confidence
- Apathy
- Urge to laugh or cry at inappropriate times
- Physical symptoms: How stress can affect your body
  - Headaches
  - Digestive problems
  - Muscle tension and pain
  - Sleep disturbances
  - Fatigue
  - Chest pain, irregular heartbeat
  - High blood pressure
  - Weight gain or loss
  - Asthma or shortness of breath
  - Skin problems
  - Decreased sex drive
- Behavioral symptoms: How stress can affect your behavior
  - Eating more or less
  - Sleeping too much or too little
  - Isolating yourself from others
  - Neglecting your responsibilities
  - Increasing alcohol and drug use
  - Nervous habits (e.g., nail biting, pacing)
  - Teeth grinding or jaw clenching
  - Overdoing activities such as exercising or shopping
  - Losing your temper
  - Overreacting to unexpected problems

Keep in mind that the signs and symptoms of stress can be caused by other psychological or physical problems, so it's important that you consult a doctor to evaluate physical symptoms. Similarly, emotional symptoms such as anxiety or depression can mask conditions other than stress. It's important to find out whether or not they are stress-related.

What are the different types of stress?

Acute stress: Acute stress is the most common and most recognizable form of stress, the kind of sudden jolt in which you know exactly why you're stressed: you were just in a car accident; the school nurse just called; a bear just ambled onto your campsite. Or it can be something scary but thrilling, such as a parachute jump. Along with obvious dangers and threats, common causes of acute stressors include noise, isolation, crowding, and hunger. Normally, your body rests when these types of stressful events cease and your life gets back to normal. Because the effects are short-term, acute stress usually doesn't cause severe or permanent damage to the body.

Episodic acute stress: Some people endure acute stress frequently; their lives are chaotic, out of control, and they always seem to be facing multiple stressful situations. They're always in a rush, always late, always taking on too many projects, handling too many demands. Unlike people for whom stress is a once-in-a-while spike, these folks are experiencing episodic acute stress.

According to the American Psychological Association [APA], those prone to episodic acute stress include driven, hard-charging "Type A" personality types and worrywarts, always anxious about the next disaster they're sure lurks around the corner. While the Type A tends to seem angry and hostile and the worrier more depressed, both are frequently over-aroused and tense, and both are susceptible to the physical manifestations of extended stress, including high blood pressure and heart disease.

If you're prone to episodic acute stress, you may not know it or admit to it. You may be wedded to a lifestyle that promotes stress. You may explain your frequent stress as temporary ("I just have a million things going on right now"), as integral to your work or home life ("Things are always crazy around here"), or as a part of your personality ("I have a lot of nervous energy, that's all"). You may blame your frequent stress on other people or outside events, or you might view it as entirely normal and unexceptional. Unfortunately, people with episodic acute stress may find it so habitual that they resist changing their lifestyles until they suffer severe physical symptoms.

Chronic stress: The APA Help Center describes chronic stress as "unrelenting demands and pressures for seemingly interminable periods of time." Chronic stress is stress that wears you down day after day and year after year, with no visible escape. It grinds away at both mental and physical health, leading to breakdown and even death.

Common causes of chronic stress include:

- poverty and financial worries;
- long-term unemployment;
- dysfunctional family relationships;
- caring for a chronically ill family member;
- feeling trapped in unhealthy relationships or career choices;
- living in an area besieged by war or violence;
- bullying or harassment; or
- perfectionism.

One of the most dangerous aspects of chronic stress is that people who suffer from it get used to it. They accept chronic stress as their lot in life, or they forget it's there. Because chronic stress is based on long-term, often intractable situations, both the mental and physical symptoms of chronic stress can be difficult to treat.

Traumatic stress: Severe stress reactions can result from a catastrophic event or intense experience such as a natural disaster, sexual assault, life-threatening accident, or participation in combat. After the initial shock and emotional fallout, many trauma victims gradually begin to recover. But for some people, the psychological and physical symptoms triggered by the trauma don't go away, the body doesn't regain its equilibrium, and life doesn't return to normal. This is a condition known as posttraumatic stress disorder (PTSD). Common symptoms include flashbacks or nightmares about the trauma, avoidance of places and things associated with the trauma, hypervigilance for signs of danger, chronic irritability and tension, and depression. PTSD is a serious disorder that requires professional intervention.

What are the long-term effects of stress?

The stress response of the body is meant to protect and support us. When faced with a threat, whether it be to our physical safety or emotional equilibrium, the body's defenses kick into high gear in a process known as the "fight or flight" response. The sympathetic nervous system pumps out adrenaline, preparing us for emergency action. Our heart rate and blood flow to the large muscles increase, the blood vessels under the skin constrict to prevent blood loss in case of injury, the pupils dilate so we can see better, and our blood sugar ramps up, giving us an energy boost.

The stress response is what helped our stone age ancestors survive, enhancing their ability to fight or flee from danger. But in the modern world, most stressors are psychological, rather than physical. Caring for a chronically ill child or getting audited by the IRS qualify as stressful situations, but neither calls for either fight or flight. Unfortunately, our bodies don't make this distinction. Like a caveman confronting a saber-tooth tiger, we go into automatic overdrive, releasing the same hormones that enabled prehistoric humans to move and think faster, hit harder, see better, hear more acutely, and jump higher than they could only seconds earlier.

The problem with the stress response is that the more it is activated, the harder it is to shut off. Instead of leveling off once the crisis has passed, your stress hormones, heart rate, and blood pressure remain elevated. Extended or repeated activation of the stress response takes a heavy toll on the body. The physical wear and tear it causes includes damage to the cardiovascular system and immune system suppression. Stress compromises your ability to fight off disease and infection, makes it difficult to conceive a baby, and stunts growth in children. It can even rewire the brain, leaving you more vulnerable to everyday pressures and mental health problems such as anxiety and depression. And, of course, the stress of living with a debilitating disease or disorder just adds to the problem.

Recent research suggests that anywhere from two thirds to 90 percent of illness is stress-related. The following text lists some of the health problems that can be caused or exacerbated by long-term stress:

Health problems linked to stress:

- Heart attack
- Hypertension
- Stroke
- Cancer
- Diabetes
- Depression
- Obesity
- Eating disorders
- Substance abuse

- Ulcers
- Irritable bowel syndrome
- Memory loss
- Autoimmune diseases (e.g., lupus)
- Insomnia
- Thyroid problems
- Infertility

What can I do to manage stress and its symptoms?

Fortunately, physicians, mental health professionals, and others have discovered many ways for people to cope with stress, repair its damages, and work on removing its sources.

Chapter 4

The Effects of Stress on the Body and Mind

Maybe it's money trouble or the burden of caring for a sick relative. Maybe it's your job. Maybe it's the traffic. Whatever the cause, everyone seems stressed out these days. People once hotly debated the idea that stress can affect your body, but we now know that stress can cause both short- and long-term changes to your body and mind. The more we understand how stress affects us, the more we learn about how to cope better.

Long before humans learned how to drive cars to work and check in with the office on handheld computers, our bodies evolved to be finely attuned to a predator's attack. When we sense danger, our bodies quickly release hormones like adrenaline into our bloodstream that increase our heart rate, focus our attention, and cause other changes to quickly prepare us for coming danger. Stress was—and still is—crucial to our survival.

The stress that we're adapted to deal with, however, is the short, intense kind—like running away before a bear can make a lunch of us. Modern life frequently gives us little time between periods of stress for our body to recuperate. This chronic stress eventually takes both a mental and physical toll.

It's long been known that blood pressure and cholesterol levels go up in people who are stressed. Studies have now linked chronic stress with cardiovascular problems like hypertension, coronary heart disease, and stroke.

"Stressed Out? Stress Affects Both Body and Mind" is from the National Institutes of Health (NIH, www.nih.gov) publication *News in Health,* January 2007.

The immune system is also affected by stress. Dr. Esther M. Sternberg at the National Institutes of Health (NIH)'s National Institute of Mental Health says it makes sense for the immune system to gear up and get ready to heal potential wounds. But chronic stress can cause the system to backfire. Research has shown that wounds in people under chronic stress heal more slowly. Caregivers of people with Alzheimer disease, who are often under great stress, are more likely to get the flu or a cold—and when they take vaccines to protect their loved ones from getting flu, their bodies don't respond as well.

Certain hormones that are released when you're stressed out, such as cortisol and catecholamines, have been tied to these long-term effects of stress. Sternberg says, "If you're pumping out a lot of cortisol and your immune cells are bathed in high levels of stress hormones, they're going to be tuned down."

Animal studies and brain imaging studies in people have shown that chronic stress can have a similar effect on the brain. Dr. Bruce S. McEwen of Rockefeller University explains, "Hyperactivity of the stress response results in changes over time in the circuitry of the brain."

Brain cells bombarded by stress signals have little recovery time and eventually start to shrink and cut connections to other brain cells. The network that coordinates our thoughts, emotions, and reactions thus starts to rearrange. Over time, entire regions of the brain can grow or shrink. That may explain why studies have linked higher levels of stress hormones with lower memory, focus, and problem-solving skills.

Not everyone deals with stress the same way, however, and why some people seem to cope better is a major area of research. McEwen says studies in animals show that early life experiences and the quality of maternal care affect how curious an animal is when it's older and how stressed it gets in a new environment.

Dr. Teresa Seeman of the University of California at Los Angeles School of Medicine points out that studies have also linked poverty and deprivation in childhood with how well people deal with stress. "There does appear to be a lingering impact," Seeman says, but adds that it's difficult to know the exact cause.

Two things that affect how much stress people feel are self-esteem and a sense of control. Workers who feel more in control at their jobs tend to feel less stress. People with low self-esteem produce more cortisol when they're asked to do something that's not easy for them, like speak in front of other people. They also don't become accustomed to the stress even after doing something several times and continue to produce high levels of cortisol.

It's not easy to change things like self-esteem and your sense of control at work, but there are things you can do to help you cope with the stresses of modern life.

"Sleep deprivation is a major issue," McEwen says. People who are stressed out tend to get less quality sleep. And sleep deprivation affects your ability to control your mood and make good decisions. It also throws the stress hormones in your body off balance.

"If you're sleep deprived," McEwen explains, "blood pressure and cortisol don't go down at night like they should." McEwen sees people who work night shifts as a window into what chronic stress does to the body over time. "They're more likely to become obese and to have diabetes, cardiovascular disease, and depression," he says.

People who are stressed out tend to do other things that make their bodies less healthy and more vulnerable to the effects of stress. Many eat more fatty comfort foods, which can lead to obesity and diabetes. They may smoke or drink more, raising the risk for cancer and other diseases. And they often feel they're just too busy to exercise.

Seeman says, "Being physically active helps keep the body's systems in better shape and thus better able to deal with any demands from other stressful conditions."

Another factor affecting how we deal with stress is the isolation of modern life. Sometimes it seems like the only time we interact with our family or coworkers is when we're having a conflict. Seeman says it's important to develop a network of people you can go to and talk with when you're confronted with difficulties in your life.

"Large studies have clearly shown," she says, "that people who have more social relationships, a larger network of people they interact with on a regular basis, live longer. Research suggests they're less likely to show declines as they're older."

All this research highlights the fact that healthy practices can complement mainstream medicine to help treat and prevent disease. Do things that make you feel good about yourself, mentally and physically. Get enough sleep. Eat a healthy diet and exercise regularly. Develop a network of people you can turn to in difficult times.

If you still find yourself too stressed out, talk to your health care professional. There are many therapies they may recommend to help you deal with stress and its consequences. The effects of being chronically stressed are too serious to simply accept as a fact of modern life.

Ways of Reducing Stress

- Get enough sleep.

- Exercise and control your diet.
- Build a social support network.
- Create peaceful times in your day.
- Try different relaxation methods until you find one that works for you.
- Don't smoke.
- Don't drink too much or abuse any other substances.

Chapter 5

Statistics on Stress: Variations among Demographic Groups

We live in a world with many sources of stress, with many things to do and to worry about. These include the pressures of life at work and at home, problems with money, health, loneliness, children, and privacy.

When shown a list of 14 different hassles that tend to be associated with stress, the hassles that are experienced by the largest numbers of people are related to money (rising prices, 74%; concerns about money for emergencies, 53% and not having enough money for basic necessities, 36%); having too many things to do (56%); having trouble sleeping (53%); concerns about health (43%); and the illness of a family member (36%).

Many, but fewer, people say they experienced having too much information to process at any one time (33%), feeling lonely (29%), or problems at work (24%). And, of course, some people experience many more hassles and experience much more stress than others.

These are some of the results of a nationwide survey of 2,747 adults surveyed online between September 7 and 13, 2006.

Variations among Different Demographic Groups

Analysis of the results of this survey shows that different demographic groups experience more or less, and different sources of, stress. The one group that stands out as having much less stress than all of

The Harris Poll® #75, October 6, 2006, "The Many Sources of Stress and the Hassles of Daily Life" Harris Interactive Inc. All rights reserved.

the others is older adults (9% of "matures," aged 61 and older, report experiencing a lot of stress in their lives, compared to 25% or more of other generations). While "baby boomers" (aged 42 to 60), like those younger than them, are subject to many sources of stress, the matures are much less stressed. They are by a wide margin less likely to worry about having too many things to do, to have concerns about money for emergencies or basic necessities, to feel that they have too much information to process at anyone time or (and this may be a surprise) to feel lonely. Indeed, the younger the people are, the more likely they are to experience loneliness. Those who say they have been lonely in the last month include 45 percent of "echo boomers" (aged 18 to 29), 31 percent of "generation Xers" (aged 30 to 41), 24 percent of baby boomers, and 18 percent of matures.

There are many other differences between different demographic groups. For example:

- Unsurprisingly, those with low household incomes are much more likely to experience problems with rising prices and to have concerns about money for emergencies and basic necessities. On the other hand, those with higher household incomes are more likely to feel that they have too many things to do, to have problems at work, or have problems with aging parents.

- Lesbians, gays, bisexuals, and transgendered (GLBT) people are more likely than heterosexuals to have concerns about their health or to worry about money and to be lonely.

- People with disabilities experience more stress and more hassles than other people in relation to money, sleeping, health, and loneliness.

Hassles Are Highly Correlated with Feeling Stressed

The survey finds very strong associations between almost all of the 14 hassles and feeling stressed. For example:

- Fully 80 percent of those who experience a lot of stress say that they have had too many things to do in the last month. This falls to only 29 percent of those who do not experience much stress.

- Fully 76 percent of those who experience a lot of stress say they had trouble sleeping compared to only 29 percent of those with little stress.

- Fully 71 percent of those who have a lot of stress say they experienced concerns about money for emergencies in the last month compared to only 30 percent among those whose lives are not much stressed.

A recent survey published in *The Journal of the American Medical Association* compared the health status of comparable groups

Table 5.1. Those Who Experienced 14 Hassles in the Last Month

"Have you experienced the following in the past month?"
Base: All Adults

	September 2006 %	2000 %	2002 %
Rising prices	74	77	69
Too many things to do	56	57	62
Trouble sleeping	53	N/A	N/A
Concerns about money for emergencies	53	51	51
Concerns about health in general	43	48	47
Illness of a family member	36	42	37
Not enough money for basic necessities	36	33	35
Too much information to process at one time	33	N/A	N/A
Being lonely	29	18	15
Problems with your work, boss or fellow workers	24	22	20
Problems with aging parents	21	22	23
Frequent or excessive noise	20	17	18
Problems with my children	19	N/A	N/A
Abuse of your personal privacy	13	15	18
Average Score (see note 3)	35	34	33

Notes:

1. The 2000 and 2002 surveys were conducted by telephone, whereas this survey was conducted online.

2. The question asked in 2000 and 2002 was slightly different. "Please tell me if (read item) has affected you in the last month or not?"

3. Average score is based on the 12 items that were asked in all three surveys.

Table 5.2. Those Who Experienced 14 Hassles—By Generation and Gender

"Have you experienced the following in the past month?": Those saying "Yes"
Base: All Adults

	Total	Generation				Gender	
		Echo Boomers (18–20)	Gen X (30–41)	Baby Boomers (42–60)	Matures (61+)	Male	Female
	%	%	%	%	%	%	%
Rising prices	74	66	79	75	74	70	77
Too many things to do	56	70	66	59	27	54	58
Trouble sleeping	53	53	62	55	41	46	60
Concerns about money for emergencies	53	51	65	60	28	46	59
Concerns about health in general	43	40	42	45	41	37	48
Illness of a family member	36	36	33	39	36	33	39
Not enough money for basic necessities	36	38	50	38	17	31	41
Too much information to process at one time	33	43	38	34	18	29	37
Being lonely	29	45	31	24	18	26	32
Problems with my work, boss, or fellow workers	24	32	28	28	5	26	22
Problems with aging parents	21	16	20	30	10	20	21
Frequent or excessive noise	20	29	22	19	11	20	20
Problems with my children	19	9	26	24	14	14	24
Abuse of my personal privacy	13	15	11	14	9	13	12

Table 5.3. Those Who Experienced 14 Hassles—By Race and Party

"Have you experienced the following in the past month?": Those saying "Yes"
Base: All Adults

	Total	Race			Party ID		
		White	Black	Hispanic	Republican	Democrat	Independent
	%	%	%	%	%	%	%
Rising prices	74	74	77	75	65	80	75
Too many things to do	56	56	53	58	56	56	54
Trouble sleeping	53	54	53	54	50	57	50
Concerns about money for emergencies	53	51	68	52	47	55	53
Concerns about health in general	43	42	51	39	36	47	43
Illness of a family member	36	35	45	40	34	40	37
Not enough money for basic necessities	36	33	53	44	31	40	33
Too much information to process at one time	33	33	25	42	31	37	30
Being lonely	29	30	25	31	25	31	28
Problems with my work, boss, or fellow workers	24	24	22	22	24	25	22
Problems with aging parents	21	19	26	25	19	23	22
Frequent or excessive noise	20	20	17	20	18	19	22
Problems with my children	19	20	23	21	17	20	19
Abuse of my personal privacy	13	10	16	14	10	13	15

Table 5.4. Those Who Experienced 14 Hassles—By Income

"Have you experienced the following in the past month?": Those saying "Yes"
Base: All Adults

	Total	Income				
		$15K–$24.9K	$25K–$34,9K	$35K–$49,9K	$50K–$74,9K	$75K+
	%	%	%	%	%	%
Rising prices	74	89	79	78	74	66
Too many things to do	56	52	53	58	59	62
Trouble sleeping	53	56	61	57	48	51
Concerns about money for emergencies	53	71	66	58	56	41
Concerns about health in general	43	50	52	42	40	37
Illness of a family member	36	41	38	32	35	37
Not enough money for basic necessities	36	61	51	43	32	21
Too much information to process at one time	33	33	31	36	33	36
Being lonely	29	34	31	33	23	22
Problems with my work, boss, or fellow workers	24	19	21	27	25	30
Problems with aging parents	21	17	21	18	19	28
Frequent or excessive noise	20	23	24	22	19	19
Problems with my children	19	19	23	25	21	19
Abuse of my personal privacy	13	13	14	13	9	12

Table 5.5. Those Who Experienced 14 Hassles—By Sexual Orientation and Disability

"Have you experienced the following in the past month?": Those saying "Yes"
Base: All Adults

	Total	Sexual Orientation		Disabilities	
		LGBT	Heterosexual	People with Disabilities	People without Disabilities
	%	%	%	%	%
Rising prices	74	74	74	80	69
Too many things to do	56	63	56	53	56
Trouble sleeping	53	55	54	63	49
Concerns about money for emergencies	53	62	53	59	48
Concerns about health in general	43	57	42	58	34
Illness of a family member	36	45	36	42	29
Not enough money for basic necessities	36	53	36	42	33
Too much information to process at one time	33	34	34	37	31
Being lonely	29	46	28	37	25
Problems with my work, boss, or fellow workers	24	25	24	18	26
Problems with aging parents	21	28	21	21	16
Frequent or excessive noise	20	33	20	22	19
Problems with my children	19	16	20	24	18
Abuse of my personal privacy	13	17	12	13	11

Table 5.6. Those Who Experienced 14 Hassles—By Children and Employment

"Have you experienced the following in the past month?": Those saying "Yes"
Base: All Adults

	Total	Children		Employment	
		Household with Children	Household without Children	Employed	Not Employed
	%	%	%	%	%
Rising prices	74	77	72	73	74
Too many things to do	56	71	49	65	42
Trouble sleeping	53	59	50	53	54
Concerns about money for emergencies	53	64	47	58	45
Concerns about health in general	43	40	44	41	46
Illness of a family member	36	37	36	35	40
Not enough money for basic necessities	36	45	32	38	34
Too much information to process at one time	33	43	28	38	26
Being lonely	29	27	30	29	28
Problems with my work, boss, or fellow workers	24	27	22	35	6
Problems with aging parents	21	22	20	23	17
Frequent or excessive noise	20	22	19	22	17
Problems with my children	19	32	13	20	18
Abuse of my personal privacy	13	13	12	14	11

60

Table 5.7. How Much Stress People Have in Their Lives

"How much stress is in your life?
Base: All Adults

	Total %
A lot	23
Some	47
Not too much	27
None at all	3

Table 5.8. Those Who Experienced "A Lot" of Stress—Demographic Variations

	%
All Adults	23
AGE	
Echo Boomers (18–29)	29
Gen. X (30–41)	28
Baby Boomers (42–60)	25
Matures (61+)	9
GENDER	
Male	18
Female	29
RACE/ETHNICITY	
White	23
Black	16
Hispanic	29
HOUSEHOLD INCOME	
Less than $15,000	25
$15,000–$24,999	23
$25,000–$34,999	29
$35,000–$49,999	24
$50,000–$74,999	21
$75,000 or more	23
DISABILITY	
People with disabilities	27
People without disabilities	19
CHILDREN	
Households with children	30
Households with no children	20
PARTY IDENTIFICATION	
Republican	22
Democrat	22
Independent	24

Table 5.9. Correlation between Experience of Hassles and Sense of Stress

"Have you experienced the following in the past month?: Those saying "Yes"
Base: All Adults

	All Adults	Amount of Stress		
		A Lot	Some	Not Too Much/None At All
	%	%	%	%
Rising prices	74	81	76	64
Too many things to do	56	80	61	29
Trouble sleeping	53	76	57	29
Concerns about money for emergencies	53	71	59	30
Concerns about health in general	43	65	42	25
Illness of a family member	36	47	38	25
Not enough money for basic necessities	36	55	40	17
Too much information to process at one time	33	58	32	16
Being lonely	29	47	29	14
Problems with your work, boss, or fellow workers	24	39	26	10
Problems with aging parents	21	28	22	12
Frequent or excessive noise	20	34	19	10
Problems with my children	19	36	17	10
Abuse of your personal privacy	13	20	12	7

(middle-aged whites) in England and the United States and found that Americans were much more likely than their English counterparts to suffer from seven common diseases including diabetes, cardiovascular diseases, stroke, and cancer. The research did not set out to explain these differences. However, one hypothesis is that Americans tend to experience more stress than the English. And, of course, a growing body of research has reported that increased stress is associated with higher incidence of a number of common diseases, including cardiovascular disease and cancer.

Methodology

The Harris Poll® was conducted online within the United States between September 7 and 13, 2006 among 2,747 adults (aged 18 and over). Figures for age, sex, race, education, region, and household income were weighted where necessary to bring them into line with their actual proportions in the population. Propensity score weighting was also used to adjust for respondents' propensity to be online.

All surveys are subject to several sources of error. These include: sampling error (because only a sample of a population is interviewed); measurement error due to question wording and/or question order, deliberately or unintentionally inaccurate responses, nonresponse (including refusals), interviewer effects (when live interviewers are used), and weighting.

With one exception (sampling error) the magnitude of the errors that result cannot be estimated. There is, therefore, no way to calculate a finite "margin of error" for any survey and the use of these words should be avoided.

With pure probability samples, with 100 percent response rates, it is possible to calculate the probability that the sampling error (but not other sources of error) is not greater than some number. With a pure probability sample of 2,747 adults one could say with a 95 percent probability that the overall results have a sampling error of +/-2 percentage points. However that does not take other sources of error into account. This online survey is not based on a probability sample and therefore no theoretical sampling error can be calculated.

These statements conform to the principles of disclosure of the National Council on Public Polls.

Chapter 6

Genes, Personality, and Anxiety-Related Traits

Finding any real "personality" genes is decades away. But researchers have a good start.

In fact, more researchers are jumping into the complex fray of behavioral genetics each year, fueled by the hope that identifying genes related to personality traits will not only help them better understand what makes people tick but also what goes wrong when normal "ticking" turns pathological.

The goal is to discover genes that affect brain functions that in turn affect how people interact with their environments. The research is slowed by the complexity of the search: Many genes are responsible for various aspects of people's temperament, and those genes appear to interact with each other in complicated ways that influence several traits at once—and then likely only in very subtle ways, with any one gene likely accounting for only 1 or 2 percent of the variance in a trait.

Researchers do, however, believe that their work will eventually pay off and they'll have a new, more comprehensive, understanding of personality and psychopathology as well as the complex play between genes and environment in shaping personality.

Progress to Date

Scientists have a strong foundation for their search for personality

Azar, B. (2002). Searching for genes that explain our personalities. *Monitor on Psychology,* 33 (8), 44–46. Copyright © 2002 by the American Psychological Association. Reprinted with permission.

genes from the years of basic psychology and neuroscience studies that have explored just exactly what personality is and how personality-related behaviors might be influenced by specific neural mechanisms. And although researchers still debate exactly how to define personality, they have identified certain core personality dimensions that are consistent across cultures, including novelty-seeking, neuroticism, and agreeableness.

Intriguing to people has been research in animals and humans that links certain neurotransmitters with some of these dimensions or traits. For example, many studies have found a connection between high levels of the neurotransmitter dopamine and behaviors related to novelty-seeking. That gives researchers a place to start looking—genes related to dopamine—among the nearly 50,000 in the human genome.

To date, there are only two real candidate genes that anyone speaks of with any confidence. The first potential link is between some behaviors related to the Big-Five trait novelty-seeking and a gene that produces the protein responsible for creating a dopamine receptor called DRD4. While some studies have failed to replicate this connection, others have identified a link between the DRD4 gene and other traits linked to novelty-seeking, such as drug abuse and attention deficit hyperactivity disorder. The indication is that this gene—or perhaps some other gene related to it—may influence all these inter-related characteristics.

The second candidate—linked to the Big-Five trait neuroticism—is commonly called the "Prozac" gene because it produces a protein related to the neurotransmitter serotonin. Also known as the serotonin transporter gene or 5-HTTLPR, it has the strongest evidence linking it to neuroticism and other anxiety-related traits, such as harm avoidance.

Even so, the gene appears to account for only about 1 to 2 percent of the variance for these traits, says National Cancer Institute molecular biologist Dean Hamer, Ph.D., one of the first scientists to search for personality genes. "If that's as good as it gets," he says, "everything else is likely worse." That means perhaps hundreds of genes influence each of our personality traits ever so slightly.

In fact, the work is so difficult from a molecular biology point of view, Hamer is all but abandoning it.

"After 10 years or so, it's quite clear to me that at least for most traits there are a very large number of genes involved," he says. The only area he'll continue working on is sexual orientation. There he feels there's a better chance of finding just a few key genes.

Blurring Lines between 'Normal' and Pathological

The difficulty of the work isn't stopping others who anticipate the promise of a greater understanding of personality as well as psychopathology. Already, research has begun to blur the traditional line delineating personality and psychopathology as separate entities.

For example, over the past decade, studies have established a connection between high scores on the standard personality trait of neuroticism and major depression. In fact, high neuroticism scores can predict whether someone will develop major depression, says Kenneth Kendler, M.D., director of the Psychiatric Genetics Research Program at Virginia Commonwealth University, who conducted some of the research showing this link. Other studies by Kendler suggest that neuroticism and depression share as much as 60 percent of their genes. In fact, most researchers in this area expect they'll find that many of the genes that influence general personality also play a role in many forms of psychopathology.

Such findings would suggest that conditions such as depression, anxiety disorders, and attention deficit hyperactivity disorder are one end of a continuum that includes normal personality traits.

"Once we get genes for psychopathology, we'll get genes for personality" and vice versa, says Robert Plomin, Ph.D., deputy director of the Social, Genetic and Developmental Psychiatry Research Centre in the Institute of Psychiatry at King's College, London. "At least for more common disorders, such as hyperactivity, all the evidence points to a continuum of traits. Activity and hyperactivity are just variants of each other."

Understanding Environment through Genes

The research could also revolutionize how psychologists define psychopathology, which is currently diagnosed by symptoms, says Plomin.

"All our concern about diagnosis based on symptoms might be off base," he says. Instead, psychopathology could be defined and diagnosed based on genes and their interaction with the environment to produce certain outcomes. This would allow clinicians to detect people at risk for a certain disorder and, perhaps, prevent symptoms from ever occurring by modifying a person's environment.

Of course, the reality of using genetic markers to diagnose psychiatric disorders—not to mention to assess personality traits—is likely decades away. In fact, some researchers think it's unlikely because of the number of genes involved in any one trait.

"One can fantasize about replacing self-report inventories with genetic assays to assess personality traits," says psychologist Jeff McCrae, Ph.D., a personality psychologist at the National Institute on Aging (NIA), "but I doubt it will ever become a reality. The link between genes and traits is too imperfect, and we would need to discover all the genes associated with each trait and how they interact in order to come up with a gene-based personality assessment." More likely—and equally important for personality researchers—is the idea that they will be able to include genetic markers among the criteria they use to validate their personality measures.

"[Genetic markers] could provide one more objective indicator against which to evaluate our instruments," says McCrae.

In addition, finding genes is sure to help researchers better understand how environment and genes interact to shape personality. That's the idea behind research by McCrae and his long-time NIA collaborator Paul Costa, Ph.D. They have developed the Five-Factor Theory, which says that personality traits themselves are genetically based, but that characteristic adaptations—habits, beliefs, values, self-concepts, roles, relationships, skills—are shaped jointly by genetically determined traits and the environment.

Once they and other researchers pin down at least some of the genetics of the traits, they could much more easily evaluate the environmental contribution to these characteristic adaptations.

"For example," says McCrae, "we might find that people high in Gene A everywhere in the world cried when they were depressed, but that they only attempted suicide in certain cultures."

That might, he says, suggest that the environment has little to do with the physiological expression of affect, but is crucial for understanding and preventing suicide.

Though concrete answers are far off, "Understanding the genes and their interactions will most certainly also help us understand environmental influences," says University of Illinois personality and social psychologist Ed Diener, Ph.D. "We will be able to see when the environment 'overrides' the genes and why. And we will be able to see how environmental variations interact with genetic variations."

—Beth Azar is a writer in Portland, Oregon.

Chapter 7

Gender Differences in Stress Management

Chapter Contents

Section 7.1

Women, Stress, and Hormones

"Hormones: How Do They Affect Anxiety in Women?" © 2004 Anxiety Disorders Association of America. All Rights Reserved. Reprinted with permission. For more information visit http://www.adaa.org or call 240-485-1001.

It is well known that, compared to men, women are more prone to develop anxiety disorders and depression. One factor that may contribute to the increased risk of anxiety in women is biology, particularly the constant fluctuations in reproductive hormones that women experience until after menopause.

What is known about hormones and how they can impact a woman's life? Understanding the effects of hormones on anxiety disorders can help women have a more informed discussion of treatment and care with their health care providers.

Do monthly changes throughout the menstrual cycle affect anxiety disorders?

Research suggests that obsessive-compulsive disorder (OCD) seems to worsen premenstrually, but panic disorder does not. Not enough is known about the effects of the menstrual cycle on social anxiety, post-traumatic stress disorder (PTSD), phobias, or generalized anxiety to suggest a relationship. Woman with premenstrual mood disorder (PMD) may experience complete relief of anxiety symptoms during the first two weeks after onset of menses.

Will the symptoms related to my anxiety disorder be affected by pregnancy?

During pregnancy, levels of many hormones rise steadily. Unfortunately, little is known about how these hormone changes during pregnancy affect women with anxiety disorders. There is evidence that many women with panic-type anxiety have a reduction in panic symptoms during pregnancy. This may occur because progesterone—which rises greatly during pregnancy—has breakdown products that have effects similar to benzodiazepine medications like clonazepam and diazepam.

The hormones oxytocin and prolactin have been shown to have antianxiety effects in animals. These hormones may help reduce panic anxiety during pregnancy. However, other hormonal changes during pregnancy, e.g., possible increases in androgen hormones, may contribute to a worsening of OCD symptoms that some women experience.

Although these hormone changes occur gradually during pregnancy, they reverse very suddenly after delivery. This abrupt drop likely contributes to postpartum worsening of anxiety and depression in some. Although pregnancy may provide some relief of panic-type anxiety, the risk of panic seems to increase after delivery.

Women who continue to experience symptoms of anxiety during pregnancy should talk to their OB/GYN [obstetrician/gynecologist] about treatments.

Will breastfeeding have beneficial affects on anxiety?

Breastfeeding may help prevent some of the sudden hormonal transitions that occur at the end of pregnancy, since oxytocin and prolactin continue to be released. If the frequency of breastfeeding decreases gradually over time, the drop in oxytocin and prolactin for the mother will also be more gradual.

Studies have shown that women who breastfeed have reduced hormonal and nervous system reactions to acute stress. There have also been reports that breastfeeding may reduce anxiety symptoms for some women, but clearly other women continue to have anxiety. High levels of anxiety postpartum can make breastfeeding difficult because anxiety and stress suppress the release of oxytocin, a hormone needed for milk release.

How does menopause affect anxiety disorders?

After age 50, women are no longer at the same two-fold increased risk of developing an anxiety disorder. However, there has been little study of the effects of menopause on anxiety or why women might experience this reduced risk.

There seems to be variations among individuals in how perimenopause and menopause affect anxiety symptoms. During perimenopause, the three- to seven-year transition period between regular menstrual cycling and the last menstrual period, hormone levels can be very erratic, sometimes reaching levels much higher than those experienced before this period. This makes it difficult to figure out the role of hormones in any symptom changes during perimenopause.

Women who do experience greater anxiety symptoms should talk with their health care provider.

Do hormonal medications affect anxiety disorders?

Symptoms related to anxiety disorders do not appear to improve or worsen with any type of hormonal contraception, e.g., birth control pills. Estrogen replacement after menopause has been shown to reduce hormonal and nervous system responses to stress. In addition, estrogen therapy has been shown to reduce symptoms of perimenopausal depression.

These studies suggest that estrogen treatment may be helpful for anxiety during perimenopause or menopause, but no studies have examined the effect of estrogen or progesterone replacement on anxiety disorder symptoms.

What other hormones can affect anxiety disorders?

High levels of thyroid hormones can cause panic attacks, tremors, insomnia, palpitations, and other symptoms of anxiety. Overactivity of the thyroid gland, or hyperthyroidism, is a well-known cause of anxiety. Women are at greater risk of thyroid illness than men, partly because 10 to 20 percent of women have "anti-thyroid" antibodies circulating in their bloodstream that have the potential to cause hyperthyroidism. Usually, these antibodies do not cause a problem. However, if women do have anti-thyroid antibodies, postpartum is a time of increased risk for autoimmune hyperthyroidism. Women with thyroid conditions who have an anxiety disorder or exhibit symptoms of anxiety should discuss these with their doctor.

Although the details are still unclear on how hormones affect anxiety disorders in women, the early evidence does indicate that connections do exist. Further study in this area of anxiety disorders research will yield more answers over time. Until then, women at every stage of life should discuss their concerns with their OB/GYN and other health care providers to ensure proper treatment.

Section 7.2

Relationship Conflicts
Stress Men More Than Women

Meyers, L. (2006). Relationship conflicts stress men more than women. *Monitor on Psychology*, 37 (5), 14. Copyright © 2006 by the American Psychological Association. Reprinted with permission.

Attachment style can predict a person's physical stress response to conflict with a romantic partner, but the specific vulnerable attachment styles are different in men and in women, according to an April [2006] study in the *Journal of Personality and Social Psychology* (Vol. 90, No. 4).

The study—part of a larger National Institute of Mental Health-funded investigation—involved 124 couples between the ages of 18 and 21 who had been together for at least two months. Powers and her team assessed participants' self-reported avoidance of intimacy and dependence on their romantic partner and anxiety about rejection and abandonment. "Secure" types had low levels of anxiety and avoidance, "anxious-ambivalent" had high levels of anxiety and low levels of avoidance, "fearful-avoidant" had high levels of both anxiety and avoidance and "dismissing-avoidant" had low anxiety and high avoidance.

After filling out the questionnaires, couples spent 15 minutes discussing an issue that caused heated and unresolved discussions in the past month. The researchers collected seven cortisol samples assessing physiological stress in anticipation of the conflict, throughout the conflict and during a 40-minute recovery period.

The researchers found that although both men and women have a physiological response to relationship conflict, the response is much more pronounced in men than in women and involves different attachment factors. Anxiety was a strong predictor for response in men, but in women, only highly avoidant types showed significant cortisol changes.

"Men and women may face different demands in the conflict-negotiation task," Powers explains. In a relationship, women are often expected to initiate and guide conflict discussions, says Powers.

For avoidant women, who prefer to distance themselves in conflict situations, the study's task may be particularly difficult, she believes. Indeed, avoidant women in the study showed high reactivity before and during the conflict, but recovered rapidly after leaving the discussion. For these women, avoiding sustained conflict appears to be physiologically rewarding.

Men, on the other hand, are often expected to be more passive participants, so Powers surmises that although they may want to resolve issues, anxious men feel particularly uncomfortable actively confronting relationship conflicts.

However, men in the study who had secure female partners showed the lowest levels of cortisol reactivity, indicating that their partners were helping to regulate their physiological stress levels. The converse was true for women—their partners' attachment style did not have a regulating effect on their stress levels.

Chapter 8

Stress at Work

Chapter Contents

Chapter 8

Stress at Work

Chapter Contents

Section 8.1

Statistics on Stress and Anxiety in the Workplace

"Workplace Stress and Anxiety Disorders Survey," © 2006 Anxiety Disorders Association of America. All Rights Reserved. Reprinted with permission. For more information visit http://www.adaa.org or call 240-485-1001.

Anxiety Disorders Association of America (ADAA)'s 2006 Stress & Anxiety Disorders Survey found the majority of working Americans experience stress or anxiety in their daily lives—no surprise. However, ADAA learned from the survey that close to half of U.S. employees report experiencing persistent stress or excessive anxiety in their daily lives. And while only 9 percent of the respondents have been diagnosed with an anxiety disorder, 24 percent have taken prescription medication to manage stress and other emotional problems.

A certain amount of stress and anxiety is normal—at work and at home. However, persistent, excessive, and irrational anxiety that interferes with everyday functioning is often an indication of a more serious problem, namely an anxiety disorder.

Snapshot of Stress, Anxiety, and Anxiety Disorders in the Workplace

Self-reporting of anxiety symptoms and prescription medication use is high among America's employees, but diagnoses of anxiety disorders are dramatically lower.

- 72 percent of people who have daily stress and anxiety say it interferes with their lives at least moderately.

- 40 percent experience persistent stress or excessive anxiety in their daily lives.

- 24 percent have taken prescription medication to manage stress, nervousness, emotional problems, or lack of sleep.

- 28 percent have had an anxiety or panic attack. However, only 9 percent have been diagnosed with an anxiety disorder.

76

Workplace Stress and Anxiety Affects Life at Work—and at Home

Professional and personal consequences of workplace stress affect America's workforce.

- **On the job:** Employees say stress and anxiety most often impacts their:
  - workplace performance (56 percent)
  - relationship with co-workers/peers (51 percent)
  - quality of work (50 percent)
  - relationships with superiors (43 percent)
- **During off time:** Over three fourths of people who say stress interferes with their work say it carries over to their personal life, particularly men (83 percent versus 72 percent for women).
- **With spouses and loved ones:** Seven in 10 of these adults report workplace stress affects their personal relationships, mainly with their spouses. Men report it affecting personal relationships more than women (79 percent versus 61 percent).
- **And the main culprits are:** According to employees, the work-related situations that cause the most stress are:
  - deadlines (55 percent)
  - interpersonal relationships (53 percent)
  - staff management (50 percent)
  - dealing with issues/problems that arise (49 percent)

Americans Use a Variety of Methods for Managing Workplace Stress

Finding relief takes many forms, some healthy, but many unhealthy.

- Dreaming of a less stressful job? The top method of managing high levels of stress at work for both men and women is to sleep more (44 percent total).
- Women and men find different ways to cope:
  - Women are significantly more likely than men to eat more (46 percent versus 27 percent) and talk to family and friends (44 percent versus 21 percent) to manage job stress.

- Men are significantly more likely than women to have sex more frequently (19 percent versus 10 percent) and use illicit drugs (12 percent versus 2 percent) to manage job stress.

- Common ground exists. Other ways both men and women cope with job stress are:
  - consuming more caffeine (31 percent)
  - smoking (27 percent)
  - exercising more frequently (25 percent)
  - taking over-the-counter or prescription medication (23 percent)
  - consuming more alcoholic beverages (20 percent)

Employees Do Not Communicate Stress Levels to Bosses and Fear Repercussions

Most employees are not comfortable discussing stress with their employer.

- **Tight-lipped workforce:** Less than half (40 percent) of employees whose stress interferes with work have talked to their employer about it, mainly because they:
  - fear their boss would interpret it as lack of interest or unwillingness to do the activity (34 percent)
  - fear being labeled as "weak" (31 percent)
  - fear it would affect promotion opportunities (22 percent)
  - fear it would go in their file (22 percent)
  - fear being laughed at or not taken seriously (20 percent)

- **Help is not always on the way:** Of those who did speak to their employer, four in 10 were offered some type of help from their employer, most often in the form of a referral to a mental health professional (26 percent) or a relaxation/stress management class (22 percent).

Persistent Stress, Excessive Anxiety, and Anxiety Disorders Prevalent among Workers

Many employees report suffering from anxiety that goes beyond normal, everyday stress in that it is persistent and excessive, and affects their ability to function. Yet many less reported suffering from an anxiety disorder—a telling inconsistency. Employees whose anxiety interferes with their everyday functioning may be suffering from an anxiety disorder, the most common mental illness in the United States.

- **Anxiety that gets in the way of life:** One in four employees reports persistent stress or excessive anxiety has impaired their ability to function in the past six months.

- **Chronic anxiety as a way of life?** Four in ten respondents agree with the statement that "persistent stress and/or excessive anxiety are a normal part of life," particularly men (44 percent versus 36 percent for women).

- **Fear of stigma remains:** Only one fourth of employees with an anxiety disorder have told their employers. Those who have not were afraid:
  - their boss would interpret it as lack of interest of unwillingness to do the activity (38 percent)
  - it would affect promotion opportunities (34 percent)
  - it would go in their file (31 percent)

- **Other reasons:** Less commonly, people with anxiety disorders did not share it with their employer because of reasons unrelated to stigma.
  - Only 14 percent did not report their anxiety disorder because they didn't want to produce a doctor's note
  - 7 percent didn't because they didn't think it was their employer's business
  - 6 percent didn't because they didn't think it was necessary
  - 3 percent didn't because they didn't want to

Anxiety Disorders Disrupt Job Functioning and Work Relationships

Employees with an anxiety disorder say it leads to a host of difficulties at work. With over 18 percent of the population suffering from an anxiety disorder, this is likely making much more of an impact on productivity and efficiency at U.S. companies than most employers realize.

- **Strained relations:** Almost half of employees with an anxiety disorder say that it interferes with their relationships with people at work, mainly by causing them to avoid social situations such as parties or eating out (73 percent), become short-tempered (53 percent), and avoid participating in meetings (43 percent).

- **Symptom triggers:** Half of employees with an anxiety disorder said their functional work responsibilities trigger symptoms of the disorder (53 percent), primarily dealing with problems and meeting deadlines. Interpersonal relationships also trigger symptoms of anxiety disorders (46 percent), as do changes to employees' work situations (37 percent)—such as leaving a job, starting a new one, or getting fired—and staff management (35 percent).

- **Trying to cope:** Employees with anxiety disorders use a variety of methods for easing their symptoms, mainly:

  - taking over-the-counter or prescription medication (52 percent)

  - sleeping more (50 percent)

  - eating more (39 percent)

  - talking to family or friends (38 percent)

  - talking to a medical or mental health professional (37 percent)

- **Differences exist:** Stark differences exist in the way some men cope compared to women:

  - Men are significantly more likely than women to try to ease their symptoms by having sex more frequently (25 percent versus 6 percent) and using illicit drugs (11 percent versus 0 percent).

Section 8.2

Causes of Job Stress and Effects on Productivity

Excerpted from the booklet "STRESS . . . at Work," by the National Institute for Occupational Safety and Health (NIOSH, www.cdc.gov/niosh), part of the Centers for Disease Control and Prevention, January 1999. NIOSH Publication: 99-101. Reviewed by David A. Cooke, M.D., April 2007.

The nature of work is changing at whirlwind speed. Perhaps now more than ever before, job stress poses a threat to the health of workers and, in turn, to the health organizations. This chapter highlights knowledge about the causes of stress at work and outlines steps that can be taken to prevent job stress.

Stress in Today's Workplace

The longer he waited, the more David worried. For weeks he had been plagued by aching muscles, loss of appetite, restless sleep, and a complete sense of exhaustion. At first he tried to ignore these problems, but eventually he became so short-tempered and irritable that his wife insisted he get a checkup. Now, sitting in the doctor's office and wondering what the verdict would be, he didn't even notice when Theresa took the seat beside him. They had been good friends when she worked in the front office at the plant, but he hadn't seen her since she left three years ago to take a job as a customer service representative. Her gentle poke in the ribs brought him around, and within minutes they were talking and gossiping as if she had never left.

"You got out just in time," he told her. "Since the reorganization, nobody feels safe. It used to be that as long as you did your work, you had a job. That's not for sure anymore. They expect the same production rates even though two guys are now doing the work of three. We're so backed up I'm working 12-hour shifts six days a week. I swear I hear those machines humming in my sleep. Guys are calling in sick just to get a break. Morale is so bad they're talking about bringing in some consultants to figure out a better way to get the job done."

81

"Well, I really miss you guys," she said. "I'm afraid I jumped from the frying pan into the fire. In my new job, the computer routes the calls and they never stop. I even have to schedule my bathroom breaks. All I hear the whole day are complaints from unhappy customers. I try to be helpful and sympathetic, but I can't promise anything without getting my boss's approval. Most of the time I'm caught between what the customer wants and company policy. I'm not sure who I'm supposed to keep happy. The other reps are so uptight and tense they don't even talk to one another. We all go to our own little cubicles and stay there until quitting time. To make matters worse, my mother's health is deteriorating. If only I could use some of my sick time to look after her. No wonder I'm in here with migraine headaches and high blood pressure. A lot of the reps are seeing the employee assistance

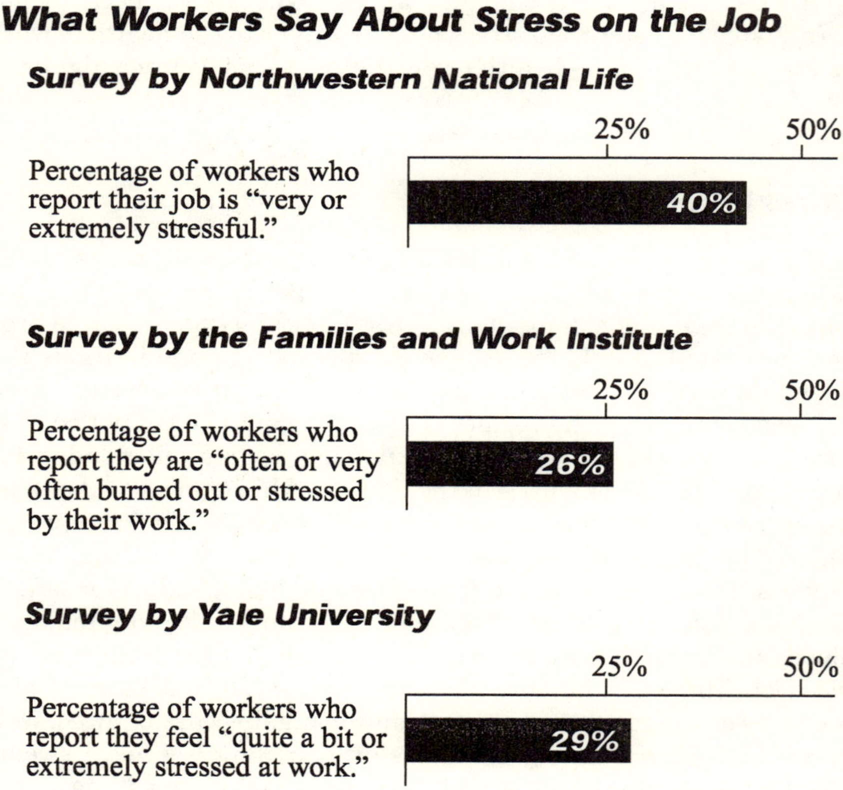

What Workers Say About Stress on the Job

Survey by Northwestern National Life

Percentage of workers who report their job is "very or extremely stressful."

Survey by the Families and Work Institute

Percentage of workers who report they are "often or very often burned out or stressed by their work."

Survey by Yale University

Percentage of workers who report they feel "quite a bit or extremely stressed at work."

Figure 8.1. Job stress is a common and costly problem in the American workplace.

counselor and taking stress management classes, which seems to help. But sooner or later, someone will have to make some changes in the way the place is run."

Scope of Stress in the American Workplace

David's and Theresa's stories are unfortunate but not unusual. Job stress has become a common and costly problem in the American workplace, leaving few workers untouched. For example, studies report the following:

- One fourth of employees view their jobs as the number one stressor in their lives. (Northwestern National Life)

- Three fourths of employees believe the worker has more on-the-job stress than a generation ago. (Princeton Survey Research Associates)

- Problems at work are more strongly associated with health complaints than are any other life stressor—more so than even financial problems or family problems. (St. Paul Fire and Marine Insurance Co.)

Fortunately, research on job stress has greatly expanded in recent years. But in spite of this attention, confusion remains about the causes, effects, and prevention of job stress. This text summarizes what is known about job stress and what can be done about it.

What Is Job Stress?

Job stress can be defined as the harmful physical and emotional responses that occur when the requirements of the job do not match the capabilities, resources, or needs of the worker. Job stress can lead to poor health and even injury.

The concept of job stress is often confused with challenge, but these concepts are not the same. Challenge energizes us psychologically and physically, and it motivates us to learn new skills and master our jobs. When a challenge is met, we feel relaxed and satisfied. Thus, challenge is an important ingredient for healthy and productive work. The importance of challenge in our work lives is probably what people are referring to when they say "a little bit of stress is good for you."

But for David and Theresa, the situation is different—the challenge has turned into job demands that cannot be met, relaxation has turned to exhaustion, and a sense of satisfaction has turned into feelings of stress. In short, the stage is set for illness, injury, and job failure.

What Are the Causes of Job Stress?

Nearly everyone agrees that job stress results from the interaction of the worker and the conditions of work. Views differ, however, on the importance of worker characteristics versus working conditions as the primary cause of job stress. These differing viewpoints are important because they suggest different ways to prevent stress at work.

According to one school of thought, differences in individual characteristics such as personality and coping style are most important in predicting whether certain job conditions will result in stress—in other words, what is stressful for one person may not be a problem for someone else. This viewpoint leads to prevention strategies that focus on workers and ways to help them cope with demanding job conditions.

Although the importance of individual differences cannot be ignored, scientific evidence suggests that certain working conditions are stressful to most people. The excessive workload demands and conflicting expectations described in David's and Theresa's stories are good examples. Such evidence argues for a greater emphasis on working conditions as the key source of job stress, and for job redesign as a primary prevention strategy.

Job Conditions That May Lead to Stress

The design of tasks: Heavy workload, infrequent rest breaks, long work hours and shift work; hectic and routine tasks that have little inherent meaning, do not utilize workers' skills, and provide little sense of control.

- *Example:* David works to the point of exhaustion. Theresa is tied to the computer, allowing little room for flexibility, self-initiative, or rest.

Management style: Lack of participation by workers in decision-making, poor communication in the organization, lack of family-friendly policies.

- *Example:* Theresa needs to get the boss's approval for everything, and the company is insensitive to her family needs.

Interpersonal relationships: Poor social environment and lack of support or help from coworkers and supervisors.

- *Example:* Theresa's physical isolation reduces her opportunities to interact with other workers or receive help from them.

Work roles. Conflicting or uncertain job expectations, too much responsibility, too many "hats to wear."

- *Example:* Theresa is often caught in a difficult situation trying to satisfy both the customer's needs and the company's expectations.

Career Concerns. Job insecurity and lack of opportunity for growth, advancement, or promotion; rapid changes for which workers are unprepared.

- *Example:* Since the reorganization at David's plant, everyone is worried about their future with the company and what will happen next.

Environmental Conditions. Unpleasant or dangerous physical conditions such as crowding, noise, air pollution, or ergonomic problems.

- *Example:* David is exposed to constant noise at work.

Job Stress and Health

Stress sets off an alarm in the brain, which responds by preparing the body for defensive action. The nervous system is aroused and hormones are released to sharpen the senses, quicken the pulse, deepen respiration, and tense the muscles. This response (sometimes called the fight or flight response) is important because it helps us defend against threatening situations. The response is preprogrammed biologically. Everyone responds in much the same way, regardless of whether the stressful situation is at work or home.

Short-lived or infrequent episodes of stress pose little risk. But when stressful situations go unresolved, the body is kept in a constant state of activation, which increases the rate of wear and tear to biological systems. Ultimately, fatigue or damage results, and the ability of the body to repair and defend itself can become seriously compromised. As a result, the risk of injury or disease escalates.

In the past 20 years, many studies have looked at the relationship between job stress and a variety of ailments. Mood and sleep disturbances, upset stomach and headache, and disturbed relationships with family and friends are examples of stress-related problems that are quick to develop and are commonly seen in these studies. These early signs of job stress are usually easy to recognize. But the effects of job stress on chronic diseases are more difficult to see because chronic diseases take a long time to develop and can be influenced by many factors other than stress. Nonetheless, evidence is rapidly accumulating to suggest that stress plays an important role in several types of chronic health problems—especially cardiovascular disease, musculoskeletal disorders, and psychological disorders.

Early Warning Signs of Job Stress

- Headache
- Sleep disturbances
- Difficulty in concentrating
- Short temper
- Upset stomach
- Job dissatisfaction
- Low morale

Job Stress and Health: What the Research Tells Us

Cardiovascular disease: Many studies suggest that psychologically demanding jobs that allow employees little control over the work process increase the risk of cardiovascular disease.

Musculoskeletal disorders: On the basis of research by the National Institute for Occupational Safety and Health (NIOSH) and many other organizations, it is widely believed that job stress increases the risk for development of back and upper-extremity musculoskeletal disorders.

Psychological disorders: Several studies suggest that differences in rates of mental health problems (such as depression and burnout) for various occupations are due partly to differences in job stress levels. (Economic and lifestyle differences between occupations may also contribute to some of these problems.)

Workplace injury: Although more study is needed, there is a growing concern that stressful working conditions interfere with safe work practices and set the stage for injuries at work.

Suicide, cancer, ulcers, and impaired immune function: Some studies suggest a relationship between stressful working conditions and these health problems. However, more research is needed before firm conclusions can be drawn. (*Encyclopaedia of Occupational Safety and Health*)

Stress, Health, and Productivity

Some employers assume that stressful working conditions are a necessary evil—that companies must turn up the pressure on workers and set aside health concerns to remain productive and profitable in today's economy. But research findings challenge this belief. Studies show that stressful working conditions are actually associated with increased absenteeism, tardiness, and intentions by workers to quit their jobs—all of which have a negative effect on the bottom line.

Recent studies of so-called healthy organizations suggest that policies benefiting worker health also benefit the bottom line. A healthy organization is defined as one that has low rates of illness, injury, and disability in its workforce and is also competitive in the marketplace. NIOSH research has identified organizational characteristics associated with both healthy, low-stress work and high levels of productivity. Examples of these characteristics include the following:

- Recognition of employees for good work performance
- Opportunities for career development
- An organizational culture that values the individual worker
- Management actions that are consistent with organizational values

What Can Be Done about Job Stress?

The examples of Theresa and David illustrate two different approaches for dealing with stress at work.

Stress management: Theresa's company is providing stress management training and an employee assistance program (EAP) to improve the ability of workers to cope with difficult work situations. Nearly one half of large companies in the United States provide some

87

type of stress management training for their workforces. Stress management programs teach workers about the nature and sources of stress, the effects of stress on health, and personal skills to reduce stress—for example, time management or relaxation exercises. (EAPs provide individual counseling for employees with both work and personal problems.) Stress management training may rapidly reduce stress symptoms such as anxiety and sleep disturbances; it also has the advantage of being inexpensive and easy to implement. However, stress management programs have two major disadvantages:

- The beneficial effects on stress symptoms are often short-lived.
- They often ignore important root causes of stress because they focus on the worker and not the environment.

Organizational change: In contrast to stress management training and EAP programs, David's company is trying to reduce job stress by bringing in a consultant to recommend ways to improve working conditions. This approach is the most direct way to reduce stress at work. It involves the identification of stressful aspects of work (e.g., excessive workload, conflicting expectations) and the design of strategies to reduce or eliminate the identified stressors. The advantage of this approach is that it deals directly with the root causes of stress at work. However, managers are sometimes uncomfortable with this approach because it can involve changes in work routines or production schedules, or changes in the organizational structure.

As a general rule, actions to reduce job stress should give top priority to organizational change to improve working conditions. But even the most conscientious efforts to improve working conditions are unlikely to eliminate stress completely for all workers. For this reason, a combination of organizational change and stress management is often the most useful approach for preventing stress at work.

Section 8.3

Burnout: The Body's Response to Constant Levels of High Stress

"Burnout: Signs, Symptoms, and Prevention," reprinted with permission from http://www.helpguide.org/mental/burnout_signs_symptoms.htm. © 2007 Helpguide.org. All rights reserved. Helpguide provides a detailed list of related references for this article, including links to information from other websites. For a complete list of Helpguide's current resources related to stress signs and symptoms, causes of stress, burnout, and stress relief and relaxation techniques, visit www.helpguide.org.

What is burnout?

Burnout is a state of emotional and physical exhaustion caused by excessive and prolonged stress. It can occur when you feel overwhelmed and unable to meet constant demands. As the stress continues, you begin to lose the interest or motivation that led you to take on a certain role in the first place. Burnout reduces your productivity and saps your energy, leaving you feeling increasingly hopeless, powerless, cynical, and resentful. The unhappiness burnout causes can eventually threaten your job, your relationships, and your health.

How can you tell if you're burning out?

Because burnout doesn't happen overnight—and it's difficult to fight once you're in the middle of it—it's important to recognize the early signs of burnout and head it off. Burnout usually has its roots in stress, so the earlier you recognize the symptoms of stress and address them, the better chance you have of avoiding burnout.

The signs of burnout tend to be more mental than physical. They can include feelings of:

- frustration and powerlessness;
- hopelessness;
- being drained of emotional energy;
- detachment, withdrawal, isolation;

- being trapped;
- having failed at what you're doing;
- irritability;
- sadness; and
- cynicism (people act out of selfishness and nothing can be done about it).

If you're burning out and the burnout expresses itself as irritability, you might find yourself always snapping at people or making snide remarks about them. If the burnout manifests itself as depression, you might want to sleep all the time or always be "too tired" to socialize. You might turn to escapist behaviors such as sex, drinking, drugs, partying, or shopping binges to try to escape from your negative feelings. Your relationships at work and in your personal life may begin to fall apart.

What is the difference between stress and burnout?

Burnout may be the result of unrelenting stress, but it isn't the same as too much stress. Stress, by and large, involves too much: too many pressures that demand too much of you physically and psychologically. Stressed people can still imagine, though, that if they can just get everything under control, they'll feel better. Burnout, on the other hand, is about not enough. Being burned out means feeling empty, devoid of motivation, and beyond caring. People experiencing burnout often don't see any hope of positive change in their situations. If excessive stress is like drowning in responsibilities, burnout is being all dried up.

Dr. Arch Hart, in an article on stress and burnout in the clergy, lists some specific differences between stress and burnout (see Table 8.1).

One other difference between stress and burnout: While you're usually aware of being under a lot of stress, you don't always notice burnout when it happens. The symptoms of burnout—the hopelessness, the cynicism, the detachment from others—can take months to surface. If someone close to you points out changes in your attitude or behavior that are typical of burnout, listen to that person.

What causes job burnout?

Most of us have days when we're bored to death with what we do at work; when our co-workers and bosses seem irremediably wrong-headed;

90

when the dozen balls we keep in the air aren't noticed, let alone rewarded; when dragging ourselves into work requires the determination of Hercules; when caring about work seems like a waste of energy; when nothing we do appears to make a difference in a workplace full of bullying supervisors, clueless colleagues, and ungrateful clients.

We all have bad days at work. But when every day is a bad day, you're flirting with burnout. Most burnout has to do with the workplace, and it's present in every occupation. Those most at risk may be service professionals, who spend their work lives attending to the needs of others, especially if their work puts them in frequent contact with the dark or tragic side of human experience, or if they're underpaid, unappreciated, or criticized for matters beyond their control.

The following scenarios can lead to workplace burnout:

- setting unrealistic goals for yourself or having them imposed upon you;

- being expected to be too many things to too many people;

- working under rules that seem unreasonably coercive or punitive;

- doing work that frequently causes you to violate your personal values;

Table 8.1. Stress vs. Burnout

Stress	Burnout
Characterized by over-engagement	Characterized by disengagement
Emotions are overreactive	Emotions are blunted
Produces urgency and hyperactivity	Produces helplessness and hopelessness
Exhausts physical energy	Exhausts motivation and drive, ideals, and hope
Leads to anxiety disorders	Leads to paranoia, detachment, and depression
Causes disintegration	Causes demoralization
Primary damage is physical	Primary damage is emotional
Stress may kill you prematurely, and you won't have enough time to finish what you started.	Burnout may never kill you, but your life may not seem worth living.

91

- boredom from doing work that never changes or doesn't challenge you; and

- feeling trapped for economic reasons by a job that fits any of the scenarios above.

Remember, workplace burnout isn't the same as workplace stress. When you're stressed, you care too much, but when you're burned out, you don't see any hope of improvement. You don't want to get to that point.

What causes caregiver burnout?

Outside the world of paid work, the people more prone to burnout than any other group are caregivers: people who devote themselves to the unpaid care of chronically ill or disabled family members. More than 7 million American households contain caregivers, and that number will probably rise as life expectancy increases and the baby boomers age. While caregiving always represents stress for the caregiver, what may be a burden to one person may be more manageable to another. When caregiving goes on indefinitely, however, burnout—the point at which the caregiving experience is not a healthy option for the caregiver or the person receiving care—is always a possibility.

The stressors of caregiving—changes in the family dynamic, household disruption, financial concerns, and the sheer amount of work involved—can be overwhelming. The Ohio State University Department of Aging reports that "people today are feeling tremendous pressure to 'do it all,' taking care of children and aging parents while maintaining career and home. Instead of having a sense of accomplishment, many people feel guilt when they run out of energy to handle all of the tasks.

Another source of caregiver burnout is the lack of hope for a happy outcome. Often the rewards of caregiving, if they come at all, are intangible and far off, and the lack of control the caregiver feels over the situation is often compounded by other factors such as lack of finances, little or no family support, or poor management and planning skills. Without support, the caregiver becomes more and more isolated and sinks further and further into frustration and despair.

Pablo Casals, the world-renowned cellist, said, "The capacity to care is the thing that gives life its deepest significance and meaning." It's essential that caregivers receive enough support that they don't lose that capacity.

Can burnout be prevented or treated?

Because burnout is related to stress, many of the methods effective in countering stress can help prevent burnout as well. For one thing, it's important to build or maintain a foundation of good physical health, so be sure to eat right, get enough sleep, and make exercise part of your daily routine.

Preventing job burnout: The most effective way to head off job burnout is to quit doing what you're doing and do something else, whether that means changing jobs or changing careers. But if that isn't an option for you, there are still things you can do to improve your situation, or at least your state of mind.

Preventing caregiver burnout: When it comes to caregiver burnout, the stakes are high, as burned-out caregivers endanger people they

Table 8.2. Ways to Prevent Job Burnout

Clarify your job description	Ask your supervisor for an updated description of your job duties and responsibilities. You may then be able to point out that some of the things you're expected to do are not part of your job description and gain a little leverage by showing that you've been putting in work over and above the parameters of your job.
Request a transfer	If your workplace is large enough, you might be able to escape a toxic environment by transferring to another department. Talk to your supervisor or court a request from another supervisor.
Ask for new duties	If you've been doing the exact same work for a long time, ask to try something new: a different grade level, a different sales territory, a different machine.
Look for a new job	Update your résumé and apply for jobs that are related to but different from what you do now.
Make a career move	Get whatever training you need to make a big move in the same field, such as practicing a new area of law or teaching high school rather than elementary.
Make a career change	If you know you want to work in a different career, start taking steps toward it now, even if it's one community-college course at a time. Find out what the requirements are for the job you really want and start meeting them little by little.
Get career advice	Consult a career counselor or use the services of an agency that offers vocational services.

care about. And caregivers are more likely to be truly isolated from others. So the first strategy for preventing burnout as a caregiver is, don't try to do it all alone.

There are services to help caregivers in most communities, and the cost may be based on ability to pay or covered by the care receiver's insurance. Check to see if these services are available through local agencies:

- adult day care centers;
- home health aides;
- home-delivered meals;
- respite care;
- transportation services; or
- skilled nursing.

Also, enlist friends and family who live near you to run errands, bring a hot meal, or "baby-sit" the care receiver so you can have a well-deserved break. Finally, be sure to reward yourself. You deserve it.

For more ways to head off caregiver burnout, see Table 8.3.

Best defense against all burnout—Being with other people: Although taking time to yourself to relax is important in reducing stress, if you are approaching burnout, it's also crucial that you cultivate relationships with other people and spend time socializing with them. Poor relationships and isolation can contribute to burnout, but positive relationships can help prevent or reduce its onset.

Here are some steps you can take to improve your relationships with others:

- Nurture your closest relationships, such as those with your partner, children or friends. These relationships can help restore energy and alleviate some of the psychological effects of burnout, such as feelings of being under-appreciated. Try to put aside what's burning you out and make the time you spend with loved ones positive and enjoyable.

- Develop casual social relationships, on and off site, with people at your workplace. "We do all kinds of things, whether it is getting together to play cards or going out to eat. It gives everyone an opportunity to relax and blow off steam," a teacher wrote to a contributors' site. Just remember to avoid hanging out with negative-minded people who do nothing but complain.

- Connect with a cause or a community group that is personally meaningful to you. Joining a religious, social, or support group can give you a place to talk to like-minded people about how to deal with daily stress—and to make new friends. If your line of work has a professional association, you can attend meetings and interact with others coping with the same workplace demands.

- Practice healthy communication. Express your feelings to others who will listen, understand, and not judge. Burnout involves feelings that fester and grow, so be sure to let your emotions out in healthy, productive ways.

In summary, to prevent or recover from burnout, learn to cultivate methods of personal renewal, self-awareness, and connection with others, and don't be afraid to acknowledge your own needs and find ways to get your needs met.

Table 8.3. Ways to Prevent Caregiver Burnout

Educate yourself	Learn as much about the care receiver's illness and about how to be a caregiver as you can. The more you know, the more effective you'll be, and the better you'll feel about your efforts.
Join a support group	Find a caregivers' support group. You'll feel better knowing that other people are in the same situation, and their knowledge can be invaluable, especially if they're dealing with the same illness you are.
Know your limits	Be realistic about how much of your time and yourself you can give, set limits, and communicate those limits to doctors, family members, and other people involved.
Accept your feelings	You might be angry toward the care receiver because your care isn't appreciated; because you feel trapped in the position of caregiver; because someone you care about is ill. And then you might feel guilty for being angry. As long as you don't compromise the well-being of the care receiver, allow yourself to feel what you feel.
Confide in others	Talk to people about what you feel; don't keep your emotions bottled up. This is where the support group comes in, but trusted friends and family members can help, too.

Chapter 9

Negative Health Effects of Financial Stress

Every New Year's Eve, millions of Americans resolve to get healthier and wealthier. Health and personal finances are related in a variety of ways. Perhaps the simplest association is the high cost of unhealthy habits. Kick a $5 a day smoking habit, for example, and you can save $1,825 annually. The U.S. Department of Health and Human Services ("Preventing Obesity and Chronic Diseases," 2003) reports that a 10% weight loss will reduce an overweight person's lifetime medical costs by $2,200 to $5,300. Other linkages between financial well-being and physical health include: overdue medical debt resulting in delayed or inadequate treatment, stress and anxiety caused by financial difficulties (Drentea & Lavrakas, 2000), and lower retirement asset accumulation (Kim, 2004) and/or a poor credit history due to high medical bills.

Some employers are starting to use incentives (e.g., cash bonuses) and/or penalties (e.g., insurance surcharges) to motivate workers to adopt healthy lifestyle habits and reduce health care costs (Andrews, 2004; Wysocki, 2004). Others, particularly smaller companies ("Despite Rising Health-Care Costs," 2004), are simply shifting more of the burden of health care costs onto their employees through higher co-payments and deductibles (Fuhrmans, 2004a). There is also evidence of another employment-related linkage between health and wealth:

"Negative Health Effects of Financial Stress" *Consumer Interests Annual,* Volume 51. © 2005 American Council on Consumer Interests. Reprinted with permission.

workers earning less than $30,000 a year are less likely to have health insurance coverage and benefits. Two of five workers in low-paying jobs reported either not filling a prescription, skipping a test, or not seeing a doctor when sick, compared to just one-fifth of high-income workers (Fuhrmans, 2004b).

This study adds to the knowledge base about associations between health and wealth by exploring the specific health effects associated with financial distress. Respondents were asked to indicate if they felt that their health had been affected by their financial problems and, if they answered yes, to explain how with an open-ended response. The population for this study was a group of financially distressed consumers who telephoned a large national non-profit credit counseling organization, seeking assistance with outstanding debt, and subsequently joined its debt management program. A total of 6,757 questionnaires were mailed in June 2003 and 3,121 respondents (46%) returned usable questionnaires.

Characteristics of the sample are as follows: 69% were employed full time and 12% part time; 53% were married, 37% single living alone, and 10% single with a partner; 40% had two or more people to support, 21% had one dependent, and 39% had none. In addition, 71% of the sample was female and 54% were homeowners. More than 6 in 10 (62%) were age 45 or younger. Almost half (47%) of the sample had an annual family income of $30,000 or less, 30% earned 30,001 to $50,000, and 23% earned above $50,000. More than half (51%) of the sample reported experiencing moderate financial stress, and 23% and 12%, severe and overwhelming financial stress, respectively.

In this study, respondents reported exactly how their health was affected by their financial distress. Four in ten respondents (1,323/3,121 = 42.4%) answered yes to the question "Do you feel your health has been affected by your financial problems? If yes, please explain"; 1,091 (82.5%) specified some type of health effect. Some listed specific physical ailments while others mentioned an inability to afford health care services or recommended health maintenance practices. The responses were examined and classified into naturally occurring categories. The frequencies for each categorized response are reported in Table 9.1. The total adds up to more than 100% because up to three health effects per respondent were recorded from their open-ended responses.

These results indicate that there are a variety of perceived impacts of financial distress upon mental and physical health. Intuitively, it makes sense that poor health and financial problems are associated. Financial problems, such as overextended credit, are one of many life events that can cause people to experience the physical manifestations of stress (e.g., insomnia, migraines, anxiety) that are associated with many health problems and/or to cut back on recommended screening, prevention, and health maintenance activities. Indeed, stress was identified as a health effect of financial problems by almost half of the survey respondents who reported their personal finances affected their health (613/1,434 = 46.3%). Conversely, poor health can result in increased medical expenses, reduced productivity and earnings, and other negative financial effects that increase debt and drain household wealth.

Several of the "other" responses alluded to debt and problems paying bills, disability, missed workdays, and a change in work hours. These findings suggest that holistic educational programs and client support services should be developed that purposely blend health and personal finance topics to meet learner needs. For example, a class

Table 9.1. Health Effects of Financial Distress

Health Effect of Financial Problems	Frequency (Percentage)
Stress/stressed out	613 (46.3%)
Worry, nerves, tension, anxiety, pressure	157 (11.9%)
Depression/depressed	132 (10.0%)
Insomnia and sleep disorders/problems	122 (9.2%)
Headaches/migraines	96 (7.3%)
High blood pressure/hypertension	95 (7.2%)
Stomach/abdominal/digestive problems	38 (2.9%)
Other aches and pains (e.g., back, chest)	16 (1.2%)
Ulcers or possible ulcers	13 (1.0%)
Appetite disorders and weight gain or loss	46 (3.5%)
Fatigue and feeling tired/weak	14 (1.1%)
Drug, alcohol, or cigarette use	4 (.3%)
General or other sicknesses	85 (6.4%)
Unable to afford or access health care services and exams	8 (.6%)
Can't afford or don't follow recommended health maintenance practices	22 (1.7%)
Other responses	111 (8.4%)

about debt reduction might also cover stress management techniques. A cancer support group might discuss coping with the financial impact of diagnosis and treatment. Credit counselors might make inquiries about their clients' physical health and make referrals to low-cost health care services where needed. All too often, financial educators and health educators operate on separate tracks (Vitt, Siegenthaler, Lyter, & Kent, 2002) that are limited solely to their area of expertise.

Research is increasingly confirming the view that financial distress plays a role in causing and aggravating different health disorders. Continued research is needed on the effects of personal finances upon health and health upon personal finances, especially with panel data over time. In addition, more study is needed about successful motivational and behavior change strategies (e.g., employer incentives) that promote good health and financial security, as well as key "success factors" such as automation, environmental influences, positive thinking, and personal control.

References

Andrews, M. (2004, Dec.). Get healthy, get wealthy. *Money,* 33(12), 57. Despite rising health-care costs, few companies have cut benefits (2004, Sept.). *HR Focus,* 81(9), 3–5.

Drentea, P. & Lavrakas, P.J. (2000). Over the limit: The association among health status, race, and debt. *Social Science and Medicine,* 50, 517–529.

Fuhrmans, V. (2004a, Sept. 23). Burden of health care grows, even for the insured. *The Wall Street Journal,* p. D2.

Fuhrmans, V. (2004b, October 6). Health-care surge set to ease. *The Wall Street Journal,* p. A2.

Kim, J.E. (2004, Nov. 2). Rising health costs hinder retirement savings. *The Wall Street Journal,* p. D2.

Preventing obesity and chronic diseases through good nutrition and physical activity (2003). *Preventing Chronic Diseases: Investing Wisely in Health.* Washington DC: U.S. Department of Health and Human Services. Retrieved October 28, 2004 from www.healthierus.gov/steps/summit/prevportfolio/PA-HHS.pdf.

Vitt, L.A., Siegenthaler, J.K., Siegenthaler, L., Lyter, D.M., & Kent, J. (2002, January). Consumer health care finances and education: Matters of values. *Issue Brief Number 241*. Washington DC: Employee Benefit Research Institute.

Wysocki, B. (2004, Oct. 12). Companies get tough with smokers, obese to trim costs. *The Wall Street Journal*, p. B1, B13.

Authors: Barbara O'Neill, Rutgers Cooperative Research and Extension; Benoit Sorhaindo, InCharge Education Foundation, Inc.; Jing Jian Xiao, University of Arizona; E. Thomas Garman, Virginia Tech University.

Chapter 10

Caregiver Stress

What is a caregiver?

Caregivers are people who take care of other adults, most often parents or spouses, who are ill or disabled. The people who receive care usually need help with basic daily tasks. Caregivers help with many things such as the following:

- grocery shopping
- house cleaning
- cooking
- shopping
- paying bills
- giving medicine
- toileting
- bathing
- dressing
- eating

Usually caregivers take care of elderly people. Less often, caregivers are grandparents who are raising their grandchildren. The terms informal caregiver and family caregiver refer to people who are

---

"Caregiver Stress" is from the National Women's Health Information Center (NWHIC, www.womenshealth.gov), January 2006.

not paid to provide care. As the American population ages, the number of caregivers and the demands placed on them will grow.

Who are our nation's caregivers?

About one in four American families or 22.4 million households care for someone over the age of 50. The number of American households involved in caregiving may reach 39 million by 2007.

- About 75% of caregivers are women.

- Two thirds of caregivers in the United States have jobs in addition to caring for another person.

- Most caregivers are middle-aged: 35–64 years old.

What is caregiver stress?

Caregiver stress is the emotional strain of caregiving. Studies show that caregiving takes a toll on physical and emotional health. Caregivers are more likely to suffer from depression than their peers. Limited research suggests that caregivers may also be more likely to have health problems like diabetes and heart disease than non-caregivers.

Caring for another person takes a lot of time, effort, and work. Plus, most caregivers juggle caregiving with full-time jobs and parenting. In the process, caregivers put their own needs aside. Caregivers often report that it is difficult to look after their own health in terms of exercise, nutrition, and doctor's visits. So, caregivers often end up feeling angry, anxious, isolated, and sad.

Caregivers for people with Alzheimer disease (AD) or other kinds of dementia are particularly vulnerable to burnout. Research shows that most dementia caregivers suffer from depression and stress. Also, studies show that the more hours spent on caregiving, the greater the risk of anxiety and depression.

Women caregivers are particularly prone to feeling stress and overwhelmed. Studies show that female caregivers have more emotional and physical health problems, employment-related problems, and financial strain than male caregivers. Other research shows that people who care for their spouses are more prone to caregiving-related stress than those who care for other family members.

It is important to note that caring for another person can also create positive emotional change. Aside from feeling stress, many caregivers say their role has had many positive effects on their lives. For example, caregivers report that caregiving has given them a sense of purpose. They say that their role makes them feel useful, capable and that they are making a difference in the life of a loved one.

How can I tell if caregiving is putting too much stress on me?

If you have any of the following symptoms, caregiving may be putting too much strain on you:

- sleeping problems—sleeping too much or too little
- change in eating habits—resulting in weight gain or loss
- feeling tired or without energy most of the time
- loss of interest in activities you used to enjoy such as going out with friends, walking, or reading
- easily irritated, angered, or saddened
- frequent headaches, stomachaches, or other physical problems

What can I do to prevent or relieve stress?

Take care of yourself. In the process, you'll become a better caregiver. Take the following steps to make your health a priority:

- Find out about community caregiving resources.
- Ask for and accept help.
- Stay in touch with friends and family. Social activities can help you feel connected and may reduce stress.
- Find time for exercise most days of the week.
- Prioritize, make lists, and establish a daily routine.
- Look to faith-based groups for support and help.
- Join a support group for caregivers in your situation (like caring for a person with dementia). Many support groups can be found in the community or on the internet.
- See your doctor for a checkup. Talk to him or her about symptoms of depression or sickness you may be having.
- Try to get enough sleep and rest.
- Eat a healthy diet rich in fruits, vegetables, and whole grains and low in saturated fat.

- Ask your doctor about taking a multivitamin.
- Take one day at a time.

Caregivers who work outside the home should consider taking some time off. If you are feeling overwhelmed, taking a break from your job may help you get back on track. Employees covered under the federal Family and Medical Leave Act may be able to take up to 12 weeks of unpaid leave per year to care for relatives. Ask your human resources office about options for unpaid leave.

What is respite care?

The term respite care means care that gives the regular caregiver some time off. Respite care gives family caregivers a much-needed break. In the process, respite care reduces caregiver stress.

Respite care may be provided by these types of personnel and facilities:

- home health care workers
- adult day-care centers
- short-term nursing homes
- assisted living homes

Respite care is essential to family caregivers. Studies show that respite care helps caregivers keep their loved ones at home for longer periods of time.

What is the National Family Caregiver Support Program (NFCSP)?

The National Family Caregiver Support Program (NFCSP) is a federally-funded program through the Older Americans Act. The NFCSP helps states provide services that assist family caregivers. To be eligible for the NFCSP, caregivers must meet one of these criteria:

- care for adults aged 60 years and older
- be grandparents or relatives caring for a child under the age of 18

Each state offers different amounts and types of services. These include the following:

- information about available services
- help accessing support services
- individual counseling and organization of support groups
- caregiver training
- respite care
- limited supplemental services to complement the care provided by caregivers

How can I find out about caregiving resources in my community?

A number of resources can help direct you to the caregiver services you need. These agencies will be able to tell you these facts:

- what kind of services are available in your community
- if these services are right for you
- if you are eligible for these services
- and whom to contact and hours of operation

People who need help caring for an older person should contact their local Area Agency on Aging (AAA). AAAs are usually listed in the government sections of the telephone directory under "Aging" or "Social Services." A listing of state and area agencies on aging is also available online at: http://www.aoa.gov/eldfam/How_To_Find/Agencies/Agencies.asp.

The National Eldercare Locator, a toll-free service of the Administration on Aging, is another good resource. They can be reached by telephone at 800-677-1116 or online at www.eldercare.gov. The Eldercare Locator can help find your local or state AAA. When contacting the Eldercare Locator, callers should have the address, zip code, and county of residence for the person needing assistance.

What kind of caregiver services can I find in my community?

There are many kinds of community care services such as the following:

- transportation
- meals

- adult day care
- home care
- cleaning and yard work services
- home modification
- senior centers
- hospice care
- support groups
- legal and financial counseling

What kind of home care help is available?

There are two kinds of home care: home health care and non-medical home care services. Both types help sick and disabled people live independently in their homes for as long as possible. Caregivers and doctors decide what services are necessary and most helpful.

Home health care includes health-related services such as the following:

- medicine assistance
- nursing services
- physical therapy

Non-medical home care services include these types of services:

- housekeeping
- cooking
- companionship

How will I pay for home health care?

Medicare, Medicaid, and some private insurance companies will cover the cost of limited home care. Coverage varies from state to state. Other times, you will have to pay out of pocket for these services.

The cost of home care depends on what types of services are used. Non-medical workers like housekeepers are much less expensive than nurses or physical therapists. Also, some home care agencies are cheaper than others.

Who is eligible for Medicare home health care services?

To get Medicare home health care, a person must meet all of the following four conditions:

- A doctor must decide that the person needs medical care in the home and make a plan for home care.

- The person must need at least one of the following: sporadic (and not full time) skilled nursing care, physical therapy, speech language pathology services, or continue to need occupational therapy.

- The person must be homebound. This means that he or she is normally unable to leave home. When the person leaves home, it must be infrequent, for a short time, or to get medical care, or to attend religious services.

- The home health agency caring for the person must be approved by the Medicare program.

To find out if a person is eligible for Medicare home health care services, call the Regional Home Health Intermediary at 800-MEDI-CARE or visit the Medicare website at: www.medicare.gov.

Will Medicaid help pay for home health care?

To qualify for Medicaid, a person must have a low income and few other assets. Medicaid coverage differs from state to state. In all states, Medicaid pays for basic home health care and medical equipment. In some cases, Medicaid will pay for a homemaker, personal care, and other services not covered by Medicare.

For more information on Medicaid coverage of home health care in your state, call your state medical assistance office. For state telephone numbers, call 800-MEDICARE.

For More Information

For more information on caregivers, call the National Women's Health Information Center at 800-994-9662 or contact the following organizations:

Administration for Children and Families
Phone: 202-401-9215
Website: www.acf.dhhs.gov

Administration on Aging
Phone: 202-619-0724
Website: www.aoa.gov

Alzheimer's Association
Phone: 800-272-3900
Website: www.alz.org

Family Caregiver Alliance
Phone: 415-434 3388
Website: www.caregiver.org

National Adult Day Services Association, Inc.
Phone: 800-558-5301
Website: www.nadsa.org

National Association of Area Agencies on Aging
Phone: 202-872-0888
Website: www.n4a.org

National Family Caregivers Association
Phone: 800-896-3650
Website: www.nfcacares.org

The National Respite Locator Service
Phone: 800-773-5433
Website: www.respitelocator.org/index.htm

Chapter 11

Social Isolation, Loneliness, and Chronic Stress

Loneliness kills, according to research dating back to the 1970s. In one classic study, published in the *American Journal of Epidemiology* (Vol. 109, No. 2, pages 186–204), socially isolated people in Alameda County, California, were between two and three times more likely to die during the nine-year study than those who had many friends.

"The increase in morbidity with social isolation is equal to that of cigarette smoking," notes Martha McClintock, Ph.D., a University of Chicago psychology professor who researches social isolation and stress.

But while the pathway from smoking to cancer is largely established, the path from loneliness and other forms of chronic stress to many health consequences—including increased risk for cancer, cardiovascular illness, and Alzheimer disease—is not, she says. In humans, some of the effect may be due to the practical benefits of having a social network, says Gretchen Hermes, a fourth-year M.D.-Ph.D. student at the University of Chicago. For instance, people with many friends might be more likely to brush their teeth and exercise. And gregarious people may have more friends who bring them food or medicine when they get sick.

Dingfelder, S. (2006). Socially isolated and sick. *Monitor on Psychology, 37* (10), 18–19. Copyright © 2006 by the American Psychological Association. Reprinted with permission.

But new animal studies suggest that there are direct, physiological pathways from loneliness and other chronic stressors to illness. And those pathways may differ depending on gender and temperament, with male and behaviorally inhibited animals being particularly susceptible, researchers are finding.

Acute Stress: An Immune Booster?

Hermes and her colleagues found that, overall, social isolation suppressed wound healing in male and female rats, according to a study published last year in the *American Journal of Physiology-Regulatory, Comparative and Integrative Physiology* (Vol. 290, No. 1, pages 273–282). However, when they also acutely stressed the rats by trapping them in a small tube, the socially isolated female rats surprised researchers with an enhanced immune response, while the socially isolated male rats showed a further suppression of the immune response.

The researchers housed 60 female and 60 male rats either in groups of five or in isolated cages for more than three months. Then they injected half of the animals with a few milligrams of seaweed, right under their skin. The substance is harmless, but the immune system identifies it as foreign and surrounds it with scar tissue before absorbing it back into the body.

Both male and female isolated rats took longer to heal the wound than their group-housed brothers and sisters, the researchers found. While rats don't often face seaweed injections in the wild, the procedure taps into an underlying defense against many common illnesses, McClintock says.

"The basic inflammatory response is involved in a whole variety of different diseases, ranging from heart disease to infectious diseases and some forms of cancer," she notes.

Though socially isolated male and female rats responded similarly to the seaweed test, differences emerged when they were also exposed to an acute stressor. Two weeks before the seaweed injection, the researchers placed half of the socially isolated animals in a restraint tube for 30 minutes, a procedure that mimics the experience of being trapped in a collapsing burrow, says Hermes.

For the female rats, the trial revved up their immune systems—and they healed faster than those who didn't spend time in the restraint tube. The acutely stressed males, conversely, showed a slowed immune response.

"The females were much more resilient," Hermes notes.

The results fit with research on humans, says McClintock.

"Men who are lonely, or bereaved, or who lose their partners are known to be more vulnerable to disease and death, whereas women are more resilient," she notes.

The differences in both rats and humans may stem from the evolutionary pressure, McClintock theorizes. To pass on their genes, male animals only need to live long enough to mate. Female animals have to make it for the long haul.

"They need to survive to deliver and to take care of their young," she notes. "You can imagine it would be beneficial for evolution to select for females who could respond to a brief stressor with augmenting their immune function."

The Cost of Inhibition

One strength of the study is that they were able to randomly assign animals to social or isolated groups, notes McClintock. "That doesn't happen in nature," she says. For instance, some rats and humans tend to seek out others, while behaviorally inhibited animals will more likely live in isolation.

Even discounting of the effect of isolation, behavioral inhibition does seem to carry a health cost, according to a study published in the July issue of *Hormones and Behavior* (Vol. 50, No. 1, pages 454–462). In fact, behaviorally inhibited rats—those that tend to explore less because they find novel environments more threatening—died of natural causes a full six months earlier than their easygoing sisters, researchers found.

Penn State biobehavioral health professor Sonia Cavigelli, Ph.D., and her colleagues tested the temperament of 81 female rats when they were 20 days old, by placing them in an unfamiliar room, which included opaque walls and novel objects. Some of the animals moved freely around the room and sniffed the objects, while others huddled in the corner.

The animals then were housed in groups of three and lived out their natural lifespan. The particular strain of rat used in the study tends to live about two years, and they usually die of cancerous tumors that begin in their mammary glands, says Cavigelli.

While all the animals tended to die of tumors over time, the gregarious animals developed them about six months later than the inhibited ones. This may be because the inhibited animals don't socialize as much as other animals, or they may just get startled more often.

"Individuals that go through the stress response more frequently go through faster wear and tear on the system," Cavigelli notes.

Both studies shed light on the intricate mechanisms through which chronic stress, due to either social isolation or hypervigilance, can kill, says McClintock.

"They really begin to get to the richness of the dynamic," she notes. "In the area of stress, immunity, social context, and sex, one shouldn't expect simple main effects."

Chapter 12

Childhood Stress

As providers and caretakers, adults tend to view the world of children as happy and carefree. After all, kids don't have jobs to keep or bills to pay, so what could they possibly have to worry about?

Plenty! Even very young children have worries and feel stress to some degree. Stress is a function of the demands placed on us and our ability (or sometimes our perceived ability) to meet them.

Sources of Childhood Stress

Pressures often come from outside sources (such as family, friends, or school), but they can also come from within. The pressure we place on ourselves can be most significant because there is often a discrepancy between what we think we ought to be doing and what we are actually doing in our lives.

Stress can affect anyone—even a child—who feels overwhelmed. A 2-year-old child, for example, may be anxious because the person he or she needs to feel good—a parent—isn't there enough to satisfy him or her. In preschoolers, separation from parents is the greatest cause of anxiety.

As children get older, academic and social pressures (especially the quest to fit in) create stress. In addition, well-meaning parents

This information was provided by KidsHealth, one of the largest resources online for medically reviewed health information written for parents, kids, and teens. For more articles like this one, visit www.KidsHealth.org, or www.TeensHealth.org. © 2005 The Nemours Foundation. This document was reviewed by David V. Sheslow, Ph.D., and Meredith Lutz Stehl, MS, June 2005.

sometimes unwittingly add to the stress in their children's lives. For example, high-achieving parents often have great expectations for their children, who may lack their parents' motivation or capabilities. Parents who push their children to excel in sports or who enroll their children in too many activities may also cause unnecessary stress and frustration if their children don't share their goals.

Many professionals feel that a number of children are too busy and do not have time to play creatively or relax after school. Kids who begin to complain about the number of activities they are involved in or refuse to go to activities may be signaling to their parents that they are too busy. It's a good idea to talk with your child about how he or she is feeling about after-school activities. If he or she complains, talk about the pros and cons of quitting one of the activities. If quitting isn't an option, talk about ways that you can help your child manage his or her time and responsibilities so that they don't create so much anxiety.

Your child's stress level may be intensified by more than just what's happening in his or her own life. Does your child hear you talking about troubles at work, worrying about a relative's illness, or fighting with your spouse about financial matters? Parents need to be careful how they discuss such issues when their children are near because children will pick up on their parents' anxieties and start to worry themselves.

The events of September 11, 2001, and the changes in our world since then also added to the stress of many children—and not just those who were directly affected by the tragedy. Children who watch replays of the disturbing images on TV or hear talk of plane crashes, war, and bioterrorism may worry about their own safety and that of the people they love. Talk to your child about what he or she sees and hears and monitor what he or she watches on TV so that you can help your child understand what's going on and reassure him or her.

Also, consider that complicating factors, such as an illness, death of a loved one, or a divorce, may be causing your child's stress. When these factors are added to the everyday pressures kids face, the stress is magnified. Even the most amicable divorce can be a difficult experience for children because their basic security system—their family—is undergoing a tough change. Separated or divorced parents should never put kids in a position of having to choose sides or expose them to negative comments about the other spouse.

Recognizing Symptoms of Stress

It's not always easy to recognize when your child is stressed out. Short-term behavioral changes, such as mood swings, acting out, changes in sleep patterns, or bedwetting, can be indicators of stress. Some children experience physical effects, including stomachaches and headaches. Others have trouble concentrating or completing schoolwork. Still others become withdrawn or spend a lot of time alone. Younger children may show signs of reacting to stress by picking up new habits like thumb sucking, hair twirling, or nose picking; older children may begin to lie, bully, or defy authority. A child who is stressed out may also have nightmares, difficulty leaving you, over-reactions to minor problems, and drastic changes in academic performance.

Reducing Your Child's Stress

How can you help your child cope with stress? Proper rest and good nutrition can help increase your child's coping skills, as can good parenting. Make time for your child each day. Whether he or she needs to talk or just be in the same room with you, make yourself available. Even as your child gets older, this "quality time" is important. It's really hard for some people to come home after work, get down on the floor, and play with their kids or just talk to them about their day—especially if they've had a stressful day themselves. But by showing interest in your child's life, regardless of your child's age, you're showing your child that he or she is important to you.

Help your child cope with stress by talking with him or her about what may be causing it. Together, you can come up with a few solutions. Some possibilities are cutting back on after-school activities, spending more time talking with parents or teachers, developing an exercise regimen, or keeping a journal.

You can also help your child by anticipating potentially stressful situations and preparing him or her for them. For example, let your child know ahead of time that there is a doctor appointment coming up and talk about what will happen there.

Remember that some level of stress is normal; let your child know that it's OK to feel angry, scared, lonely, or anxious. Let him or her know that other people share his or her feelings.

Working through the Stress with Your Child

When children are unwilling or have trouble discussing these issues, it may be helpful to talk with your child about your own concerns. This will help your child see that you are willing to discuss these issues and allow him or her to feel like he or she has someone to talk with when he or she is ready. If your child continues to show symptoms that concern you and is unwilling to talk, it might be helpful to see a counselor or another type of mental health care specialist.

Books are a great way to allow young children to identify with characters in stressful situations and learn how they cope. Some titles include *Alexander and the Terrible, Horrible, No Good, Very Bad Day* by Judith Viorst; *Tear Soup* by Pat Schweibert, Chuck DeKlyen, and Taylor Bills; and *Dinosaurs Divorce* by Marc Brown and Laurene Krasny Brown.

Most parents have the skills necessary to deal with their child's stress. The time to seek professional attention is when any change in behavior persists, when your child's stress is causing serious anxiety, or when the behavior is causing significant problems with your child's functioning at school or at home.

If you are unsuccessful after several attempts to get to the source of your child's troubles, see your child's doctor and talk to the counselors and teachers at your child's school. These sources can lead you to competent professional help.

Chapter 13

Adolescent Stress

Adults commonly tell young people that the teenage years are the "best years of your life." The rosy remembrance highlights happy groups of high school students energetically involved at a dance or sporting event, and a bright-eyed couple holding hands or sipping sodas at a local restaurant. This is only part of the picture. Life for many young people is a painful tug-of-war filled with mixed messages and conflicting demands from parents, teachers, coaches, employers, friends, and oneself. Growing up—negotiating a path between independence and reliance on others—is a tough business. It creates stress, and it can create serious depression for young people ill-equipped to cope, communicate, and solve problems.

A study and a survey conducted recently in Minnesota provide information about the prevalence of adolescent stress and depression. The study and survey point out some of the stressful events young people experience, describe how young people deal with stress, and indicate the risk factors for young people most vulnerable to stress, depression, and self-destructive behavior. This major research project provides data on adolescent stress, depression, and suicide collected from nearly 4,300 high school students in 52 rural Minnesota counties. (Garfinkel, et al., 1986).

Adults need to be familiar with the family, biological, and personality factors that predispose a young person to depression. They can

"Adolescent Stress and Depression," by Joyce Walker, © 2005 University of Minnesota Extension. Reprinted with permission.

learn to recognize the kinds of psychological, behavioral, and social events that most often signal trouble. Awareness of the way these risk factors "pile up" helps any adult living and working with adolescents to be sensitive when stress and depression are imminent.

Stress and Depression Are Real

Stress and depression are serious problems for many teenagers, as the 1986 study of Minnesota high school students reveals. Although 61 percent of the students are not depressed and seem to handle their problems in constructive ways, 39 percent suffer from mild to severe depression. These young people often rely on passive or negative behaviors in their attempts to deal with problems.

Stress is characterized by feelings of tension, frustration, worry, sadness, and withdrawal that commonly last from a few hours to a few days. Depression is both more severe and longer lasting. Depression is characterized by more extreme feelings of hopelessness, sadness, isolation, worry, withdrawal, and worthlessness that last for two weeks or more. The finding that 9 percent of high school students are severely depressed is important since depression is the most important risk factor for suicide. The Minnesota Study found that 88 percent of the youth who reported making suicide attempts were depressed. Approximately 6 percent of the students reported suicide attempts in the previous six months.

Common Causes and Responses to Stress

Young people become stressed for many reasons. The Minnesota study presented students with a list of 47 common life events and asked them to identify those they had experienced in the last six months that they considered to be "bad." The responses indicated that they had experienced an average of two negative life events in the last six months. The most common of these were:

1. Break up with boy/girlfriend;
2. Increased arguments with parents;
3. Trouble with brother or sister;
4. Increased arguments between parents;
5. Change in parents' financial status;
6. Serious illness or injury of family member;

7.   Trouble with classmates;

8.   Trouble with parents.

These events are centered in the two most important domains of a teenager's life: home and school. They relate to issues of conflict and loss. Loss can reflect the real or perceived loss of something concrete such as a friend or money, and it can mean the loss of such intrinsic things as self-worth, respect, friendship, or love.

In a more informal survey of 60 young people (Walker, 1985), the primary sources of tension and trouble for teens and their friends were: relationships with friends and family; the pressure of expectations from self and others; pressure at school from teachers, coaches, grades, and homework; financial pressures; and tragedy in the lives of family and friends (described as death, divorce, cancer).

Most teenagers respond to stressful events in their lives by doing something relaxing, trying positive and self-reliant problem-solving, or seeking friendship and support from others. Common examples include listening to music, trying to make their own decisions, day-dreaming, trying to figure out solutions, keeping up friendships, watching television, and being close to people they care about. These behaviors are appropriate for adolescents who are trying to become independent, take responsibility for themselves, and draw on friends and family for support.

Troubled Youth Respond Differently

The majority of young people face the stress of negative life events, find internal or external resources to cope, and move on. But for others, the events pile up and the stressors are too great. In the Minnesota study teens who reported that they had made a suicide attempt had five additional "bad" events on their list: parents' divorce, loss of a close friend, change to a new school, failing grades, and personal illness or injury. It is significant that the young people who showed high degrees of depression and who had made suicide attempts reported over five of these "bad" events in the past six months, more than twice as many as the rest of the group.

The actions in response to stress were also different for those who reported serious depression or a suicide attempt. Young people who are depressed are at much greater risk of attempting suicide than non-depressed youth—although not all youth who attempt suicide are depressed. These young people report exhibiting much more anger and ventilation; avoidance and passivity; and aggressive, antisocial behavior.

They describe yelling, fighting, and complaining; drinking, smoking, and using doctor-prescribed drugs more frequently; and sleeping, riding around in cars, and crying more often. They are less inclined to do things with their family or to go along with parents' rules and requests.

A Closer Look at High-Risk Youth

It is important not to overreact to isolated incidents. Young people will have problems and will learn, at their own rate, to struggle and deal with them. But it is critical for parents and helping adults to be aware of the factors that put a youth at particular risk, especially when stressful events begin to accumulate for these vulnerable individuals. A good starting point for identifying and intervening with highly troubled and depressed young people is the careful study of suicidal adolescents.

Family history and biology can create a predisposition for dealing poorly with stress. These factors make a person susceptible to depression and self-destructive behavior.

- history of depression and/or suicide in the family;
- alcoholism or drug use in the family;
- sexual or physical abuse patterns in the family;
- chronic illness in oneself or family;
- family or individual history of psychiatric disorders such as eating disorders, schizophrenia, manic-depressive disorder, conduct disorders, or delinquency;
- death or serious loss in the family;
- learning disabilities or mental/physical disabilities;
- absent or divorced parents; inadequate bonding in adoptive families; and
- family conflict; poor parent/child relationships.

Personality traits, especially when they change dramatically, can signal serious trouble. These traits include:

- impulsive behaviors, obsessions, and unreal fears;

- aggressive and antisocial behavior;
- withdrawal and isolation; detachment;
- poor social skills resulting in feelings of humiliation, poor self-worth, blame, and feeling ugly;
- over-achieving and extreme pressure to perform; and
- problems with sleeping and/or eating.

Psychological and social events contribute to the accumulation of problems and stressors, such as:

- loss experience such as a death or suicide of a friend or family member; broken romance, loss of a close friendship or a family move;
- unmet personal or parental expectation such as failure to achieve a goal, poor grades, social rejection;
- unresolved conflict with family members, peers, teachers, or coaches that results in anger, frustration, rejection;
- humiliating experience resulting in loss of self-esteem or rejection; or
- unexpected events such as pregnancy or financial problems.

Predispositions, stressors, and behaviors weave together to form a composite picture of a youth at high risk for depression and self-destructive behavior. Symptoms such as personal drug and alcohol use, running away from home, prolonged sadness and crying, unusual impulsivity or recklessness, or dramatic changes in personal habits are intertwined with the family and personal history, the individual personality, and the emotional/social events taking place in a person's life.

It is not always easy for one person to see the whole picture. That's why it is essential that people who have hunches that something is wrong take the lead to gather perspectives from other friends, family members, and professionals who know the young person. It is all too often true that the survivors of an adolescent suicide only put the pieces together after the fact, when they sit together and try to figure out what happened. How fortunate a troubled young person is to have a caring adult take the initiative to look more closely before something serious happens.

Several common themes run through these two. First, young people must learn and practice coping skills to get them through an immediate conflict or problem. Coping strategies must emphasize self-responsibility to find positive, non-destructive ways to find relief. Second, communication skills are important. This involves being able to talk and selecting a good listener. It is important to express feelings, vent emotions, and talk about the problems and issues. Peers are good sympathizers, but it often takes an adult perspective to begin to plan how to make changes for the better. Third, young people need help to learn problem-solving skills. Sorting out the issues, setting goals, and making plans to move forward are skills that can be taught and practiced.

Ultimately, most young people will develop and assume the responsibility for their own protection and peace of mind. But during the years of learning and practice, parents, teachers, and helping adults need to be aware of the signs and patterns that signal danger. Awareness of adolescent stress and depression opens the door for adults to begin constructive interventions and stimulate emotional development.

References

Garfinkel, B. *Suicidal Behavior in Children and Adolescents*. Manuscript submitted for publication, 1985.

Garfinkel, B., Hoberman, H., Parsons, J., and Walker, J. *Adolescent Stress, Depression and Suicide: Minnesota study*. Unpublished raw data, 1986.

Fairfax County Public Schools. *The Adolescent Suicide Prevention Program: A Guide for Schools and Communities*. Fairfax, VA: Department of Student Services and Special Education, 1985.

Lewinsohn, P., and Teri, L. The Selection of Depressed and Non-depressed Subjects on the Basis of Self-report Data. Extended version of article in *Journal of Consulting and Clinical Psychology,* 1982, 50, 590–591.

Teri, L. The Use of the Beck Depression Inventory with Adolescents. *Journal of Abnormal Child Psychology,* 1982, 10, 227–284.

Select Committee on Aging, House of Representatives. *Suicide and Suicide Prevention* (Comm. Pub. No. 98497). Washington, DC: U.S. Government Printing Office, 1985.

Walker, J. Identification of Adolescent Stressors. Unpublished raw data, 1985.

Chapter 14

Stress and Aging

Increasing scientific evidence suggests that prolonged psychological stress takes its toll on the body, but the exact mechanisms by which stress influences disease processes had remained elusive, until recently. Now, scientists report that psychological stress may exact its toll—at least in part—by affecting molecules believed to play a key role in biological aging and, possibly, disease development.

In a landmark research study published in the December 1, 2004 issue of the *Proceedings of the National Academies of Sciences,* health psychologist Elissa Epel, Ph.D. and her colleagues found evidence to support the long suspected association between stress and cellular aging. According to Epel, Assistant Professor, Department of Psychiatry, University of California, San Francisco, both a prolonged objectively stressful situation and the perception of stress had an impact on three specific biological factors—oxidative stress, lower telomerase activity, and shorter telomere length—all of which are related to cell longevity and disease.

The results of the study, which involved 58 women, all of whom were biological mothers either of a chronically ill child (39 women, so-called "caregivers") or a healthy child (19 women, or "controls") were dramatic.

In one of the study's key findings, the duration of caregiving, after controlling for the age of the women, proved critical. The more years

"Stress and Aging," reprinted with permission from the American Federation for Aging Research. © 2005. For further information, visit www.infoaging.org.

of caregiving, the shorter the length of the telomeres, the lower the telomerase activity, and the greater the oxidative stress. The authors first looked at perceived stress. When they found a relationship, co-author Richard Cawthon said, "If there truly is a relationship with chronic stress, it should come out with years of caregiving." For that reason the research team examined years of caregiving in relation to cell aging, and the effect was almost identical to that of perceived stress.

Telomeres are the protective structures at the end of chromosomes. Like the caps of a shoelace, telomeres prevent the DNA [deoxyribonucleic acid] strands from unraveling. They also promote genetic stability. Each time a cell divides, a portion of telomeric DNA dwindles away by a few base pairs. After many rounds of cell division, so much DNA has diminished that the aged cell stops dividing. Thus, telomeres play a critical role in determining the health and life span of cells, as well as whatever tissues those particular cells may form.

According to Epel, both kinds of stress also affected the cellular enzyme telomerase, which replenishes a portion of telomeres with each round of cell division, thus protecting these structures. We already knew that oxidative stress hastens the shortening of telomeres in cell culture. In our study, we found that oxidative stress was related to shorter telomeres in people, as well. Oxidative stress is related to an overabundance of free radical toxins in the body. Free radicals damage lipids, proteins, and DNA—including the DNA of telomeres.

The perception of being stressed correlated in both the caregiver and control groups with the biological markers. In fact, in the most stunning result, telomeres of women with the highest perceived psychological stress—across both groups—had undergone the equivalent of approximately 10 years of additional aging compared with women across both groups who had the lowest perception of being stressed.

The highest stress group also had significantly decreased telomerase activity and higher oxidative stress than the lowest-stress group. This is the first evidence that psychological stress—and how a person perceives stress—may damp down telomerase and have a significant impact on the length of telomeres, suggesting that chronic stress may modulate the rate of cellular aging.

There was much variation among the caregivers' health and cell aging, which suggests that being a caregiver does not doom someone to developing short telomeres or lower levels of telomerase. Rather, it increases an individual's predisposition to these differences in telomere length and telomerase levels. Stress, therefore, is simply a risk factor for disease, rather than a direct marker of disease.

This new work quantifies a physiological price to feeling highly stressed. It emphasizes the importance of having some respite—that means taking time out to get one's own needs met. These may include sleep, social connections, exercise, and having some free time.

Part Two

The Physical Effects of Stress

Chapter 15

How Stress Affects the Body: The Link to Serious, Life-Threatening Diseases

Whether from a charging lion, or a pending deadline, the body's response to stress can be both helpful and harmful. The stress response gives us the strength and speed to ward off or flee from an impending threat. But when it persists, stress can put us at risk for obesity, heart disease, cancer, and a variety of other illnesses.

Perhaps the greatest understanding of stress and its effects has resulted from a theory by George Chrousos, M.D., Chief of the Pediatric and Reproductive Endocrinology Branch at the National Institute of Child Health and Human Development (NICHD), and Philip Gold, M.D., of the Clinical Neuroendocrinology Branch at the National Institute of Mental Health (NIMH).

Introduction

A threat to your life or safety triggers a primal physical response from the body, leaving you breathless with heart pounding and mind racing. From deep within your brain, a chemical signal speeds stress hormones through the bloodstream, priming your body to be alert and ready to escape danger. Concentration becomes more focused, reaction time faster, and strength and agility increase. When the stressful situation ends, hormonal signals switch off the stress response and the body returns to normal.

"Stress System Malfunction Could Lead to Serious, Life Threatening Disease," from the National Institutes of Health (NIH, www.nih.gov), September 9, 2002.

But in our modern society, stress doesn't always let up. Many of us now harbor anxiety and worry about daily events and relationships. Stress hormones continue to wash through the system in high levels, never leaving the blood and tissues. And so, the stress response that once gave ancient people the speed and endurance to escape life-threatening dangers runs constantly in many modern people and never shuts down.

Research now shows that such long-term activation of the stress system can have a hazardous, even lethal effect on the body, increasing risk of obesity, heart disease, depression, and a variety of other illnesses.

Much of the current understanding of stress and its effects has resulted from the theory by Drs. Chrousos and Gold. Their theory explains the complex interplay between the nervous system and stress hormones—the hormonal system known as the hypothalamic-pituitary-adrenal (HPA) axis. Over the past 20 years, Dr. Chrousos and his colleagues have employed the theory to understand a variety of stress-related conditions, including depression, Cushing syndrome, anorexia nervosa, and chronic fatigue syndrome.

The Stress Circuit

The HPA axis is a feedback loop by which signals from the brain trigger the release of hormones needed to respond to stress. Because of its function, the HPA axis is also sometimes called the "stress circuit."

Briefly, in response to a stress, the brain region known as the hypothalamus releases corticotropin-releasing hormone (CRH). In turn, CRH acts on the pituitary gland, just beneath the brain, triggering the release of another hormone, adrenocorticotropin (ACTH) into the bloodstream. Next, ACTH signals the adrenal glands, which sit atop the kidneys, to release a number of hormonal compounds.

These compounds include epinephrine (formerly known as adrenaline), norepinephrine (formerly known as noradrenaline), and cortisol. All three hormones enable the body to respond to a threat. Epinephrine increases blood pressure and heart rate, diverts blood to the muscles, and speeds reaction time. Cortisol, also known as glucocorticoid, releases sugar (in the form of glucose) from the body reserves so that this essential fuel can be used to power the muscles and the brain.

Normally, cortisol also exerts a feedback effect to shut down the stress response after the threat has passed, acting upon the hypothalamus and causing it to stop producing CRH.

This stress circuit affects systems throughout the body. The hormones of the HPA axis exert their effect on the autonomic nervous system, which controls such vital functions as heart rate, blood pressure, and digestion.

The HPA axis also communicates with several regions of the brain, including the limbic system, which controls motivation and mood, with the amygdala, which generates fear in response to danger, and with the hippocampus, which plays an important part in memory formation as well as in mood and motivation. In addition, the HPA axis is also connected with brain regions that control body temperature, suppress appetite, and control pain.

Similarly, the HPA axis also interacts with various other glandular systems, among them those producing reproductive hormones, growth hormones, and thyroid hormones. Once activated, the stress response switches off the hormonal systems regulating growth, reproduction,

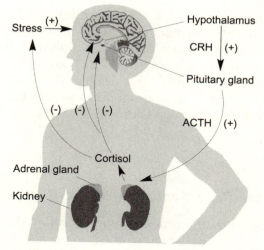

Regulation of the stress response by the hypothalamus-pituitary-adrenal (HPA) axis.

ACTH = adrenocorticotropic hormone; CRH = corticotropin-releasing hormone; + = stimulates; - = inhibits.

Figure 15.1. *The body's response to stressors. (Source: From "Understanding Stress: Characteristics and Caveats," in the National Institute of Alcohol Abuse and Alcoholism (NIAAA) journal* Alcohol Research & Health, *Volume 23, Number 4, 1999.)*

metabolism, and immunity. Short term, the response is helpful, allowing us to divert biochemical resources to dealing with the threat.

Stress, Heredity, and the Environment

According to Dr. Chrousos, this stress response varies from person to person. Presumably, it is partially influenced by heredity. For example, in most people the HPA axis probably functions appropriately enough, allowing the body to respond to a threat, and switching off when the threat has passed. Due to differences in the genes that control the HPA axis, however, other people may fail to have a strong enough response to a threat, while still others may over respond to even minor threats.

Beyond biological differences, the HPA axis also can alter its functioning in response to environmental influences. The HPA axis may permanently be altered as a result of extreme stress at any time during the life cycle—during adulthood, adolescence, early childhood, or even in the womb.

If there are major stresses in early childhood, the HPA feedback loop becomes stronger and stronger with each new stressful experience. This results in an individual who, by adulthood, has an extremely sensitive stress circuit in place. In life threatening situations—such as life in an area torn by war—this exaggerated response would help an individual to survive. In contemporary society, however, it usually causes the individual to overreact hormonally to comparatively minor situations.

Effects on the Body

Stress and the Reproductive System

Stress suppresses the reproductive system at various levels, says Dr. Chrousos. First, CRH prevents the release of gonadotropin releasing hormone (GnRH), the "master" hormone that signals a cascade of hormones that direct reproduction and sexual behavior. Similarly, cortisol and related glucocorticoid hormones not only inhibit the release of GnRH, but also the release of luteinizing hormone, which prompts ovulation and sperm release. Glucocorticoids also inhibit the testes and ovaries directly, hindering production of the male and female sex hormones testosterone, estrogen, and progesterone.

The HPA overactivity that results from chronic stress has been shown to inhibit reproductive functioning in anorexia nervosa and in starvation, as well as in highly trained ballet dancers and runners. For example, in one study, Chrousos found that men who ran more than 45 miles per week produced high levels of ACTH and cortisol in response to the stress of extreme exercise. These male runners had low LH and testosterone levels. Other studies have shown that women undertaking extreme exercise regimens had ceased ovulating and menstruating.

However, the interaction between the HPA axis and the reproductive system is also a two-way street. The female hormone estrogen exerts partial control of the gene that stimulates CRH production. This may explain, why, on average, women have slightly elevated cortisol levels. In turn, higher cortisol levels, in combination with other, as yet unknown, factors, may be the reason why women are more vulnerable than men to depression, anorexia nervosa, panic disorder, obsessive-compulsive disorder, and autoimmune diseases like lupus and rheumatoid arthritis.

Growth and Stress

The hormones of the HPA axis also influence hormones needed for growth. Prolonged HPA activation will hinder the release of growth hormone and insulin-like growth factor 1 (IGF-1), both of which are essential for normal growth. Glucocorticoids released during prolonged stress also cause tissues to be less likely to respond to IGF-1. Children with Cushing syndrome—which results in high glucocorticoid levels—lose about 7.5 to 8.0 centimeters from their adult height.

Similarly, premature infants are at an increased risk for growth retardation. The stress of surviving in an environment for which they are not yet suited, combined with the prolonged stress of hospitalization in the intensive care unit, presumably activates the HPA axis. Growth retarded fetuses also have higher levels of CRH, ACTH, and cortisol, probably resulting from stress in the womb or exposure to maternal stress hormones.

Old research has also shown that the stress from emotional deprivation or psychological harassment may result in the short stature and delayed physical maturity of the condition known as psychosocial short stature (PSS).

PSS was first discovered in orphanages, in infants who failed to thrive and grow. When these children were placed in caring environments in which they received sufficient attention, their growth resumed. The children's cortisol levels were abnormally low, a seeming contradiction, which Chrousos investigated by studying a small, non-human primate, the common marmoset. These monkeys live in small family groups in which infants are cared for by both parents. As in human society, the infants are sometimes well cared for, but sometimes abused. Like humans, the abused monkeys showed evidence of PSS.

The researchers determined that the stressed and abused monkeys appeared to respond normally to stress, but seemed unable to "switch off" the stress response by secreting appropriate cortisol levels, thereby remaining in a state of prolonged stress arousal as compared to their peers.

The Gastrointestinal Tract and Stress

As many of us know, stress can also result in digestive problems. The stress circuit influences the stomach and intestines in several ways. First, CRH directly hinders the release of stomach acid and emptying of the stomach. Moreover, CRH also directly stimulates the colon, speeding up the emptying of its contents. In addition to the effects of CRH alone on the stomach, the entire HPA axis, through the autonomic nervous system, also hinders stomach acid secretion and emptying, as well as increasing the movement of the colon.

Also, continual, high levels of cortisol—as occur in some forms of depression, or during chronic psychological stress—can increase appetite and lead to weight gain. Rats given high doses of cortisol for long periods had increased appetites and had larger stores of abdominal fat. The rats also ate heavily when they would normally have been inactive. Overeating at night is also common among people who are under stress.

The Immune System and Stress

The HPA axis also interacts with the immune system, making you more vulnerable to colds and flu, fatigue, and infections.

In response to an infection, or an inflammatory disorder like rheumatoid arthritis, cells of the immune system produce three substances that cause inflammation: interleukin 1 (IL-1), interleukin 6 (IL-6), and tumor necrosis factor (TNF). These substances, working either singly or in combination with each other, cause the release of CRH. IL-6 also promotes the release of ACTH and cortisol. Cortisol and other compounds then suppress the release of IL-1, IL-6, and TNF, in the process switching off the inflammatory response.

Ideally, stress hormones damp down an immune response that has run its course. When the HPA axis is continually running at a high level, however, that damping down can have a downside, leading to decreased ability to release the interleukins and fight infection.

In addition, the high cortisol levels resulting from prolonged stress could serve to make the body more susceptible to disease, by switching off disease-fighting white blood cells. Although the necessary studies have not yet been conducted, Dr. Chrousos considers it possible that this same deactivation of white blood cells might also increase the risk for certain types of cancer.

Conversely, there is evidence that a depressed HPA axis, resulting in too little corticosteroid, can lead to a hyperactive immune system and increased risk of developing autoimmune diseases—diseases in which the immune system attacks the body's own cells. Over-activation of the antibody-producing B cells may aggravate conditions like lupus, which result from an antibody attack on the body's own tissues.

Stress-Related Disorders

One of the major disorders characteristic of an overactive HPA axis is melancholic depression. Chrousos' research has shown that people with depression have a blunted ability to "counter-regulate," or adapt to the negative feedback of increases in cortisol. The body turns on the "fight or flight" response, but is prevented from turning it off again. This produces constant anxiety and overreaction to stimulation, followed by the paradoxical response called "learned helplessness," in which victims apparently lose all motivation.

Hallmarks of this form of depression are anxiety, loss of appetite, loss of sex drive, rapid heart beat, high blood pressure, and high cholesterol and triglyceride levels. People with this condition tend to produce higher-than-normal levels of CRH. The high levels of CRH are probably due to a combination of environmental and hereditary causes, depending on the person affected.

However, rather than producing higher amounts of ACTH in response to CRH, depressed people produce smaller amounts of this substance, presumably because their hippocampuses have become less sensitive to the higher amounts of CRH. In an apparent attempt to switch off excess CRH production, the systems of people with melancholic depression also produce high levels of cortisol. However, by-products of cortisol, produced in response to high levels of the substance, also depress brain cell activity. These byproducts serve as sedatives, and perhaps contribute to the overall feeling of depression.

Other conditions are also associated with high levels of CRH and cortisol. These include anorexia nervosa, malnutrition, obsessive-compulsive disorder, anxiety disorder, alcoholism, alcohol and narcotic withdrawal, poorly controlled diabetes, childhood sexual abuse, and hyperthyroidism.

The excessive amount of the stress hormone cortisol produced in patients with any of these conditions is responsible for many of the observed symptoms. Most of these patients share psychological symptoms including sleep disturbances, loss of libido, and loss of appetite as well as physical problems such as an increased risk for accumulating abdominal fat and hardening of the arteries and other forms of cardiovascular disease. These patients may also experience suppression of thyroid hormones, and of the immune system. Because they are at higher risk for these health problems, such patients are likely to have their life spans shortened by 15 to 20 years if they remain untreated.

Although many disorders result from an overactive stress system, some result from an underactive stress system. For example, in the case of Addison disease, lack of cortisol causes an increase of pigment in the skin, making the patient appear to have a tan. Other symptoms include fatigue, loss of appetite, weight loss, weakness, loss of body hair, nausea, vomiting, and an intense craving for salt. Lack of the hormone CRH also results in the feelings of extreme tiredness common to people suffering from chronic fatigue syndrome. Lack of CRH is also central to seasonal affective disorder (SAD), the feelings of fatigue and depression that plague some patients during winter months.

Chrousos and his team, showed that sudden cessation of CRH production may also result in the depressive symptoms of postpartum depression. In response to CRH produced by the placenta, the mother's system stops manufacturing its own CRH. When the baby is born, the sudden loss of CRH may result in feelings of sadness or even severe depression for some women.

Recently, Dr. Chrousos and his coworkers uncovered evidence that frequent insomnia is more than just having difficulty falling asleep. The researchers found that, when compared to a group of people who did not have difficulty falling asleep, the insomniacs had higher ACTH and cortisol levels, both in the evening and in the first half of the night. Moreover, the insomniacs with the highest cortisol levels tended to have the greatest difficulty falling asleep.

The researchers theorized that, in many cases, persistent insomnia may be a disorder of the stress system. From their ACTH and cortisol levels, it appears that the insomniacs have nervous systems that are on overdrive, alert and ready to deal with a threat, when they should otherwise be quieting down. Rather than prescribing drugs known as hypnotics to regulate the sleep system, the researchers suggested that physicians might have more success prescribing antidepressants, to help calm an overactive stress system. Behavior therapy, to help insomniacs relax in the evening, might also be useful.

After conducting many years of research into the functioning of the HPA axis, Dr. Chrousos concluded that chronic stress should not be taken lightly or accepted as a fact of life.

"Persistent, unremitting stress leads to a variety of serious health problems," Dr. Chrousos said. "Anyone who suffers from chronic stress needs to take steps to alleviate it, either by learning simple techniques to relax and calm down, or with the help of qualified therapists."

Chapter 16

Stress and Sleep

Sleep is an essential part of our daily lives and well-being. Lost sleep robs us of the opportunity to restore ourselves physically, emotionally, and even cognitively. Lost sleep and the resulting daytime sleepiness affect our mood, behavior, and performance. In effect, we are how we sleep. How we sleep at night affects who we are, what we do, and how we do it during the day, although we are not always aware of many signs and symptoms as well as the costs and consequences caused by sleep disruptions. A night of seven to nine hours of restful, uninterrupted sleep becomes particularly important during times of high stress and anxiety.

"Not getting enough sleep impairs our work performance, increases the risk for injuries, and makes it more difficult to get along with others," says Mark Rosekind, Ph.D., an expert on fatigue and performance issues. "Without sufficient sleep it is more difficult to concentrate, make careful decisions, and follow instructions, we are more likely to make mistakes or errors, and are more prone to being impatient and lethargic. Our attention, memory, and reaction time are all affected. But while we may recognize these symptoms, we do not always associate them as being symptoms of sleep loss," he adds.

Dr. Rosekind also notes that while one night of significant sleep loss can affect alertness the next day, accumulated sleep loss over multiple nights is a problem that must be dealt with. Dr. Rosekind, president and chief scientist of Alertness Solutions in Cupertino, California, is a

"Sleep is Important When Stress and Anxiety Increase, Says NSF" © 2003 National Sleep Foundation (www.sleepfoundation.org). All rights reserved. Reprinted with permission.

member of the National Sleep Foundation's board of directors. He is former director of NASA's Fatigue Countermeasures Program.

In order to help people address their need for sleep and sleep problems, the National Sleep Foundation (NSF) offers the following information about sleep problems and symptoms that can signal inadequate sleep and tips for helping people maximize the sleep they do get during these times of high stress and anxiety:

- Don't expect to fall asleep immediately after hearing or watching disturbing news. Stop watching or listening to news programs at least an hour before trying to go to sleep. Leave the war news (or other bad news on the TV or radio) in the living room or den and out of the bedroom.

- Engage in a relaxing, non-alerting activity at bedtime such as reading or listening to music. For some people, soaking in a warm bath or hot tub can be helpful. Avoid activities that are mentally or physically stimulating.

- Do not eat or drink too much before bedtime. Alcohol is not a sleep aid; don't use it to try to help you sleep.

- Only get into bed when you're tired. If you don't fall asleep within 15 minutes, get out of bed, go to another room and engage in a relaxing activity such as reading. Return to your bed when you're sleepy.

- Create a sleep-promoting environment that is quiet, dark, cool, and comfortable.

During the Day

- Consume less or no caffeine. Excess caffeine has the potential to disturb sleep at night. If you feel tired during the day, substitute a short nap of about 15 to 20 minutes for caffeine. Naps can relieve acute sleepiness and restore alertness, but for people suffering from insomnia, daytime naps should be avoided.

- Avoid alcohol and nicotine, especially close to bedtime.

- Exercise, but not within 3 hours before bedtime.

Anytime

- Talk to other people. Many people think their symptoms of sleeplessness are unique to them. If you talk to others, you will find that many share your problems. Learning how others have coped can be helpful.

- Seek professional help. If you are unable to deal with the sleeplessness and it is becoming a problem for you, you might benefit from professional help. Your family doctor will know about medications that can help you fall asleep without a hangover the following day.

- Remember—sleeplessness associated with an acute stressful situation usually improves on its own. Be patient.

Common Sleep Problems during Times of Stress

- Insomnia is characterized by difficulty falling asleep, waking up frequently during the night, waking up too early, or feeling unrefreshed upon awakening. If these symptoms persist for more than a few days, seek help from a physician or other health care provider. Be cautious about self-treatments such as alcoholic beverages that may worsen the problem or not be effective.

- Nightmares can increase during periods of great stress for all people, though they occur most frequently in children age 3 to 6. Avoid eating or taking high-dose vitamins before bed, which can increase brain activity and the onset of nightmares. Also avoid alcohol, caffeine, and other stimulants. Exercise and relaxation techniques may be helpful.

- Excessive daytime sleepiness (EDS) and fatigue, with symptoms such as difficulty concentrating or dozing off while watching TV or reading, are best handled by stopping what you are doing and taking a nap or retiring early and going to sleep. Be cautious about treating EDS with caffeine or over-the-counter stimulants as they temporarily mask sleep loss and can cause sleep disruption. If EDS persists for more than a few days, speak to a physician or other health care provider.

Symptoms That Can Signal Inadequate Sleep

- Dozing off while engaged in an activity such as reading, watching TV, sitting in meetings, or sitting in traffic

- Slowed thinking and reacting

- Difficulty listening to what is said or understanding directions

- Difficulty remembering or retaining information
- Frequent errors or mistakes
- Narrowing of attention or missing important changes in a situation
- Depression or negative mood
- Impatience or being quick to anger
- Frequent blinking, difficulty focusing eyes, or heavy eyelid

Helping Children

At times of acute stress or trauma, parents and guardians should expect children to experience sleep problems, regardless of their age. It may take a few weeks for them to get back to their normal routines, but if the problems continue beyond that time, consider seeking further help from your child's physician or other health care provider, the school psychologist, or your child's teacher.

There are things parents can do to help minimize the impact of stressful events on their children, and help them get a restful night's sleep.

For All Children

- Your child's anxiety may affect falling asleep. Find out about his/her concerns and talk about them. While you should try to avoid these conversations at bedtime, don't shut off the conversation; talk briefly and offer to continue the conversation tomorrow.
- To avoid insomnia, try to maintain your child's usual bedtime and bedtime routines.
- Avoid foods and beverages containing caffeine at least four hours before bedtime, and exposure to news broadcasts at least an hour before bedtime.

Middle School and Younger Children

- If your child has trouble falling asleep alone, avoid a drastic response (e.g., everyone sleeping together). Stay near until your child falls asleep. Provide reassurance by telling him/her you will check in.

- Turn on a light in the hallway or next room, but not the bedroom. Music can provide some soothing noise. The presence of a family pet in the bedroom (even a goldfish!) is often reassuring.

- If your child has nightmares and wakes up in the middle of the night, don't have a long discussion about the dream; be reassuring and help your child fall back to sleep. In the morning, if he or she tells you about a bad dream, that's a good time to talk either about the dream or the events that may have precipitated it.

- If your child is significantly anxious at bedtime, relaxation techniques (familiar tapes, deep breathing exercises) can be distracting and anxiety reducing.

Adolescents

Teens may be more affected by events than we realize and, therefore, at higher risk for sleep problems. Their greater understanding of events can be accompanied by a greater degree of worrying, making them more at risk for insomnia than younger children.

- Show teens the extra support, doting, and soothing that is given to younger children.

- Teens may experience insomnia or phase delay, such as going to bed later than usual because of talking on the phone, watching television, or e-mailing friends. Parents must set limits on this behavior, and keep their teen on a normal bedtime routine.

Chapter 17

The Dietary and Weight Consequences of Stress

Chapter Contents

Section 17.1

Stress: The Number-One Emotional Eating Trigger

"The Number One Predictor of Diet Failure—and How to Beat It" is from the National Women's Health Information Center's Pick Your Path to Health Campaign, 1995–2001. Reviewed by David A. Cooke, M.D., March 2007.

The single most common emotional eating trigger and the number-one predictor of weight loss relapse is stress, according to obesity expert Dr. John P. Foreyt of Baylor College of Medicine.

Being "stressed out" is a common expression nowadays. You hear this phrase often and perhaps even utter it from time to time yourself. However, do you really know what being stressed out means?

It is commonly used in a negative sense, and when translated it usually means you are beyond your comfort or tolerance level—physically and/or psychologically.

Stress isn't necessarily a bad thing. It's a natural part of living. Life without any stress is impossible. When you're working hard, tired, hungry, emotionally charged, or sick with the flu, your body secretes hormones in response to these stressors in order to reestablish your body's stability. That's the inside chemistry of stress. Your challenge is to try to maintain a comfortable amount of stress that you can manage.

Recognizing Stress

"I don't know. I start feeling anxious. My temper gets short. I feel hopeless. I know when I'm getting stressed out," says Kathy Dyer of Bowie, Maryland, mother of three ranging in age from 5 months to 13 years old, and full-time policy analyst and attorney for the federal government. Kathy is ahead of the game by the mere fact that she realizes when she has stress and can take measures to handle the situation.

Research has shown that African-American women have higher levels of adrenaline in their systems as they are stressed and this can result in high blood pressure and even premature death.

The first step in managing stress is to recognize that it exists. The big stressors are easy to identify—natural disasters, illness, death, births, marriage, moving, and job changes. But daily life, the low-grade, day-to-day responsibilities—and yes, even things you enjoy doing that need your constant attention—are stressors and can eventually take a toll on your health. Debra Churos of Alexandria, Virginia, mother of an 8-year-old daughter and part-time office worker, identified some of the following symptoms when she is stressed.

- anxiety
- short temper
- eating—anything and everything
- feeling hopeless
- crying
- irritability
- headaches
- breathing heavier and heart pounding
- more emotional/stressed around menstrual cycle

According to the American Medical Women's Association, Debra's symptoms are common. Whether you have these symptoms or not, you can be pretty sure that stress has some role and effect on your life and health, and it can play havoc with your weight-control efforts.

Strategies to Deal with It

Stress happens. And when it does, you will react to it. The most common reaction is to eat. Actually, it's not a bad idea to eat when feeling stressed. But what you will probably do is to eat something that makes you feel good. You know what those feel-good-foods are: ice cream, potato chips, macaroni and cheese, and peach cobbler. This is especially true if you grew up using food as a stress releaser. Instead of reaching for the ice cream, try using these alternatives to release stress.

- Try healthy comfort-food alternatives: Low-fat proteins (yogurt, turkey), vegetables, and fruit. If you have a refrigerator at the office, keep some of these at the office for when you get hungry. If that's not an option, have some fruit or cut-up raw vegetables in a plastic bag in your purse or at your desk.

- Don't sweat the small stuff: Manage your time better. Make a list of what needs to be done and prioritize them. As Debra says, "I ask myself what's the most important thing to accomplish and what can wait."

- Find time to relax and unwind: Go to a place just for yourself (bathroom, the park, a special place in your home). Find 10 to 20 minutes each day to relax and to just give your mind a break.

- Pray, meditate, yoga: It works for many people.

- Exercise.

- Establish a support system: Join a woman's group of any kind where you will get support and a chance to relate to others.

- Reduce environmental stressors: Dislike your job? Find another one.

- Noisy neighbors getting on your nerves? Move. Sometimes we can't control our environment, but when we can, it can make all the difference.

- Ask for help when you need it: Ask and you shall receive.

As you pick your path to a more stress-manageable and healthy life, keep in mind every woman needs a break.

Section 17.2

The Perils of Stress Eating

"Perils of Stress Eating, Snacks, and Soft Drinks," by Nancy Kuppersmith, M.S., R.D., and Cynthia Kennedy, M.S., R.D., University of Louisville Department of Family and Geriatric Medicine. © University of Louisville Research Foundation. Reprinted with permission. This document is undated.

The scene: you are stressed. Before you know it, there is food in your mouth. How did that food get there?

You Are Not Hungry

You know you shouldn't be eating the food. All of a sudden, you feel guilty, angry at yourself, and you want to eat more, even though you know you shouldn't.

Meanwhile the Calories Are Adding Up

This situation happens over and over in the lives of many people. The reason why people eat when stressed is complex but stress eating can be stopped. First we need to become aware that we are doing it.

Eating will not:

- pay the bills;
- make a problem better;
- save a relationship; or
- solve any problem except hunger.

However, stress eating can cause weight gain. This can lead to more stress. Don't get trapped in the stress eating cycle—get relief some other way. Call a friend, join a support group, read a book, or get help from a counselor who specializes in the stress eating cycle.

If snacking is a problem for you, the more you learn to manage your snacking, the easier it will be to manage your health and weight. Avoid

151

temptations by planning ahead. Stay focused on living a life that is healthiest for you.

Stop Stress Eating

Before you eat anything, ask yourself: am I really hungry?

- If the answer is yes, go ahead and eat.
- If the answer is no, do not eat. Find something else to do, like taking a walk, working on a hobby, cleaning, or talking.

If you find yourself in the process of eating, stop, calm down, and try to figure out what is wrong instead of eating.

Remember, eating will not control the stress around you. In fact, it will add to your stress. Instead of eating, try doing something else with the problem that is causing the stress.

Snacks: Solid and Liquid

Mindless snacking and drinking sugared beverages can add unnecessary calories and cause what seems like overnight weight gain. Here are some day-to-day temptations to avoid:

- Vending machines
- Leftovers in the refrigerator
- Goodies being passed around the office
- Tasting food while cooking a meal
- Drinking a caffeinated soft drink in the car to avoid getting sleepy while driving
- Using food as a "crutch"
- Munching while watching TV, using the computer, or playing a video game

Tempting Snack Situations

- At work, food is either there or brought in for a meal. We can be tempted to eat before even thinking about our hunger because the sights and smells are hard to resist.
- Grocery stores often have candy bars, soft drinks, and cookies on sale, and the price is too good.

- TV food commercials can be so tempting that we are mindlessly led to the kitchen to reach for the first available food or drink.

- Vending machines are everywhere and we are tempted again.

- Fast food signs on the road tempt us to pull in and get a quick drink or bite to eat.

- Banks and restaurants often have pieces of candy, and since they are free, we help ourselves.

- Bad news—before we know it, food or drink is in our mouth!

Avoiding the Perils

- Eat meals at regular times every day and plan ahead for snacks by packing them from home.

- Have plenty of water, diet soft drinks, sugar-free iced tea, or other sugar-free beverages available to drink, rather than drinks with sugar added.

- Don't skip a meal or two to allow you to eat more at a party or gathering. Your hunger may make it difficult to control portion size. Instead, if you're hungry, eat a healthy snack before going to a gathering so you will have control over how much you choose to eat.

- Pack your lunch so you know ahead of time what you will be having and you can eat it, or part of it, instead of being tempted by foods that are brought in.

- Take up a hobby such as working on a puzzle, knitting, sewing, or crocheting while watching television so you have something to do with your hands besides eat.

- Instead of eating at the gas station, get out of the car and take a short walk to energize you for the rest of the trip.

Section 17.3

Binge Behavior and Addiction Linked to Stress

"Binge behavior/addiction linked to stress, tripling desire for sugar,"
April 13, 2006, University of Michigan News Service. © 2006 Regents
of the University of Michigan. Reprinted with permission.

Stressed individuals might be particularly prone to binge eating or drug addiction because of high levels of a hormone mechanism in their brain, according to University of Michigan (U-M) and Georgetown University research.

"There are lots of reasons why stressed people might over eat or gamble or chase after hedonic rewards. Unfortunately this new result reveals another one," said U-M psychology professor Kent Berridge. "People who feel bad during stress cope in part by overeating or pursuing other incentives.

"Now it turns out a stress chemical also activates the same brain mechanism that goes wrong in drug addiction to make us excessively want pleasurable things."

The study, published in the [April 13, 2006 issue of the] journal *BMC Biology*, shows that rats with levels of corticotropin-releasing factor (CRF) in their brain similar to the levels experienced by humans when they are stressed show an exaggerated craving for a reward—some sugar—whenever presented with a cue that had previously been associated with that reward.

"The brain stress substance tripled the intensity of desire for sugary treats normally triggered by cues for those treats," Berridge said.

This result explains why stressed individuals might be more likely to experience strong cravings for rewards and compulsively indulge in pleasurable activities such as eating or taking drugs.

U-M psychology researcher Susana Peciña and Berridge from U-M collaborated with Georgetown University physiology and biophysics professor Jay Schulkin to painlessly inject rats with either a high dose (500ng/0.2 ml) or a low dose (250ng/ 0.2 ml) of CRF, part of the brain's internal stress-signaling system that serves as a brain stress neurotransmitter.

They injected the rats in a part of the brain called nucleus accumbens, known to be involved in the mediation of both pleasurable rewards and stress signals in humans as well as rats.

They observed the rats' behavior in response to a cue—a 30-second tone—that had previously been associated with the release of a reward, in the form of sugar pellets.

When they heard the cue, the rats pressed on a lever that they expected to release more sugar pellets. The authors made sure that the rats did not experience stress due to CRF itself or to other factors in the experimental set-up.

Their results show that injection of a high dose of CRF tripled the intensity of bursts of sugar craving, measured by the pressing on the sugar-associated lever.

The lever-pressing activity was only enhanced if the injection of CRF was followed by the cue—it did not increase following the injection alone. The low dose of CRF, or an empty injection, also failed to enhance the lever-pressing activity significantly.

"When CRF reaches the nucleus accumbens it creates a special window of vulnerability to temptation," Berridge said. "This could trap individuals into chasing incentives they could normally resist, pulled in by tempting cues or images that become more powerfully wanted."

Section 17.4

Night Eating Syndrome
Caused or Triggered by Stress

"Night eating syndrome" is information used with permission of
ANRED: Anorexia Nervosa and Related Eating Disorders, Inc.,
http://www.anred.com.

There are at least two problems that involve disordered eating primarily at night: night eating syndrome (NES), which is discussed here, and nocturnal sleep-related eating disorder.

Signs and Symptoms

- The person has little or no appetite for breakfast. Delays first meal for several hours after waking up. Is not hungry or is upset about how much was eaten the night before.

- Eats more food after dinner than during that meal.

- Eats more than half of daily food intake during and after dinner but before breakfast. May wake up and leave the bed to snack at night. May not be aware at the time of what they are doing.

- This pattern has persisted for at least two months.

- Person feels tense, anxious, upset, or guilty while eating.

- NES is thought to be stress related and is often accompanied by depression. Especially at night the person may be moody, tense, anxious, nervous, agitated, etc.

- Has trouble falling asleep or staying asleep. Wakes frequently and then often eats.

- Foods ingested are often carbohydrates: sugary and starchy.

- Behavior is not like binge eating, which is done in relatively short episodes. Night eating syndrome involves continual eating throughout evening hours.

- This eating produces guilt and shame, not enjoyment.

How Many People Have Night Eating Syndrome?

Perhaps only one to two percent (1% to 2%) of adults in the general population have this problem, but research at the University of Pennsylvania School of Medicine suggests that about six percent of people who seek treatment for obesity have NES. Another study suggests that more than a quarter (27%) of people who are overweight by at least 100 pounds have the problem.

Discussion

Night eating syndrome has not yet been formally defined as an eating disorder. Underlying causes are being identified, and treatment plans are still being developed. It seems likely that a combination of biological, genetic, and emotional factors contribute to the problem.

One theory postulates that people with this condition are under stress, either recognized or hidden. Their bodies are flooded with cortisol, a stress hormone. Eating may be the body's attempt to neutralize cortisol or slow down its production. More research needs to be done before this explanation can be accepted or rejected. In any event, stress appears to be a cause or trigger of NES, and stress-reduction programs, including mental health therapy, seem to help.

Researchers are especially interested in the foods chosen by night eaters. The heavy preference for carbohydrates, which trigger the brain to produce so-called "feel-good" neurochemicals, suggests that night eating may be an unconscious attempt to self-medicate mood problems and relieve stress.

NES may run in families. At this time it appears to respond to treatment with the selective serotonin reuptake inhibitor (SSRI) sertraline, a prescription medication. NES is remarkable for characteristic disturbances in the circadian rhythm of food intake while circadian sleep rhythms remain normal.

If you are seeking help for night eating syndrome, you would be wise to schedule a complete physical exam with your physician and also an evaluation with a counselor experienced in the treatment of eating disorders and also sleep disorders. In addition, a dietitian can help develop meal plans that distribute intake more evenly throughout the day so that you are not so vulnerable to caloric loading in the evening.

Evaluation in a sleep laboratory could be worthwhile. Most large hospitals have such facilities. It is not yet clear whether night eating is an eating disorder or sleep disorder or both. The more information available to the person and treatment team, the greater the chances are of developing an effective treatment plan.

Chapter 18

Stress and Headaches

Chapter Contents

159

Section 18.1

Stress, Mood, and Headaches

Reprinted from the website of the American Council for Headache Education (www.achenet.org). Copyright © 2004, American Council for Headache Education. All rights reserved.

Stress is by far the most common headache "trigger." Both female and male headache sufferers report that headaches are more likely to occur during or after periods of stress. Major life-changing events like marriage, birth of a child, or career changes all are sources of stress. However, research has found that it is actually the day-to-day stress or chronic "hassles" that are important in triggering headache. Compared to men, women often experience more of the types of stress that provoke headache.

Identifying the Most Common Stresses

Multiple-Role Stress

Women are likely to have "multiple-role," which is stress due to managing many different roles and responsibilities. Common roles include being a mother, wife, professional working woman, and care-taker of the home. Often these important roles conflict with one another, and women are forced to make tough choices between competing demands. Sometimes, women overextend themselves trying to do it all. Other times, women suffer disappointment and guilt if they are not able to meet all of the demands of family, home, and work.

Workplace Stress

The majority of women in America today work outside the home. Although some women hold high-status and powerful positions, many more women have jobs with high demands and low control. These jobs can lead a woman to feel "helpless" in the workplace. Helplessness worsens the physical and emotional effects of stress and also prevents individuals from even trying to improve their situation.

Financial Stress

Women on average earn less money than men and have a lower overall standard of living. Therefore, women often feel pressures from inadequate housing, poor access to health care, and fear of unexpected expenses. In such cases, women also have fewer opportunities for recreation and escape from day-to-day stress.

Caregiver Stress

Women are likely to be the primary caretaker in the family. Though many men are taking active roles in parenting, women still provide the majority of child care. There are great joys in parenting, but it can also be a physically and emotionally taxing responsibility. Women also are more likely to be the primary caregiver for aging parents and ill family members. Providing family care does not end at the close of a 40-hour workweek. Instead, the caretaker sometimes needs to provide 24-hour care on a daily basis.

Learn to Make Time for Yourself

Women that overextend themselves might find it helpful to actually schedule time for themselves (yes, mark it on the calendar, and put it in the daily planner). One easy way to do this is to make an appointment with "yourself", and show up on time as one would with any other appointment. Should someone ask for "this or that," the answer is: "I am sorry, I have an appointment." Women with migraine do not need to make themselves more important than anyone else, but they need to consider themselves at least as important as everyone else.

Stress Management

Headache sufferers can learn skills to identify the stress that triggers their headaches. Sometimes the stress can be removed or resolved. In cases where the stress is uncontrollable, a woman can learn to change her own physical and emotional reactions to stressful situations. Individuals learn to recognize and change their own reactions to stress through a variety of stress-management techniques. Techniques such as biofeedback and relaxation training are effective in reducing headache frequency and pain in many sufferers.

Other techniques can help cope with headaches while they are occurring such as taking charge of headache. This involves keeping track of headaches, monitoring success and failure of therapies, identifying and monitoring things that may "trigger" headache, and making and keeping appointments with health care providers.

The Impact of Mood on Headaches

Headache and Psychological Symptoms

Personality: Headache is not a psychological disorder, and the majority of headache sufferers do not have significant psychological problems. Physicians in the 1800s and early 1900s suggested that headaches were related to a particular personality pattern. Headache researchers have now collected over 200 scientific studies examining the personality and behavior of headache sufferers.

In most studies, headache sufferers tend to have increased daily stress, more difficulty coping with stress, and more mild symptoms of depression. However, there is no good evidence for a particular headache-prone personality.

Depression: Women have a higher risk for depression than men. In fact, women are three times more likely to experience an episode of depression than men are. The reason for the increased risk is not entirely clear, but may relate to a combination of biological (such as hormones, pregnancy, genetic predisposition) and environmental factors (stress, allergies, sleep).

Depression also is known to occur more often in headache sufferers than non-headache sufferers. The stress of coping with a chronic painful medical condition, like headache, increases the risk of depression. Even low levels of depression can reduce the effectiveness of medication and behavioral (biofeedback or relaxation training) or cognitive (behavioral) treatments for headache. Therefore, it is very important to recognize the signs of depression and discuss them with the physician. This information can help the physician select treatments that can relieve symptoms of both headache and depression.

Symptoms of possible depression:

- Sad, depressed, or irritable mood

- Loss of interest or pleasure in activities

- Weight loss (when not dieting) or weight gain

- Sleep disturbance (insomnia, early morning awakenings, increased sleeping)

- Feeling agitated or feeling sluggish
- Feelings of worthlessness
- Inability to concentrate
- Recurrent thoughts of death or suicide

Anxiety: As with depression, women are at a greater risk than men are for anxiety. Anxiety involves a state of tension or fear that occurs without clear cause. Anxiety can lower one's threshold to stress so that even small amounts of stress can be difficult for these sufferers to manage. Anxiety also can increase the level of pain or reduce the pain tolerance threshold during a headache that can undermine the effectiveness of traditional headache treatments. For some sufferers, it is necessary to treat both the anxiety and the headaches in order to get both under control.

Symptoms of possible anxiety:

- Feeling restless, keyed up, or on edge
- Being easily fatigued
- Difficulty concentrating or mind going blank
- Muscle tension
- Sleep disturbance (difficulty falling asleep or staying asleep)

Treatment

If depression or anxiety are present in a patient with migraine, both disorders need to be treated. It is generally not true that treating the depression will make the headaches go away, or that headache improvement will lead to an improvement in mood. Specific treatment for both migraine and depression exists and will produce the best outcome.

Section 18.2

Tension Headaches Often Caused by Stress

From "Headache: Hope Through Research," from the
National Institute of Neurological Disorders and Stroke
(NINDS, www.ninds.nih.gov), October 16, 2006.

Introduction

For 2 years, Jim suffered the excruciating pain of cluster headaches. Night after night he paced the floor, the pain driving him to constant motion. He was only 48 years old when the clusters forced him to quit his job as a systems analyst. One year later, his headaches are controlled. The credit for Jim's recovery belongs to the medical staff of a headache clinic. Physicians there applied the latest research findings on headache, and prescribed for Jim a combination of new drugs.

Joan was a victim of frequent migraine. Her headaches lasted 2 days. Nauseous and weak, she stayed in the dark until each attack was over. Today, although migraine still interferes with her life, she has fewer attacks and less severe headaches than before. A specialist prescribed an antimigraine program for Joan that included improved drug therapy, a new diet, and relaxation training.

An avid reader, Peggy couldn't put down the new mystery thriller. After 4 hours of reading slumped in bed, she knew she had overdone it. Her tensed head and neck muscles felt as if they were being squeezed between two giant hands. But for Peggy, the muscle-contraction headache and neck pain were soon relieved by a hot shower and aspirin.

Understanding why headaches occur and improving headache treatment are among the research goals of the National Institute of Neurological Disorders and Stroke (NINDS). As the leading supporter of brain research in the Federal Government, the NINDS also supports and conducts studies to improve the diagnosis of headaches and to find ways to prevent them.

Why Does It Hurt?

What hurts when you have a headache? The bones of the skull and tissues of the brain itself never hurt, because they lack pain-sensitive nerve fibers. Several areas of the head can hurt, including a network of nerves which extends over the scalp and certain nerves in the face, mouth, and throat. Also sensitive to pain, because they contain delicate nerve fibers, are the muscles of the head and blood vessels found along the surface and at the base of the brain.

The ends of these pain-sensitive nerves, called nociceptors, can be stimulated by stress, muscular tension, dilated blood vessels, and other triggers of headache. Once stimulated, a nociceptor sends a message up the length of the nerve fiber to the nerve cells in the brain, signaling that a part of the body hurts. The message is determined by the location of the nociceptor. A person who suddenly realizes "My toe hurts," is responding to nociceptors in the foot that have been stimulated by the stubbing of a toe.

A number of chemicals help transmit pain-related information to the brain. Some of these chemicals are natural painkilling proteins called endorphins, Greek for "the morphine within." One theory suggests that people who suffer from severe headache and other types of chronic pain have lower levels of endorphins than people who are generally pain free.

When Should You See a Physician?

Not all headaches require medical attention. Some result from missed meals or occasional muscle tension and are easily remedied. But some types of headache are signals of more serious disorders and call for prompt medical care. These include:

- sudden, severe headache;
- sudden, severe headache associated with a stiff neck;
- headache associated with fever;
- headache associated with convulsions;
- headache accompanied by confusion or loss of consciousness;
- headache following a blow on the head;
- headache associated with pain in the eye or ear;
- persistent headache in a person who was previously headache free;
- recurring headache in children; and
- headache that interferes with normal life.

A headache sufferer usually seeks help from a family practitioner. If the problem is not relieved by standard treatments, the patient may then be referred to a specialist—perhaps an internist or neurologist. Additional referrals may be made to psychologists.

What Tests Are Used to Diagnose Headache?

Diagnosing a headache is like playing Twenty Questions. Experts agree that a detailed question-and-answer session with a patient can often produce enough information for a diagnosis. Many types of headaches have clear-cut symptoms which fall into an easily recognizable pattern.

Patients may be asked: How often do you have headaches? Where is the pain? How long do the headaches last? When did you first develop headaches? The patient's sleep habits and family and work situations may also be probed.

Most physicians will also obtain a full medical history from the patient, inquiring about past head trauma or surgery, eye strain, sinus problems, dental problems, difficulties with opening and closing of the jaw, and the use of medications. This may be enough to suggest strongly that the patient has migraine or cluster headaches. A complete and careful physical and neurological examination will exclude many possibilities and the suspicion of aneurysm, meningitis, or certain brain tumors. A blood test may be ordered to screen for thyroid disease, anemia, or infections which might cause a headache.

A test called an electroencephalogram (EEG) may be given to measure brain activity. EEG's can indicate a malfunction in the brain, but they cannot usually pinpoint a problem that might be causing a headache. A physician may suggest that a patient with unusual headaches undergo a computed tomographic (CT) scan and/or a magnetic resonance imaging (MRI) scan. The scans enable the physician to distinguish, for example, between a bleeding blood vessel in the brain and a brain tumor, and are important diagnostic tools in cases of headache associated with brain lesions or other serious disease. CT scans produce X-ray images of the brain that show structures or variations in the density of different types of tissue. MRI scans use magnetic fields and radio waves to produce an image that provides information about the structure and biochemistry of the brain.

If an aneurysm—an abnormal ballooning of a blood vessel—is suspected, a physician may order a CT scan to examine for blood and then an angiogram. In this test, a special fluid which can be seen on an X-ray is injected into the patient and carried in the bloodstream to the brain to reveal any abnormalities in the blood vessels there.

A physician analyzes the results of all these diagnostic tests along with a patient's medical history and examination in order to arrive at a diagnosis.

Headaches are diagnosed as:

- vascular;
- muscle contraction (tension);
- traction; or
- inflammatory.

Vascular headaches—a group that includes the well-known migraine—are so named because they are thought to involve abnormal function of the brain's blood vessels or vascular system. Muscle contraction headaches appear to involve the tightening or tensing of facial and neck muscles. Traction and inflammatory headaches are symptoms of other disorders, ranging from stroke to sinus infection. Some people have more than one type of headache.

What Are Migraine Headaches?

The most common type of vascular headache is migraine. Migraine headaches are usually characterized by severe pain on one or both sides of the head, an upset stomach, and at times disturbed vision.

Former basketball star Kareem Abdul-Jabbar remembers experiencing his first migraine at age 14. The pain was unlike the discomfort of his previous mild headaches.

"When I got this one I thought, 'This is a headache'," he says. "The pain was intense and I felt nausea and a great sensitivity to light. All I could think about was when it would stop. I sat in a dark room for an hour and it passed."

Symptoms of Migraine

Abdul-Jabbar's sensitivity to light is a standard symptom of the two most prevalent types of migraine-caused headache: classic and common.

The major difference between the two types is the appearance of neurological symptoms 10 to 30 minutes before a classic migraine attack. These symptoms are called an aura. The person may see flashing lights or zigzag lines or may temporarily lose vision. Other classic

167

symptoms include speech difficulty, weakness of an arm or leg, tingling of the face or hands, and confusion.

The pain of a classic migraine headache may be described as intense, throbbing, or pounding and is felt in the forehead, temple, ear, jaw, or around the eye. Classic migraine starts on one side of the head but may eventually spread to the other side. An attack lasts 1 to 2 pain-wracked days.

Common migraine—a term that reflects the disorder's greater occurrence in the general population—is not preceded by an aura. But some people experience a variety of vague symptoms beforehand, including mental fuzziness, mood changes, fatigue, and unusual retention of fluids. During the headache phase of a common migraine, a person may have diarrhea and increased urination, as well as nausea and vomiting. Common migraine pain can last 3 or 4 days.

Both classic and common migraine can strike as often as several times a week, or as rarely as once every few years. Both types can occur at any time. Some people, however, experience migraines at predictable times—for example, near the days of menstruation or every Saturday morning after a stressful week of work.

The Migraine Process

Research scientists are unclear about the precise cause of migraine headaches. There seems to be general agreement, however, that a key element is blood flow changes in the brain. People who get migraine headaches appear to have blood vessels that overreact to various triggers.

Scientists have devised one theory of migraine that explains these blood flow changes and also certain biochemical changes that may be involved in the headache process. According to this theory, the nervous system responds to a trigger such as stress by causing a spasm of the nerve-rich arteries at the base of the brain. The spasm closes down or constricts several arteries supplying blood to the brain, including the scalp artery and the carotid or neck arteries.

As these arteries constrict, the flow of blood to the brain is reduced. At the same time, blood-clotting particles called platelets clump together—a process that is believed to release a chemical called serotonin. Serotonin acts as a powerful constrictor of arteries, further reducing the blood supply to the brain.

Reduced blood flow decreases the brain's supply of oxygen. Symptoms signaling a headache, such as distorted vision or speech, may then result, similar to symptoms of stroke.

Reacting to the reduced oxygen supply, certain arteries within the brain open wider to meet the brain's energy needs. This widening or dilation spreads, finally affecting the neck and scalp arteries. The dilation of these arteries triggers the release of pain-producing substances called prostaglandins from various tissues and blood cells. Chemicals that cause inflammation and swelling, and substances that increase sensitivity to pain, are also released. The circulation of these chemicals and the dilation of the scalp arteries stimulate the pain-sensitive nociceptors. The result, according to this theory: a throbbing pain in the head.

Women and Migraine

Although both males and females seem to be equally affected by migraine, the condition is more common in adult women. Both sexes may develop migraine in infancy, but most often the disorder begins between the ages of 5 and 35.

The relationship between female hormones and migraine is still unclear. Women may have "menstrual migraine"—headaches around the time of their menstrual period—which may disappear during pregnancy. Other women develop migraine for the first time when they are pregnant. Some are first affected after menopause.

The effect of oral contraceptives on headaches is perplexing. Scientists report that some women with migraine who take birth control pills experience more frequent and severe attacks. However, a small percentage of women have fewer and less severe migraine headaches when they take birth control pills. And normal women who do not suffer from headaches may develop migraines as a side effect when they use oral contraceptives. Investigators around the world are studying hormonal changes in women with migraine in the hope of identifying the specific ways these naturally occurring chemicals cause headaches.

Triggers of Headache

Although many sufferers have a family history of migraine, the exact hereditary nature of this condition is still unknown. People who get migraines are thought to have an inherited abnormality in the regulation of blood vessels.

"It's like a cocked gun with a hair trigger," explains one specialist. "A person is born with a potential for migraine and the headache is triggered by things that are really not so terrible."

These triggers include stress and other normal emotions, as well as biological and environmental conditions. Fatigue, glaring or flickering lights, changes in the weather, and certain foods can set off migraine. It may seem hard to believe that eating such seemingly harmless foods as yogurt, nuts, and lima beans can result in a painful migraine headache. However, some scientists believe that these foods and several others contain chemical substances, such as tyramine, which constrict arteries—the first step of the migraine process. Other scientists believe that foods cause headaches by setting off an allergic reaction in susceptible people.

While a food-triggered migraine usually occurs soon after eating, other triggers may not cause immediate pain. Scientists report that people can develop migraine not only during a period of stress but also afterwards when their vascular systems are still reacting. For example, migraines that wake people up in the middle of the night are believed to result from a delayed reaction to stress.

Other Forms of Migraine

In addition to classic and common, migraine headache can take several other forms.

Patients with **hemiplegic migraine** have temporary paralysis on one side of the body, a condition known as hemiplegia. Some people may experience vision problems and vertigo—a feeling that the world is spinning. These symptoms begin 10 to 90 minutes before the onset of headache pain.

In **ophthalmoplegic migraine**, the pain is around the eye and is associated with a droopy eyelid, double vision, and other problems with vision.

Basilar artery migraine involves a disturbance of a major brain artery at the base of the brain. Preheadache symptoms include vertigo, double vision, and poor muscular coordination. This type of migraine occurs primarily in adolescent and young adult women and is often associated with the menstrual cycle.

Benign exertional headache is brought on by running, lifting, coughing, sneezing, or bending. The headache begins at the onset of activity, and pain rarely lasts more than several minutes.

Status migrainosus is a rare and severe type of migraine that can last 72 hours or longer. The pain and nausea are so intense that people who have this type of headache must be hospitalized. The use of certain drugs can trigger status migrainosus. Neurologists report that many of their status migrainosus patients were depressed and anxious before they experienced headache attacks.

Headache-free migraine is characterized by such migraine symptoms as visual problems, nausea, vomiting, constipation, or diarrhea. Patients, however, do not experience head pain. Headache specialists have suggested that unexplained pain in a particular part of the body, fever, and dizziness could also be possible types of headache-free migraine.

How Is Migraine Headache Treated?

During the Stone Age, pieces of a headache sufferer's skull were cut away with flint instruments to relieve pain. Another unpleasant remedy used in the British Isles around the ninth Century involved drinking "the juice of elderseed, cow's brain, and goat's dung dissolved in vinegar." Fortunately, today's headache patients are spared such drastic measures.

Drug therapy, biofeedback training, stress reduction, and elimination of certain foods from the diet are the most common methods of preventing and controlling migraine and other vascular headaches. Joan, the migraine sufferer, was helped by treatment with a combination of an antimigraine drug and diet control.

Regular exercise, such as swimming or vigorous walking, can also reduce the frequency and severity of migraine headaches. Joan found that whirlpool and yoga baths helped her relax.

During a migraine headache, temporary relief can sometimes be obtained by applying cold packs to the head or by pressing on the bulging artery found in front of the ear on the painful side of the head.

Drug Therapy

There are two ways to approach the treatment of migraine headache with drugs: prevent the attacks or relieve symptoms after the headache occurs.

For infrequent migraine, drugs can be taken at the first sign of a headache in order to stop it or to at least ease the pain. People who get occasional mild migraine may benefit by taking aspirin or acetaminophen at the start of an attack. Aspirin raises a person's tolerance to pain and also discourages clumping of blood platelets. Small amounts of caffeine may be useful if taken in the early stages of migraine. But for most migraine sufferers who get moderate to severe headaches, and for all cluster headache patients, stronger drugs may be necessary to control the pain.

Several drugs for the prevention of migraine have been developed in recent years, including serotonin agonists, which mimic the action of this key brain chemical. One of the most commonly used drugs for the relief of classic and common migraine symptoms is sumatriptan, which binds to serotonin receptors. For optimal benefit, the drug is taken during the early stages of an attack. If a migraine has been in progress for about an hour after the drug is taken, a repeat dose can be given.

Physicians caution that sumatriptan should not be taken by people who have angina pectoris, basilar migraine, severe hypertension, or vascular or liver disease.

Another migraine drug is ergotamine tartrate, a vasoconstrictor that helps counteract the painful dilation stage of the headache. Other drugs that constrict dilated blood vessels or help reduce blood vessel inflammation also are available.

For headaches that occur three or more times a month, preventive treatment is usually recommended. Drugs used to prevent classic and common migraine include methysergide maleate, which counteracts blood vessel constriction; propranolol hydrochloride, which stops blood vessel dilation; amitriptyline, an antidepressant; valproic acid, an anticonvulsant; and verapamil, a calcium channel blocker.

Antidepressants called MAO [monoamine oxidase] inhibitors also prevent migraine. These drugs block an enzyme called monoamine oxidase, which normally helps nerve cells absorb the artery-constricting brain chemical, serotonin. MAO inhibitors can have potentially serious side effects—particularly if taken while ingesting foods or beverages that contain tyramine, a substance that constricts arteries.

Many antimigraine drugs can have adverse side effects. But like most medicines they are relatively safe when used carefully and under a physician's supervision. To avoid long-term side effects of preventive medications, headache specialists advise patients to reduce the dosage of these drugs and then stop taking them as soon as possible.

Biofeedback and Relaxation Training

Drug therapy for migraine is often combined with biofeedback and relaxation training. Biofeedback refers to a technique that can give people better control over such body function indicators as blood pressure, heart rate, temperature, muscle tension, and brain waves. Thermal biofeedback allows a patient to consciously raise hand temperature. Some patients who are able to increase hand temperature can reduce the number and intensity of migraines. The mechanisms underlying these self-regulation treatments are being studied by research scientists.

"To succeed in biofeedback," says a headache specialist, "you must be able to concentrate and you must be motivated to get well."

A patient learning thermal biofeedback wears a device that transmits the temperature of an index finger or hand to a monitor. While the patient tries to warm his hands, the monitor provides feedback either on a gauge that shows the temperature reading or by emitting a sound or beep that increases in intensity as the temperature increases. The patient is not told how to raise hand temperature, but is given suggestions such as "Imagine your hands feel very warm and heavy."

"I have a good imagination," says one headache sufferer who traded in her medication for thermal biofeedback. The technique decreased the number and severity of headaches she experienced.

In another type of biofeedback called electromyographic or EMG training, the patient learns to control muscle tension in the face, neck, and shoulders.

Either kind of biofeedback may be combined with relaxation training, during which patients learn to relax the mind and body.

Biofeedback can be practiced at home with a portable monitor. But the ultimate goal of treatment is to wean the patient from the machine. The patient can then use biofeedback anywhere at the first sign of a headache.

The Antimigraine Diet

Scientists estimate that a small percentage of migraine sufferers will benefit from a treatment program focused solely on eliminating headache-provoking foods and beverages.

Other migraine patients may be helped by a diet to prevent low blood sugar. Low blood sugar, or hypoglycemia, can cause headache. This condition can occur after a period without food: overnight, for example, or when a meal is skipped. People who wake up in the morning with a headache may be reacting to the low blood sugar caused by the lack of food overnight.

Treatment for headaches caused by low blood sugar consists of scheduling smaller, more frequent meals for the patient. A special diet designed to stabilize the body's sugar-regulating system is sometimes recommended.

For the same reason, many specialists also recommend that migraine patients avoid oversleeping on weekends. Sleeping late can change the body's normal blood sugar level and lead to a headache.

Besides Migraine, What Are Other Types of Vascular Headaches?

After migraine, the most common type of vascular headache is the toxic headache produced by fever. Pneumonia, measles, mumps, and tonsillitis are among the diseases that can cause severe toxic vascular headaches. Toxic headaches can also result from the presence of foreign chemicals in the body. Other kinds of vascular headaches include "clusters," which cause repeated episodes of intense pain and headaches resulting from a rise in blood pressure.

Chemical Culprits

Repeated exposure to nitrite compounds can result in a dull, pounding headache that may be accompanied by a flushed face. Nitrite, which dilates blood vessels, is found in such products as heart medicine and dynamite, but is also used as a chemical to preserve meat. Hot dogs and other processed meats containing sodium nitrite can cause headaches.

Eating foods prepared with monosodium glutamate (MSG) can result in headache. Soy sauce, meat tenderizer, and a variety of packaged foods contain this chemical, which is touted as a flavor enhancer.

Headache can also result from exposure to poisons, even common household varieties like insecticides, carbon tetrachloride, and lead. Children who ingest flakes of lead paint may develop headaches. So may anyone who has contact with lead batteries or lead-glazed pottery.

Artists and industrial workers may experience headaches after exposure to materials that contain chemical solvents. These solvents, like benzene, are found in turpentine, spray adhesives, rubber cement, and inks.

Drugs such as amphetamines can cause headaches as a side effect. Another type of drug-related headache occurs during withdrawal from long-term therapy with the antimigraine drug ergotamine tartrate.

Jokes are often made about alcohol hangovers but the headache associated with "the morning after" is no laughing matter. Fortunately, there are several suggested treatments for the pain. The hangover headache may also be reduced by taking honey, which speeds alcohol metabolism, or caffeine, a constrictor of dilated arteries. Caffeine, however, can cause headaches as well as cure them. Heavy coffee drinkers often get headaches when they try to break the caffeine habit.

Cluster Headaches

Cluster headaches are a rare form of headache notable for their extreme pain and their pattern of occurring in "clusters," usually at the same time(s) of the day for several weeks. A cluster headache usually begins suddenly with excruciating pain on one side of the head, often behind or around one eye. In some individuals, it may be preceded by a migraine-like "aura." The pain usually peaks over the next 5 to 10 minutes, and then continues at that intensity for up to an hour or two before going away.

People with cluster headaches describe the pain as piercing and unbearable. The nose and the eye on the affected side of the face may also get red, swollen, and runny, and some people will experience nausea, restlessness and agitation, or sensitivities to light, sound, or smell. Most affected individuals have one to three cluster headaches a day and two cluster periods a year, separated by periods of freedom from symptoms.

A small group of people develop a chronic form of the disorder, characterized by bouts of cluster headaches that can go on for years with only brief periods (2 weeks or less) of remission.

Cluster headaches generally begin between the ages of 20 and 50, although the syndrome can also start in childhood or late in life. Males are much more likely then females to develop cluster headaches. Alcohol (especially red wine) provokes attacks in more than half of those with cluster headaches, but has no effect once the cluster period ends. Cluster headaches are also strongly associated with cigarette smoking.

Scientists aren't sure what causes the disorder. The tendency of cluster headaches to occur during the same time(s) from day to day, and more often at night than during the daylight hours, suggests they could be caused by irregularities in the body's circadian rhythms, which are controlled by the brain and a family of hormones that regulate the sleep-wake cycle.

There are medications available to lessen the pain of a cluster headache and suppress future attacks. Oxygen inhalation and triptan drugs (such as those used to treat migraine) administered as a tablet, nasal spray, or injection can provide quick relief from acute cluster headache pain. Lidocaine nasal spray, which numbs the nose and nostrils, may also be effective. Ergotamine and corticosteroids such as prednisone and dexamethasone may be prescribed to break the cluster cycle and then tapered off once headaches end. Verapamil may be used preventively to decrease the frequency and pain level of attacks.

175

Lithium, valproic acid, and topiramate are sometimes also used preventively.

Painful Pressure

Chronic high blood pressure can cause headache, as can rapid rises in blood pressure like those experienced during anger, vigorous exercise, or sexual excitement.

The severe "orgasmic headache" occurs right before orgasm and is believed to be a vascular headache. Since sudden rupture of a cerebral blood vessel can occur, this type of headache should be evaluated by a doctor.

What Are Muscle-Contraction Headaches?

It's 5:00 p.m. and your boss has just asked you to prepare a 20-page briefing paper. Due date: tomorrow. You're angry and tired and the more you think about the assignment, the tenser you become. Your teeth clench, your brow wrinkles, and soon you have a splitting tension headache.

Tension headache is named not only for the role of stress in triggering the pain, but also for the contraction of neck, face, and scalp muscles brought on by stressful events. Tension headache is a severe but temporary form of muscle-contraction headache. The pain is mild to moderate and feels like pressure is being applied to the head or neck. The headache usually disappears after the period of stress is over. Ninety percent of all headaches are classified as tension/muscle contraction headaches.

By contrast, chronic muscle-contraction headaches can last for weeks, months, and sometimes years. The pain of these headaches is often described as a tight band around the head or a feeling that the head and neck are in a cast. "It feels like somebody is tightening a giant vise around my head," says one patient. The pain is steady, and is usually felt on both sides of the head. Chronic muscle-contraction headaches can cause sore scalps—even combing one's hair can be painful.

In the past, many scientists believed that the primary cause of the pain of muscle-contraction headache was sustained muscle tension. However, a growing number of authorities now believe that a far more complex mechanism is responsible.

Occasionally, muscle-contraction headaches will be accompanied by nausea, vomiting, and blurred vision, but there is no preheadache syndrome as with migraine. Muscle-contraction headaches have not been linked to hormones or foods, as has migraine, nor is there a strong hereditary connection.

Research has shown that for many people, chronic muscle-contraction headaches are caused by depression and anxiety. These people tend to get their headaches in the early morning or evening when conflicts in the office or home are anticipated.

Emotional factors are not the only triggers of muscle-contraction headaches. Certain physical postures that tense head and neck muscles—such as holding one's chin down while reading—can lead to head and neck pain. So can prolonged writing under poor light, or holding a phone between the shoulder and ear, or even gum-chewing.

More serious problems that can cause muscle-contraction headaches include degenerative arthritis of the neck and temporomandibular joint dysfunction, or TMD. TMD is a disorder of the joint between the temporal bone (above the ear) and the mandible or lower jaw bone. The disorder results from poor bite and jaw clenching.

Treatment for muscle-contraction headache varies. The first consideration is to treat any specific disorder or disease that may be causing the headache. For example, arthritis of the neck is treated with anti-inflammatory medication and TMD may be helped by corrective devices for the mouth and jaw.

Acute tension headaches not associated with a disease are treated with analgesics like aspirin and acetaminophen. Stronger analgesics, such as propoxyphene and codeine, are sometimes prescribed. As prolonged use of these drugs can lead to dependence, patients taking them should have periodic medical checkups and follow their physicians' instructions carefully.

Nondrug therapy for chronic muscle-contraction headaches includes biofeedback, relaxation training, and counseling. A technique called cognitive restructuring teaches people to change their attitudes and responses to stress. Patients might be encouraged, for example, to imagine that they are coping successfully with a stressful situation. In progressive relaxation therapy, patients are taught to first tense and then relax individual muscle groups. Finally, the patient tries to relax his or her whole body. Many people imagine a peaceful scene—such as lying on the beach or by a beautiful lake. Passive relaxation does not involve tensing of muscles. Instead, patients are encouraged to focus on different muscles, suggesting that they relax. Some people might think to themselves, "Relax" or "My muscles feel warm."

People with chronic muscle-contraction headaches may also be helped by taking antidepressants or MAO inhibitors. Mixed muscle-contraction

177

and migraine headaches are sometimes treated with barbiturate compounds, which slow down nerve function in the brain and spinal cord.

People who suffer infrequent muscle-contraction headaches may benefit from a hot shower or moist heat applied to the back of the neck. Cervical collars are sometimes recommended as an aid to good posture. Physical therapy, massage, and gentle exercise of the neck may also be helpful.

When Is Headache a Warning of a More Serious Condition?

Like other types of pain, headaches can serve as warning signals of more serious disorders. This is particularly true for headaches caused by traction or inflammation.

Traction headaches can occur if the pain-sensitive parts of the head are pulled, stretched, or displaced, as, for example, when eye muscles are tensed to compensate for eyestrain. Headaches caused by inflammation include those related to meningitis as well as those resulting from diseases of the sinuses, spine, neck, ears, and teeth. Ear and tooth infections and glaucoma can cause headaches. In oral and dental disorders, headache is experienced as pain in the entire head, including the face. These headaches are treated by curing the underlying problem. This may involve surgery, antibiotics, or other drugs.

Characteristics of the various types of more serious traction and inflammatory headaches vary by disorder:

- **Brain tumor:** Brain tumors are diagnosed in about 11,000 people every year. As they grow, these tumors sometimes cause headache by pushing on the outer layer of nerve tissue that covers the brain or by pressing against pain-sensitive blood vessel walls. Headache resulting from a brain tumor may be periodic or continuous. Typically, it feels like a strong pressure is being applied to the head. The pain is relieved when the tumor is treated by surgery, radiation, or chemotherapy.

- **Stroke:** Headache may accompany several conditions that can lead to stroke, including hypertension or high blood pressure, arteriosclerosis, and heart disease. Headaches are also associated with completed stroke, when brain cells die from lack of sufficient oxygen. Many stroke-related headaches can be prevented by careful management of the patient's condition through diet, exercise, and medication. Mild to moderate headaches are associated with transient ischemic attacks (TIAs), sometimes called mini-strokes, which result from a temporary lack of blood supply to the brain. The head pain occurs near the clot or lesion that blocks blood flow. The similarity between migraine and symptoms of TIA can cause problems in diagnosis. The rare person under age 40 who suffers a TIA may be misdiagnosed as having migraine; similarly, TIA-prone older patients who suffer migraine may be misdiagnosed as having stroke-related headaches.

- **Spinal tap:** About one fourth of the people who undergo a lumbar puncture or spinal tap develop a headache. Many scientists believe these headaches result from leakage of the cerebrospinal fluid that flows through pain-sensitive membranes around the brain and down to the spinal cord. The fluid, they suggest, drains through the tiny hole created by the spinal tap needle, causing the membranes to rub painfully against the bony skull. Since headache pain occurs only when the patient stands up, the "cure" is to remain lying down until the headache runs its course—anywhere from a few hours to several days.

- **Head trauma:** Headaches may develop after a blow to the head, either immediately or months later. There is little relationship between the severity of the trauma and the intensity of headache pain. In most cases, the cause of the headache is not known. Occasionally the cause is ruptured blood vessels, which result in an accumulation of blood called a hematoma. This mass of blood can displace brain tissue and cause headaches as well as weakness, confusion, memory loss, and seizures. Hematomas can be drained to produce rapid relief of symptoms.

- **Temporal arteritis:** Arteritis, an inflammation of certain arteries in the head, primarily affects people over age 50. Symptoms include throbbing headache, fever, and loss of appetite. Some patients experience blurring or loss of vision. Prompt treatment with corticosteroid drugs helps to relieve symptoms.

- **Meningitis and encephalitis headaches** are caused by infections of meninges—the brain's outer covering—and in encephalitis, inflammation of the brain itself.

- **Trigeminal neuralgia:** Trigeminal neuralgia, or tic douloureux, results from a disorder of the trigeminal nerve. This nerve supplies the face, teeth, mouth, and nasal cavity with feeling and also enables the mouth muscles to chew. Symptoms are headache and

179

intense facial pain that comes in short, excruciating jabs set off by the slightest touch to or movement of trigger points in the face or mouth. People with trigeminal neuralgia often fear brushing their teeth or chewing on the side of the mouth that is affected. Many trigeminal neuralgia patients are controlled with drugs, including carbamazepine. Patients who do not respond to drugs may be helped by surgery on the trigeminal nerve.

- **Sinus infection:** In a condition called acute sinusitis, a viral or bacterial infection of the upper respiratory tract spreads to the membrane that lines the sinus cavities. When one or more of these cavities are filled with fluid from the inflammation, they become painful. Treatment of acute sinusitis includes antibiotics, analgesics, and decongestants. Chronic sinusitis may be caused by an allergy to such irritants as dust, ragweed, animal hair, and smoke. Research scientists disagree about whether chronic sinusitis triggers headache.

What Causes Headache in Children?

Like adults, children experience the infections, trauma, and stresses that can lead to headaches. In fact, research shows that as young people enter adolescence and encounter the stresses of puberty and secondary school, the frequency of headache increases.

Migraine headaches often begin in childhood or adolescence. According to recent surveys, as many as half of all schoolchildren experience some type of headache.

Children with migraine often have nausea and excessive vomiting. Some children have periodic vomiting, but no headache—the so-called abdominal migraine. Research scientists have found that these children usually develop headaches when they are older.

Physicians have many drugs to treat migraine in children. Different classes that may be tried include analgesics, antiemetics, anticonvulsants, beta-blockers, and sedatives. A diet may also be prescribed to protect the child from foods that trigger headache. Sometimes psychological counseling or even psychiatric treatment for the child and the parents is recommended.

Childhood headache can be a sign of depression. Parents should alert the family pediatrician if a child develops headaches along with other symptoms such as a change in mood or sleep habits. Antidepressant medication and psychotherapy are effective treatments for childhood depression and related headache.

Conclusion

If you suffer from headaches and none of the standard treatments help, do not despair. Some people find that their headaches disappear once they deal with a troubled marriage, pass their certifying board exams, or resolve some other stressful problem. Others find that if they control their psychological reaction to stress, the headaches disappear.

"I had migraines for several years," says one woman, "and then they went away. I think it was because I lowered my personal goals in life. Today, even though I have 100 things to do at night, I don't worry about it. I learned to say no."

For those who cannot say no, or who get headaches anyway, today's headache research offers hope. The work of NINDS-supported scientists around the world promises to improve our understanding of this complex disorder and provide better tools to treat it.

Section 18.3

Medications and Stress Management Most Effective for Treating Tension Headaches

From the press release titled "Drugs and Stress Management Together Best Manage Chronic Tension Headache: Clinical Trial Proves Benefit of Combined Therapies " from the National Institute of Neurological Disorders and Stroke (NINDS, www.ninds.nih.gov), part of the National Institutes of Health, May 1, 2001. Reviewed by David A. Cooke, M.D., March 2007.

Stress management techniques such as relaxation and biofeedback can help treat chronic tension headaches, especially in combination with medicine, according to research funded by the National Institute of Neurological Disorders and Stroke (NINDS). Results of the first placebo-controlled trial comparing medicines alone vs. medicine plus stress management appeared in the May 2, 2001, issue of the *Journal of the American Medical Association*.

Tension-type headaches affect some 2 to 3 percent of the nation's population on a chronic basis, with twice as many women affected as men. Most people use over-the-counter analgesics to treat their headaches but overuse can make the headache worse and unresponsive to treatment. Stress management therapy for headache is a cognitive behavioral approach that teaches people to recognize and manage early headache signs, cope with pain and address stress-generating issues, and possibly prevent headache.

Kenneth Holroyd, Ph.D., of Ohio University in Athens, and colleagues enrolled 203 adults (with a mean of 26 chronic tension headaches a month) in an 8-month trial to study the effectiveness of behavioral and pharmacological therapies for chronic tension headache. Patients were randomly assigned to one of four treatments: tricyclic antidepressant medication (the primary drug therapy for chronic tension-type headaches), placebo, stress management therapy plus placebo, and stress management therapy plus antidepressant medication. Patients recorded headache activity and the use of analgesic and study medications in a daily diary, as well as measures of disability caused by headaches.

According to Dr. Holroyd and his colleagues, three of the four treatments—tricyclic drugs alone, tricyclics plus stress management, and stress management plus placebo—reduced chronic tension-type headache activity, analgesic use, and headache related disability. Combined drug and behavioral therapy produced a clinically significant reduction (greater than or equal to 50%) in the Headache Index (a measure of overall headache activity) for more patients than did either therapy alone. Patients who took placebos throughout the trial did not report any reduction in headache activity.

The study provides the first evidence that chronic tension-type headaches respond to brief behavioral therapy to the same degree as antidepressant medication alone. However, behavioral techniques may need to be repeated for several months before they have an impact on daily headaches.

John R. Marler, M.D., Associate Director for Clinical Trials at the NINDS, said "This study establishes the effectiveness of tricyclic medication for chronic tension headache and provides new information about the benefits of the combined medication and behavioral treatment. These findings suggest new avenues of research in the prevention and treatment of other types of headache."

Tension headache is caused by prolonged tightening of muscles in the head and neck. This most common form of headache is classified two ways: episodic, with fewer than 15 attacks per month typically triggered by some form of environmental or internal stress, and chronic, occurring on 15 or more days a month, with varied pain throughout the day. Symptoms include a dull ache on both sides of the head, tightness or sensations of pressure around the scalp or neck, and depression. Many sufferers also find it difficult to sleep.

Holroyd, Kenneth A.; O'Donnell, Francis J.; Stensland, Michael; Lipchik, Gay L.; Cordingley, Gary E.; Carlson, Bruce W. "Management of Chronic Tension-Type Headache With Tricyclic Antidepressant Medication, Stress Management Therapy, and Their Combination." *Journal of the American Medical Association*, May 2, 2001, Vol. 285, No. 17, 2208–2215.

Chapter 19

Stress and Chronic Pain

Chapter Contents

Section 19.1

Stress and Arthritis Pain

Reprinted with permission from www.allaboutarthritis.com, an informational website from DePuy Orthopaedics, Inc., a Johnson & Johnson company. © 2007 DePuy Orthopaedics, Inc. All rights reserved.

Stress is a normal part of life. It's the body's natural response to changes and challenges. It can be very helpful in the right situation. However, when the stress response is inappropriate or prolonged, it can take its toll on emotional and physical health. For people suffering from arthritis pain, stress makes it harder to cope. Luckily, the body has a natural way to counteract stress: the relaxation response. With practice, you can learn to bring on the relaxation response at will to better control your stress and arthritis pain.

The Stress-Arthritis Pain Cycle

The stress response is also called the fight-or-flight response. It's the body's way of gearing up to fight or flee when it encounters danger. Heart rate, blood pressure, breathing rate, metabolism, and muscle tension all increase. These changes would come in handy if you were being attacked or chased. Unfortunately, the body can't distinguish between the threat of a predator in the wild and that of a past due notice on a bill, so it goes into the same state of high physiological alert. Over time, this can contribute to a host of health problems, including trouble sleeping, fatigue, headaches, digestive problems, and reduced resistance to infection. It also can lead to an increased risk of anxiety and depression.

If you suffer from arthritis you need to be especially aware of stress, since it can make it harder to manage your symptoms. Unfortunately, having arthritis is a stressful experience. It's easy to get into a vicious cycle in which stress at home or work leads you to forget your medication or skip your exercise, which leads to more arthritis pain and fatigue, which leads to more stress about not being able to do the things you want, and so on.

Breaking the Vicious Cycle

"Relaxation and stress reduction techniques are designed to break this destructive cycle," says Robert Jamison, Ph.D., director of the pain management program at Brigham and Women's Hospital in Boston. But this is no one-size-fits-all solution. "Different approaches work better or worse for different individuals," says Jamison.

Some people find that learning to control their negative thoughts and attitudes is very helpful. Others benefit from better organizing their lives to head off sources of stress and frustration. Others are helped by learning how to intentionally call up the relaxation response with deep breathing, meditation, imagery, and similar methods. This means more than just doing things that make you feel happy, such as listening to music or reading a book. It involves bringing on the physiological state that is the exact opposite of the stress response. In this state, heart rate, blood pressure, breathing rate, metabolism, and muscle tension decrease, thereby undoing many of the harmful effects of stress.

Section 19.2

Mood and Stress Predict Pain in Children with Arthritis

"Mood and Stress Predict Pain in Children with Arthritis," April 4, 2005, Duke University Medical Center News Office. © 2005 University Health System. Reprinted with permission.

For children with arthritis, increases in stress and depressed mood worsen disease symptoms and predict cutbacks in social and school activities, according to a Duke University Medical Center study.

The researchers found mood was a key predictor of flare-ups in symptoms such as pain, stiffness, and fatigue. An analysis of daily pain diaries kept by children with arthritis showed as mood worsened, reporting of disease symptoms increased. Similarly, rising daily stress was linked to increased fatigue and pain. The diaries showed that children felt pain, stiffness, and fatigue during most days of the two-month study, even with treatment meant to reduce inflammation and pain.

However, the children reported positive mood on more than 90 percent of days despite these symptoms. Even so, because of their disease symptoms, many skipped social activities and, more rarely, school attendance or activities.

"Doctors should aggressively treat pain, stiffness and fatigue in children, because cutting back on play or school can exacerbate feelings of isolation, depression, and poor quality-of-life—emotions common in kids with chronic illness," said lead author Laura Schanberg, M.D. "This aggressive treatment may not mean changing or adding medication, but rather more effective application of cognitive behavioral therapy, relaxation and stress management," said Schanberg, a pediatric rheumatologist and associate professor of pediatrics at Duke.

The study was published in the April 2005 issue of *Arthritis & Rheumatism*. The research was supported by the Arthritis Foundation; the National Institute of Arthritis and Musculoskeletal and Skin Diseases of the National Institutes of Health; and the Fetzer Institute.

The Duke study was designed to analyze the daily patterns of stress, mood, and disease symptoms in children with polyarticular arthritis, in which the disease affects many joints at once. The 51 study participants, ages 8 through 18 years old, were recruited from the Duke Children's Hospital pediatric rheumatology clinic. Most children were taking a non-steroidal anti-inflammatory drug (NSAID) and/or methotrexate—both common drug treatments for arthritis.

The kid-friendly daily diary included standardized measures of disease symptoms, stress, mood, and function designed to elicit accurate, truthful responses from children. For example, daily mood was assessed with the "Facial Affective Scale," which consists of nine faces that vary in levels of expressed distress. Children were asked to "Please mark the face that looks like how you felt deep down inside today—not just how your face looked, but how you really felt inside."

The children's ratings of their daily stress, mood, pain, stiffness, and fatigue varied significantly from day to day. A drop in mood and an increase in pain symptoms played a role in predicting a reduction in social activities. However, only mood and stiffness were crucial predictors of a cutback in school attendance, the researchers found.

The diaries showed that children were more likely to cut back on social activities than skip school. Although this difference may reflect an appropriate emphasis on the importance of school, the significance of this finding should not be minimized, because reducing social activities could contribute to feelings of social isolation and worsen the quality of life for children, Schanberg said. As Schanberg explains, research has documented that children with arthritis are at increased risk for feelings of loneliness and other difficulties with peer relationships. Limited involvement in social activities and poor school attendance can hinder academic progress and social and emotional development, leading to depression and anxiety, she said.

"Comprehensive care of children with arthritis includes more than medications to treat pain and immune system dysfunction. It means helping children and families cope with routine stresses and strains of life—not the extraordinary issues, but just the normal day-to-day vagaries of life," Schanberg said.

Other members of the research team are Karen Gil of the University of North Carolina at Chapel Hill and Kelly Anthony, Eric Yow, and James Rochon of Duke.

Section 19.3

Depression and Stress Linked to Neck, Shoulder, and Back Pain in Teens

This information was provided by KidsHealth, one of the largest resources online for medically reviewed health information written for parents, kids, and teens. For more articles like this one, visit www.KidsHealth.org, or www.TeensHealth.org. © 2006 The Nemours Foundation. This information was reviewed by Steven Dowshen, M.D., March 2006.

Muscular pain in the neck, shoulders, and back plagues many American adults and is one of the leading causes of disability and missed work. But the number of teens with musculoskeletal pain has increased in recent years, too.

To find out more about the occurrence and causes of pain in teens, researchers from the Netherlands surveyed 3,485 12- to 16-year-olds from Amsterdam about how often they experienced pain in their arms, neck, shoulders, and low back. Teens also noted how much time they spent using the computer, how much time they spent exercising or playing sports, and how much time they spent in inactive pursuits, such as watching TV or playing video games. In addition, the teens reported whether they had symptoms of depression and whether they had experienced stress within the last week.

Neck and shoulder pain proved most common among teens—about 12% of teens complained of aching or pain in the neck and shoulders four or more days in the past month. About 8% of teens noted low back pain, and about 4% of teens reported having arm pain 4 or more days in the past month. In addition, girls were more likely to report neck and shoulder pain and low back pain, and rates of neck and shoulder pain were higher in teens who did not live with both parents.

The amount of time teens spent using the computer, watching TV or playing video games, or playing sports or exercising wasn't linked to arm, neck, shoulder, or back pain. However, teens who reported more symptoms of depression were more likely to experience neck/shoulder pain, low back pain, and arm pain. Also, stressed teens tended to experience more neck, shoulder, and low back pain.

What this means to you: The results of this study indicate that stressed and depressed teens may be prone to pain in the neck, shoulders, back, and arms. Even though a direct link to pain was not proven by this study, the American Academy of Pediatrics (AAP) recommends that parents limit their children's screen time (including TV and video and computer games) to no more than 1 to 2 hours a day. If your son or daughter complains of pain in the back, shoulders, neck, or arms, talk to your child's doctor. Some teens with unexplained or chronic pain may find relief through behavioral therapy to help them cope with stress and depression.

Source: A.C.M. Diepenmaat, MSC; M.F. van der Wal, Ph.D.; H.C.W. de Vet, Ph.D.; R. A. Hirasing, Ph.D.; *Pediatrics,* February 2006.

Chapter 20

Stress and the Brain and Nervous System

Chapter Contents

Section 20.1

Stress and the Developing Brain

From the National Institute of Mental Health (NIMH, www.nimh.nih.gov), part of the National Institutes of Health, NIH Publication No. 01-4603, updated February 2, 2006.

It is well-known that the early months and years of life are critical for brain development. But the question remains: just how do early influences act on the brain to promote or challenge the developmental process? Research has suggested that both positive and negative experiences, chronic stressors, and various other environmental factors may affect a young child's developing brain. And now, studies involving animals are revealing in greater detail how this may occur.

One important line of research has focused on brain systems that control stress hormones—cortisol, for example.[1,2] Cortisol and other stress hormones play an important role in emergencies: they help our bodies make energy available to enable effective responses, temporarily suppress the immune response, and sharpen attention. However, a number of studies conducted in people with depression indicate that excess cortisol released over a long time span may have many negative consequences for health.[3,4,5] Excess cortisol may cause shrinking of the hippocampus, a brain structure required for the formation of certain types of memory.

In experiments with animals, scientists have shown that a well-defined period of early postnatal development may be an important determinant of the capacity to handle stress throughout life.[2] In one set of studies, rat pups were removed each day from their mothers for a period as brief as 15 minutes and then returned. The natural maternal response of intensively licking and grooming the returned pup was shown to alter the brain chemistry of the pup in a positive way, making the animal less reactive to stressful stimuli. While these pups are able to mount an appropriate stress response in the face of threat, their response does not become excessive or inappropriate. Rat mothers who spontaneously lick and groom their pups with the same intensity even without human handling of the pups also produce pups that have a similarly stable reaction, including an appropriate stress hormone response.[6]

Striking differences were seen in rat pups removed from their mothers for periods of 3 hours a day, a model of neglect compared to pups that were not separated. After 3 hours, the mother rats tended to ignore the pups, at least initially, upon their return. In sharp contrast to those pups that were greeted attentively by their mothers after a short absence, the "neglected" pups were shown to have a more profound and excessive stress response in subsequent tests. This response appeared to last into adulthood.[7,8]

The implications of these animal studies are worrisome. However, research is in progress to determine the extent to which the hypersensitive or dysregulated stress response of "neglected" rat pups can be reversed if, for example, foster mothers are provided who will groom the pups more intensely, or if the animals are raised in an "enriched" environment following their separation. An enriched setting may include, for example, a diverse and varied diet, a running wheel, mazes, and changes of toys.

Animal investigators are well aware of another kind of long-term change, again rooted in the first days of life. Laboratory rats are often raised in shoebox cages with few sources of stimulation. Scientists have compared these animals to rats raised in an enriched environment and found that the "privileged" rats consistently have a thicker cerebral cortex and denser networks of nerve cells than the "deprived" rats.[9,10]

Another study recently reported that infant monkeys raised by mothers who experienced unpredictable conditions in obtaining food showed markedly high levels of corticotropin-releasing factor (CRF) in their cerebrospinal fluid and, as adults, abnormally low levels of cerebrospinal fluid cortisol.[11] This is a pattern often seen in humans with posttraumatic stress disorder and depression.[5] The distressed monkey mothers, uncertain about finding food, behaved inconsistently and sometimes neglectfully toward their offspring. The affected young monkeys were abnormally anxious when confronted with separations or new environments. They were also less social and more subordinate as adult animals.

It is far too early to draw firm conclusions from these animal studies about the extent to which early life experience produces a long-lived or permanent set point for stress responses, or influences the development of the cerebral cortex in humans. However, animal models that show the interactive effect of stress and brain development deserve serious consideration and continued study.

References

1. McEwen BS. Allostasis and allostatic load: implications for neuropsychopharmacology. *Neuropsychopharmacology,* 2000; 22(2): 108–24.

2. Liu D, Diorio J, Tannenbaum B, Caldji C, Francis D, Freedman A, Sharma S, Pearson D, Plotsky PM, Meaney MJ. Maternal care, hippocampal glucocorticoid receptors, and hypothalamic-pituitary-adrenal responses to stress. *Science,* 1997; 277(5332): 1659–62.

3. Sheline YI, Sanghavi M, Mintun MA, Gado MH. Depression duration but not age predicts hippocampal volume loss in medically healthy women with recurrent major depression. *Journal of Neuroscience,* 1999; 19(12): 5034–43.

4. Brown ES, Rush AJ, McEwen BS. Hippocampal remodeling and damage by corticosteroids: implications for mood disorders. *Neuropsychopharmacology,* 1999; 21(4): 474–84.

5. Heim C, Newport DJ, Heit S, Graham YP, Wilcox M, Bonsall R, Miller AH, Nemeroff CB. Pituitary-adrenal and autonomic responses to stress in women after sexual and physical abuse in childhood. *Journal of the American Medical Association,* 2000; 284(5): 592–7.

6. Francis D, Diorio J, Liu D, Meaney MJ. Nongenomic transmission across generations of maternal behavior and stress responses in the rat. *Science,* 1999; 286(5442): 1155–8.

7. Plotsky PM, Meaney MJ. Early, postnatal experience alters hypothalamic corticotropin-releasing factor (CRF) mRNA, median eminence CRF content and stress-induced release in adult rats. *Brain Research. Molecular Brain Research,* 1993; 18(3): 195–200.

8. Ladd CO, Huot RL, Thrivikraman KV, Nemeroff CB, Meaney MJ, Plotsky PM. Long-term behavioral and neuroendocrine adaptations to adverse early experience. *Progress in Brain Research,* 2000; 122: 81–103.

9. Jones TA, Klintsova AY, Kilman VL, Sirevaag AM, Greenough WT. Induction of multiple synapses by experience in the visual cortex of adult rats. *Neurobiology of Learning and Memory,* 1997; 68(1): 13–20.

10.   Green EJ, Greenough WT, Schlumpf BE. Effects of complex or isolated environments on cortical dendrites of middle-aged rats. *Brain Research,* 1983; 264(2): 233–40.

11.   Coplan JD, Andrews MW, Rosenblum LA, Owens MJ, Friedman S, Gorman JM, Nemeroff CB. Persistent elevations of cerebrospinal fluid concentrations of corticotropin-releasing factor in adult nonhuman primates exposed to early-life stressors: implications for the pathophysiology of mood and anxiety disorders. *Proceedings of the National Academy of Sciences* USA, 1996; 93(4): 1619–23.

Section 20.2

The Latest Research on Stress and Stroke Risk

"The latest research on stress and stroke risk," reprinted with permission from the American Federation for Aging Research. © 2004. For further information, visit www.infoaging.org.

Many of the risk factors for stroke are known. Researchers have asked if some of those risk factors are associated with other lesser known risks. For example, high blood pressure is known to be a risk factor for stroke, but what of stress, known to raise blood pressure?

A group of Swedish researchers looked at a group of 238 men all born in 1914, who had high blood pressure. They were observed from 1982 through 1996. They were subjected to an examination called the Color-Word Test, which asks questions that are progressive in difficulty. The subjects were found to have varying abilities to master the test. Those who were successful performed the test in stabilized patterns, those with more difficulty were described as producing cumulative patterns of responses, some who had varying degrees of difficulty with parts of the test were labeled as having dissociative patterns, and those whose results both fluctuated and showed an increase with increasing difficulty were labeled cumulative-dissociative. Strokes were observed in 43 of the subjects, and the risk of stroke was found to increase with the amount of difficulty the men had in performing the stressful Color-Word Test. Those with a stabilized pattern had strokes at a rate of 12.6 (per thousand person-years, a statistical means of comparing results); those with the cumulative pattern had a stroke rate of 14.3; those with a dissociative pattern had a stroke rate of 16.2, and those with the cumulative-dissociative pattern had a rate of 31.2. Thus the risk of stroke was highest in men with high blood pressure whose responses to stress were the least adaptive.

Section 20.3

Distress-Prone People More Likely to Develop Alzheimer's Risk

"Study: Distress-Prone People More Likely to Develop Alzheimer's Disease" is from *FDA Consumer* magazine (www.fda.gov/fdac), a publication of the U.S. Food and Drug Administration (FDA), January-February 2004.

People who tend to experience psychological distress are more likely to develop Alzheimer disease than those who are less prone to experience distress, a study indicates.

In the study, published in the Dec. 9, 2003, issue of *Neurology,* people who most often experience negative emotions such as depression and anxiety were twice as likely to develop Alzheimer disease as those who were least prone to experience negative emotions. The research is part of a larger study of older Catholic nuns, priests, and brothers called the Religious Orders study.

"People differ in their tendency to experience psychological distress, and this is a stable personality trait throughout adulthood," says study author Robert S. Wilson, Ph.D., of Rush University Medical Center in Chicago. "Since chronic stress has been associated with changes in the hippocampal area of the brain and problems with learning and memory, we wanted to test the theory that psychological distress may affect the risk of developing Alzheimer's disease."

Wilson says the findings are important because evidence has shown that many of the adverse effects of stress on the brain can be blocked

196

by drugs, including antidepressants. "But much more research is needed before we can determine whether the use of antidepressants could help reduce the risk of Alzheimer disease," he says.

In the study, 797 people with an average age of 75 were evaluated when they started the study and then on a yearly basis. Participants were evaluated on their level of proneness to stress with a rating scale that has been proven reliable. Participants rate their level of agreement (strongly disagree, disagree, etc.) with statements such as "I am not a worrier," "I often feel tense and jittery," and "I often get angry at the way people treat me."

During an average of 4.9 years of follow-up, 140 people in the study developed Alzheimer disease. Those high in proneness to stress—in the 90th percentile—were twice as likely to develop Alzheimer disease as those in the 10th percentile.

To investigate whether proneness to distress was an early sign of Alzheimer disease rather than a risk factor for the disease, the researchers studied the brains of 141 study participants who died during the course of the study. Of those, 57 met the criteria for probable Alzheimer disease. The researchers found that proneness to distress was not related to measures of Alzheimer disease pathology, such as plaques and tangles in the brain.

"This result suggests that stress proneness is a co-factor leading to dementia in Alzheimer's disease, but these results need to be confirmed," said John C. S. Breitner, M.D., M.P.H., of the VA Puget Sound Health Care System and the University of Washington in Seattle, who wrote an editorial accompanying the study.

Section 20.4

Stress and Multiple Sclerosis

Excerpted from "Taming Stress in Multiple Sclerosis," by Frederick Foley, Ph.D., with Jane Sarnoff, © 2005 National Multiple Sclerosis Society. Reprinted with permission.

Brought to You by Evolution

When our ancestors were taking a morning stroll and met a tiger, they could run or fight. Either action demanded that their bodies adjust rapidly to meet the emergency, and they experienced stress as part of the process.

Without stress, we would not be able to act in times of danger. In fact, without some stress to get us to focus on a problem we might do almost nothing. Many people perform best while under stress. But sometimes people are immobilized by the pressure that stress creates. Then stress makes it hard to concentrate and stops people from doing what needs to be done.

Today's Tigers

Stress can be caused by both pleasant and unpleasant demands and changes. People can be just as stressed by getting a promotion as by not getting one.

Stress usually begins with alarm, the modern equivalent of noticing a tiger. However, our options are rarely as simple as running away or fighting. For example, most people are very stressed at the prospect of having to use a cane or wheelchair. Many eventually experience relief or accept the benefits of the aid once the stressor—the idea of using a cane or other assistive device—has been sufficiently worked through.

Stress and MS

Having any chronic illness increases stress. MS [multiple sclerosis] is no exception. In fact, there are many stressful situations that are common with MS:

- Diagnostic uncertainties (before the definite MS diagnosis)
- The unpredictability of MS
- The invisibility of the symptoms (which can cause people with MS to question the reality of their own experience)
- The visibility of the symptoms, particularly newly emerging ones (to which others may react before the person has had time to adjust)
- The need to adjust and readjust to changing abilities
- Financial stress and concerns about employment
- The presence—or possibility—of cognitive impairment
- Loss of control (e.g., bladder dysfunction)
- The need to make decisions about disease-modifying treatment and adjusting to the treatment if it is chosen.

Does stress increase the risk of attacks or affect the long-term course of MS?

Many people with MS feel that there is a definite connection between stress and MS. Others believe that controlling stress can have a beneficial impact on MS. And still others believe that neither stress nor controlling stress has any effect on MS. Scientifically speaking, the jury is still out.

A relationship between stress and the onset of MS or MS relapses is considered possible, but hasn't been powerfully demonstrated in studies. Can a stressful event cause nerve damage or lesions? Can nerve damage or lesions increase someone's experience of stress? More research is needed to answer these questions.

Can stress make MS symptoms feel worse?

Many people with MS say yes. They experience more symptoms during stressful times. When the stress abates, their symptoms seem less troubling or less severe. This could be understood by looking at the stress and coping process.

During times of stress, more energy is required to think, problem-solve, and handle daily life. For example, one's ability to be patient with family members often wanes after a tough day. At stressful or demanding times, symptoms may be experienced more strongly, because the energy to deal with them and get on with life has been drained.

We all have finite reservoirs of coping ability. At demanding times, our supply may temporarily run dry. Any difficulty, including MS symptoms, is more challenging at these moments.

Stress can't be—and shouldn't be—totally avoided. But we can learn to reduce its intensity and to use it to work for, not against, us.

Chapter 21

The Cardiovascular Consequences of Stress

Chapter Contents

Section 21.1

Stress and Heart Disease

"Stress," is reprinted with permission from The Zena and Michael A. Wiener Cardiovascular Institute and the Marie-Josée and Henry R. Kravis Center for Cardiovascular Health at The Mount Sinai Medical Center, www.mssm.edu/cvi. © 2006 Mount Sinai School of Medicine. All rights reserved.

There is no simple definition of stress. Some health experts define it by focusing on the physiological changes in the body. Some focus on the symptoms you experience. Still others focus on the situations that trigger these responses.

Health experts do agree that some stress is essential for human survival. Stress can raise your energy level, make you feel challenged, and cause the physiological changes required to deal with the situation. This is called positive stress.

What are my body's reactions to stress?

When you perceive or anticipate a threatening or stressful situation, part of your nervous system (the sympathetic nervous system) becomes activated. and releases a number of chemicals including adrenaline and noradrenalin to get you geared up for action.

The sympathetic nervous system raises your blood pressure. It directs blood flow away from your fingers, skin, and toes and more to the large muscles in your arms and legs where it is needed for action.

The released chemicals also increase your heartbeat and breathing rates. This ensures that additional oxygen—which is necessary for fast action—is delivered to your body. As a result, you may feel pumped up. Sometimes chronic stress has the opposite effect: you feel fatigued. In extreme cases, you may temporarily feel dizzy or confused or experience blurred vision or numbing of your fingers and toes.

When your body no longer needs this level of activation, another part of the nervous system (the parasympathetic nervous system) takes over and restores a relaxed feeling. If this restoration does not happen immediately, don't worry. It sometimes takes a little time.

What is negative stress?

Some people define "negative stress" as what you experience when you have faced the physical and emotional challenges, but you remain geared up and your stress responses continue beyond normal or necessary levels. Others define "negative stress" as an experience in which the demands of the situation exceed the perceived ability to cope with them.

Negative stress can be furthered by poor stress management and ineffective coping skills.

What is the relationship between stress and heart disease?

Less is known about how stress affects heart disease than about some of the other risk factors, which include cigarette smoking, hypertension, cholesterol levels, family history, diabetes, obesity, and physical inactivity.

Whether stress acts as an independent risk factor or merely aggravates the other risk factors has yet to be determined. Nevertheless, health experts agree that stress increases the risk of heart disease.

Adrenaline and the other hormones that help you to spring into action during stress can also increase muscle tension, slow digestion, constrict and dilate your body's arteries, and cause your liver to deliver cholesterol and fat (triglyceride) into the bloodstream. The levels of a certain hormone (testosterone) may increase, which can reduce HDL cholesterol ("good" cholesterol) levels.

Repeated release of these chemicals over time may cause wear and tear on your heart and blood vessels and eventually lead to heart disease and stroke.

The rise in heart rate and blood pressure during stress may increase your heart's need for oxygen while simultaneously reducing its supply. The heart's arteries (coronary arteries) usually dilate during stress in order to deliver blood to needed body parts as quickly as possible. If you suffer from atherosclerosis ("hardening of the arteries"), your coronary arteries may be unable to dilate sufficiently under stress.

Stress may promote several of the factors that lead to blood clots (thrombosis) of the arteries leading to the heart (coronary arteries).

Certain chronic responses to stress have been associated with heart disease. Two of these responses are hostility and cynicism. If you are chronically hostile and/or cynical, you are more likely to manifest larger increases in heart rate, blood pressure, and stress hormones in response to non-social stressors than are individuals with low hostility.

Depression, and to a lesser extent, anxiety, have been associated with coronary artery disease. Health experts are revising their previously held image of the coronary-prone individual as time-pressured, impatient, and work-driven. Now, they view people who harbor negative emotions, such as depression, anxiety, hostility, or aggression, at higher risk for heart disease.

If you have recent, short-lived depression, you are at a lower risk than someone who has long-standing depression. Your risk may be lowered if you have the support of family and friends.

How can I control negative stress?

The stressful events in your life and your behavioral reactions are unique to you. You can learn to modify your appraisal of potentially stressful situations and how you deal with them. You can even exercise some control over your physical reactions. These changes can lead to enhanced health and well-being.

If you would like to manage stress in a healthful way, you must be able to recognize it. First, you should identify which events trigger stress-related symptoms in you. Next, you can ascertain your habitual ways of responding to stress. Then you can learn to develop and substitute more effective coping skills when needed.

The first step to healthy management of stress is to identify your personal stressors. The American Heart Association notes the following events and situations as potential triggers of stress:

- **Life events:** marriage, death of a family member or close friend, moving or relocating, birth or adoption of a baby, major financial setback, new job, being fired or laid off, major change in job demands (promotion or demotion), retirement, natural disaster, divorce or separation, crime, major illness of self of family member, major change in spouse's job, and changed living arrangements (addition or subtraction of family members).

- **Physical stressors:** pollution, excessive noise, physical disability or handicap, weather extremes, sleep deprivation, physical injury, lack of rest or relaxation, smoking, excessive drinking, inappropriate drug use, obesity, overeating or junk food, rapid dieting or under-eating, excessive exercise, chronic pain, excessive travel (airplanes, time zones, heavy luggage, unfamiliar bed).

- **Daily hassles:** time pressure, too many responsibilities, traffic or commute, deadlines, conflicts with co-workers, conflicts with spouse, difficulties with children, difficulties with elderly parents, being disorganized at work or home, home upkeep or maintenance, car upkeep or maintenance, household chores, financial problems.

What are typical physical symptoms of stress?

One approach to help you identify your personal stressors is to pay close attention to your body's reactions. Potential reactions to stress include: migraine or tension headaches; back, neck, shoulder aches or tension; fatigue, fingernail biting or nervous tics, insomnia, restlessness (foot-tapping, finger-drumming); lowered sex drive, digestive upsets (acid, gas, diarrhea, constipation); breathing changes ("air hunger," shallow breathing, sighing); teeth grinding or jaw clenching; sweaty or cold hands; and excess perspiration.

What are other signs of stress?

Another approach to determining your personal stressors is to pay attention to your thinking. Are you forgetful, distracted? Do you have trouble concentrating? Are your thoughts pessimistic? Are you less creative, indecisive, and inefficient? Are you cynical or hostile? Is your self-esteem or morale low?

Next, assess your feelings. How does the situation make you feel? Are you frustrated, depressed, anxious, bored, angry, resentful, apathetic, irritable, intolerant?

Finally, consider your behavior. Are you getting into accidents? Are you abusing substances? Are you withdrawn, disorganized, unable to function as before? Are you engaging in compulsive behaviors (inappropriate eating, shopping, gambling, sex, television watching)?

What are common coping approaches to stress?

The following is a list of coping responses suggested by the American Heart Association. To cope with stress, you can:

- listen to music, watch TV, movies, or read;
- write (journal, lists);
- get information or ask for help;
- attend a play, lecture, or the symphony;

- play sports, walk, run or other exercise, or stretch;
- practice active problem-solving;
- pray, meditate, or do yoga;
- engage in a hobby;
- look on the bright side;
- go outdoors or enjoy nature;
- engage in humor, laughter, or play;
- get more rest or get a massage;
- straighten or organize your environment;
- confront the situation;
- get away (vacation, trip, camping);
- engage in deep breathing;
- talk it over with friends;
- talk to a therapist, listen to relaxation tapes, or read self-help books;
- bathe, shower, or go in a hot tub.

Are there drugs I can take to manage stress?

Your doctor may prescribe a medication for relief of stress. These medications include Valium (diazepam) and Xanax (alprazolam). Tranquilizers are advisable only for short periods of time, because they are habit forming. You run the risk of becoming dependent on them.

Your doctor may suggest an antidepressant for stress and anxiety such as Tofranil, Elavil, or Nardil.

What can I do to better manage stress?

You can manage stress by attacking one or more of its components. You can remove or alter the stressor; you can change your perception of the stressful event; you can reduce your physiological reactions; or you can employ alternative coping strategies.

Common stress reduction techniques include: relaxation training, biofeedback assisted relaxation (heart rate feedback), cognitive and behavior therapies, progressive muscle relaxation, meditation, and breathing exercises. If you utilize a combination of approaches you increase your chance of successfully managing stress.

What is progressive muscle relaxation?

Progressive muscle relaxation is a technique you can use to relax your body. This is an effective coping strategy that also impacts on your physiological reactions. The American Heart Association suggests the following technique:

Get into a comfortable position with your head and neck supported. Close your eyes and tense each muscle group listed below to about 25%–50% of maximum tension. Hold the tension for a few seconds as you continue to breathe, then slowly release the tension as you focus on the pleasant contrast between tight and relaxed muscles: (1) hands and arms; (2) face; (3) neck and shoulders; (4) stomach and abdomen; (5) buttocks and thighs; (6) calves; (7) toes. Then, sit quietly for several minutes and enjoy the feeling of a relaxed body before you slowly open your eyes.

What is relaxed breathing?

Relaxed, deep, or abdominal breathing is a technique that helps you to calm down emotionally.

1. Lie down on your back. Loosen tight clothing.

2. Inhale through your mouth. Exhale through your nose.

3. As you inhale, extend your abdomen. As you exhale, pull it in.

4. As you inhale, mentally count slowly from one to four. As you exhale count from one to six or eight.

Initially, you may want to place your hand on your abdomen to actually feel the inhalations and exhalations, until your deep breathing comes naturally.

Relaxation techniques (muscle relaxation, deep breathing, and meditation) reduce your likelihood of suffering from certain heart disease (ischemic heart disease) and the likelihood of undergoing a fatal heart attack.

If you have undergone heart surgery (coronary artery bypass surgery and coronary angioplasty), you can use these relaxation techniques to enhance and improve your emotional recovery.

Section 21.2

Mental Stress Increases Risk of Death in People with Heart Disease

"New study says people take mental stress to heart" is reproduced with permission from www.americanheart.org. © 2002, American Heart Association. Reviewed by David A. Cooke, M.D., March 2007.

Mental stress can trigger a lack of blood flow to the heart and increase the risk of death in people with coronary artery disease, researchers report in *Circulation: Journal of the American Heart Association.*

"Patients who had ischemia in response to mental stress had a three-fold increase in the risk of death compared to people without mental stress," says David S. Sheps, M.D., lead author and associate chief of the division of cardiovascular medicine, University of Florida Health Sciences Center, Gainesville. "This adds to a growing body of evidence that links mental stress and bad outcomes in individuals with coronary artery disease."

Previous studies have shown that reduced blood flow during mental stress tests is linked to significantly higher rates of adverse cardiac events. These studies weren't designed to detect differences in death rates, however.

Researchers used an imaging test called radionuclide angiography to detect "wall motion" abnormalities in the heart's pumping during ischemia, which occurs when there is not enough blood flow in the coronary arteries. Radionuclide angiography involves injecting a dye to label red blood cells. This lets researchers view the working heart.

"Wall motion abnormalities are specific markers of ischemia," Sheps says. "Radionuclide imaging provides us a motion picture of the heart beating. Normally there is a nice symmetrical motion of the heart. With ischemia, certain portions will contract less vigorously or bulge out."

Mental stress increases oxygen demand because blood pressure and heart rate are elevated, he says. Vascular resistance and coronary artery constriction during mental stress also decrease the blood supply.

Psychological factors such as depression or anxiety didn't increase the patients' incidence of death in this study. They have been shown to be risk factors in other studies.

The 196 patients in this study—Psychophysiological Investigations of Myocardial Ischemia (PIMI)—had documented coronary artery disease and exercise-induced ischemia. Patients had a more than 50 percent narrowing in at least one major coronary artery or a previous heart attack. Follow-up was done at 3.5 and 5.2 years.

Patients were excluded if they had a serious noncardiac illness, unstable angina, neurological disease, were unable to discontinue medications that influence cardiac function, or had undergone coronary surgery or angioplasty.

An exercise stress test, radionuclide imaging of the heart and a psychological stress test were conducted at the start of the study. In the psychological stress test patients were asked to talk for five minutes on an assigned topic. The topic required role-playing in which a close relative was being mistreated in a nursing home.

The radionuclide test detected abnormalities in the heart's pumping ability during the speech test in 20 percent of patients. Patients with abnormalities were more often female (24 percent versus 12 percent) and were more likely to have a history of diabetes (27 percent versus 12 percent).

Patients with wall motion abnormalities during the speech test had a 2.8 times higher death rate than those without abnormalities. All of the 17 deaths were men. Forty percent of those who died had new or worsened abnormalities during the speech test compared with 19 percent of the survivors.

Sheps says further study is needed, since this was not a prospectively designed study. While the study did show increased deaths in people with wall motion abnormalities under mental stress, it was not designed to collect complete data on nonfatal events. There also were not resources to classify deaths by cause, so the researchers analyzed associations with total mortality rather than cardiac death.

He says research should focus on reproducing this finding and searching for an inexpensive replacement for myocardial imaging, which would make mental stress testing more attractive for routine and widespread clinical use.

"It is important to find out which patients are at risk and to learn ways to tailor treatment to those at risk. It may be that we can alter the lifestyles of people at risk and get them to respond differently to the stress," he says.

According to the American Heart Association, managing stress makes sense for a person's overall health, but current data do not yet support specific recommendations using stress management as a therapy for cardiovascular disease.

Co-authors include: Robert P. McMahon, Ph.D.; Lewis Becker, M.D.; Robert M. Carney, Ph.D.; Kenneth E. Freedland, Ph.D.; Jerome D. Cohen, M.D.; David Sheffield, Ph.D.; A. David Goldberg, M.D.; Mark. W. Ketterer, Ph.D.; Carl J. Pepine, M.D.; James M. Raczynski, Ph.D.; Kathleen Light, Ph.D.; David S. Krantz, Ph.D.; Peter H. Stone, M.D.; Genell L. Knatterud, Ph.D.; and Peter G. Kaufmann, Ph.D.

Section 21.3

Does Stress Cause High Blood Pressure?

From "Your Guide to Lowering High Blood Pressure," a publication of the National Heart, Lung and Blood Institute (NHLBI, www.nhlbi.nih.gov), part of the National Institutes of Health, May 2003. Text under the heading "Does stress cause high blood pressure?" is also published by NHLBI.

What are high blood pressure and prehypertension?

Blood pressure is the force of blood against the walls of arteries. Blood pressure rises and falls during the day. When blood pressure stays elevated over time, it is called high blood pressure.

The medical term for high blood pressure is hypertension. High blood pressure is dangerous because it makes the heart work too hard and contributes to atherosclerosis (hardening of the arteries). It increases the risk of heart disease and stroke, which are the first- and third-leading causes of death among Americans. High blood pressure also can result in other conditions, such as congestive heart failure, kidney disease, and blindness.

A blood pressure level of 140/90 mmHg or higher is considered high. About two thirds of people over age 65 have high blood pressure. If your blood pressure is between 120/80 mmHg and 139/89 mmHg, then you have prehypertension. This means that you don't have high blood pressure now but are likely to develop it in the future. You can take steps to prevent high blood pressure by adopting a healthy lifestyle.

Those who do not have high blood pressure at age 55 face a 90 percent chance of developing it during their lifetimes. So high blood pressure is a condition that most people have at some point in their lives.

Both numbers in a blood pressure test are important, but for people who are 50 or older, systolic pressure gives the most accurate diagnosis of high blood pressure. Systolic pressure is the top number in a blood pressure reading. It is high if it is 140 mmHg or above.

What is systolic blood pressure?

Systolic pressure is the force of blood in the arteries as the heart beats. It is shown as the top number in a blood pressure reading. High blood pressure is 140 and higher for systolic pressure. Diastolic pressure does not need to be high for you to have high blood pressure. When that happens, the condition is called "isolated systolic hypertension," or ISH.

Is isolated systolic high blood pressure common?

Yes. It is the most common form of high blood pressure for older Americans. For most Americans, systolic blood pressure increases with age, while diastolic increases until about age 55 and then declines. About 65 percent of hypertensives over age 60 have ISH. You may have ISH and feel fine. As with other types of high blood pressure, ISH often causes no symptoms. To find out if you have ISH—or any type of high blood pressure—see your doctor and have a blood pressure test. The test is quick and painless.

Is isolated systolic high blood pressure dangerous?

Any form of high blood pressure is dangerous if not properly treated. Both numbers in a blood pressure test are important, but, for some, the systolic is especially meaningful. That's because, for those persons middle aged and older, systolic pressure gives a better diagnosis of high blood pressure.

If left uncontrolled, high systolic pressure can lead to stroke, heart attack, congestive heart failure, kidney damage, blindness, or other conditions. While it cannot be cured, once it has developed, ISH can be controlled.

Clinical studies have proven that treating a high systolic pressure saves lives, greatly reduces illness, and improves the quality of life. Yet, most Americans do not have their high systolic pressure under control.

Does it require special treatment?

Treatment options for ISH are the same as for other types of high blood pressure, in which both systolic and diastolic pressures are high. ISH is treated with lifestyle changes and/or medications. The key for any high blood pressure treatment is to bring the condition under proper control. Blood pressure should be controlled to less than 140/90 mmHg. If yours is not, then ask your doctor why. You may just need a lifestyle or drug change, such as reducing salt in your diet or adding a second medication.

What is diastolic blood pressure?

Diastolic pressure is the force of blood in the arteries as the heart relaxes between beats. It's shown as the bottom number in a blood pressure reading.

The diastolic blood pressure has been and remains, especially for younger people, an important hypertension number. The higher the diastolic blood pressure the greater the risk for heart attacks, strokes and kidney failure. As people become older, the diastolic pressure will begin to decrease and the systolic blood pressure begins to rise and becomes more important. A rise in systolic blood pressure will also increase the chance for heart attacks, strokes, and kidney failure. Your physician will use both the systolic and the diastolic blood pressure to determine your blood pressure category and appropriate prevention and treatment activities.

Does stress cause high blood pressure?

Stress can make blood pressure go up for a while, and it has been thought to contribute to high blood pressure. But the long-term effects of stress are as yet unclear. Stress management techniques do not seem to prevent high blood pressure. However, such techniques may have other benefits, such as making you feel better or helping you to control overeating.

Section 21.4

Stress Raises Cholesterol Levels

"Mental Stress May Be Another Culprit in Raising Cholesterol Levels in Healthy Adults, According to Study," Copyright © 2005 by the American Psychological Association. Reprinted with permission.

There is good evidence to show that stress can increase a person's heart rate, lower the immune system's ability to fight colds, and increase certain inflammatory markers, but can stress also raise a person's cholesterol? It appears so for some people, according to a new study that examines how reactions to stress over a period of time can raise a person's lipid levels.

This finding is reported in the November [2005] issue of *Health Psychology,* published by the American Psychological Association (APA). In a sample of 199 healthy middle-aged men and women, researchers Andrew Steptoe, D.Sc., and Lena Brydon, Ph.D., of University College London examined how individuals react to stress and whether this reaction can increase cholesterol and heighten cardiovascular risk in the future. Changes in total cholesterol, including low-density lipoprotein (LDL) and high-density lipoprotein (HDL), were assessed in the participants before and three years after completing two stress tasks.

Our study found that individuals vary in their cholesterol responses to stress, said Dr. Steptoe. "Some of the participants show large increases even in the short term, while others show very little response. The cholesterol responses that we measured in the lab probably reflect the way people react to challenges in everyday life as well. So the larger cholesterol responders to stress tasks will be large responders to emotional situations in their lives. It is these responses in everyday life that accumulate to lead to an increase in fasting cholesterol or lipid levels three years later. It appears that a person's reaction to stress is one mechanism through which higher lipid levels may develop."

The stress testing session involved examining the participants' cardiovascular, inflammatory, and hemostatic functions before and after their responses to performance on moderately stressful behavioral tasks. The stress tasks used were computerized color-word interference and mirror tracing. The color-word task involved flashing a series of target color words in incongruous colors on a computer screen (for example, yellow letters spelling the color blue). At the bottom of the computer screen, four names of colors were displayed in incorrect colors. The object of the task was to match the name of the color to the target word. The other task used was mirror tracing, which required the participant to trace a star seen in a mirror image. The participants were told to focus more on accuracy than on speed in both tasks.

At the follow-up three years later, cholesterol levels in all the participants in the study had gone up, as might be expected through passage of time. However, individuals with larger initial stress responses had substantially greater rises in cholesterol than those with small stress responses. The people in the top third of stress responders were three times more likely to have a level of 'bad' (low-density lipoprotein) cholesterol above clinical thresholds than were people in the bottom third of stress responders. These differences were independent of their baseline levels of cholesterol levels, gender, age, hormone replacement, body mass index, smoking, or alcohol consumption.

The authors found no sex differences among the participants in their cholesterol levels and response to stress. Steptoe and Brydon speculate on the reasons why acute stress responses may raise fasting serum lipids. One possibility may be that stress encourages the body to produce more energy in the form of metabolic fuels—fatty acids and glucose. These substances require the liver to produce and secrete more LDL, which is the principal carrier of cholesterol in the blood. Another reason may be that stress interferes with lipid clearance and a third possibility could be that stress increases production of a number of inflammatory processes like, interleukin 6, tumor necrosis factor, and C-Reactive protein that also increase lipid production.

Even though these lipid responses to stress were not large, said Dr. Steptoe, "the levels are something to be concerned about. It does give us an opportunity to know whose cholesterol may rise in response to stress and give us warning for those who may be more at risk for coronary heart disease."

Source: "Associations Between Acute Lipid Stress Responses and Fasting Lipid Levels 3 Years Later," Andrew Steptoe, D.Sc., and Lena Brydon, Ph.D., University College London; *Health Psychology,* Vol. 24, No. 6.

Chapter 22

Stress, Diabetes, and Related Syndromes

Chapter Contents

Section 22.1

Chronic Stress Increases Risk of Diabetes and Related Disorders

"Stress and Your Health," © 2006 The Hormone Foundation. Reprinted with permission. For additional information, visit www.hormone.org.

What is stress?

Generally speaking, stress means pressure or strain. Life constantly subjects us to pressures. In people, stress can be physical (e.g., disease), emotional (e.g., grief), or psychological (e.g., fear).

Individuals vary in their ability to cope with stress. How you see a situation and your general physical health are the two major factors that determine how you will respond to a stressful event or to repeated stress.

Genes and things that happen to you early in life (e.g., child abuse or neglect), even when in the womb, can affect how you handle stressful situations, possibly making you more likely to over-react. Overeating, smoking, drinking, and not exercising, which can often result from being under stress, can also add to the negative effects of stress.

What is the stress response?

Allostasis is the process of how the body responds to stress, whether it is acute (short-term) or chronic (long-term).

The best-known acute stress response is the "fight or flight" reaction that happens when you feel threatened. In this case, the stress response causes the body to release several stress hormones (e.g., cortisol and adrenalin) into the bloodstream. These hormones intensify your concentration, ability to react, and strength. Also, your heart rate and blood pressure increase, and your immune system and memory are sharper. After you have dealt with the short-term stress, your body returns to normal.

Chronic or long-term stress, however, poses a problem. If you repeatedly face challenges and your body is constantly producing higher levels of stress hormones, it does not have time to recover.

216

These hormones build up in the blood and, over time, can cause serious health problems.

How does chronic stress affect your health?

The bodily changes that happen during moments of stress can be very helpful when they happen for a short time. But when this happens for a long period of time, producing too many stress hormones can affect your health. The long-term effect of chronic stress (called allostatic load) causes wear and tear on the body. Health problems can include:

- **Digestive system:** Stomachache is common due to a slowdown in the emptying of the stomach; also diarrhea due to more activity in the colon.

- **Obesity:** Increase in appetite, which can lead to weight gain. (Being overweight or obese puts you at risk for diabetes and cardiovascular disease.)

- **Immune system:** Weakening of the immune system so that you are more likely to have colds or other infections.

- **Nervous system:** Anxiety, depression, loss of sleep, and lack of interest in physical activity. Memory and decision making can also be affected.

- **Cardiovascular system:** Increase in blood pressure, heart rate, and the level of fats in your blood (cholesterol and triglycerides). Also, increase in blood sugar levels (especially in the evening) and appetite (which contributes to weight gain). All of these are risk factors for heart disease, atherosclerosis (hardening of the arteries), stroke, obesity, and diabetes.

How do you know you're stressed out?

When you experience short-term stress you may feel anxious, nervous, distracted, worried, and pressured. If your stress level increases or lasts for a longer time, you might experience other physical or emotional effects:

- fatigue or depression;
- chest pain or pressure or fast heartbeat;
- dizziness, shakiness, or difficulty breathing;

- irregular menstrual periods, erectile dysfunction (impotence), or loss of libido (sex drive).

These symptoms may also lead to loss of appetite, overeating, and poor sleep, all of which can have serious consequences for your health.

Usually these symptoms are minor and may be relieved through coping skills such as learning to relax, removing yourself for a time from the things that stress you out, and exercising. If the symptoms are severe, however, you may need medical help to find the source of your stress and the best way to manage it.

What should you do with this information?

There are practical steps you can take to cut back on stress. Regular, moderate exercise improves thought process and mood. So does relaxing, getting a good night's sleep, and seeking emotional support from family and friends. You can also reduce the long-term effects of chronic stress by eating a healthy, low-fat diet and avoiding smoking and drinking too much alcohol. However, if your symptoms continue or get worse, you should see your doctor.

Resources

- Find-an-Endocrinologist: www.hormone.org or call 800-HOR-MONE (800-467-6663)

- Medline Plus (NIH): www.nlm.nih.gov/medlineplus/stress.html

- U.S. Dept. of Health and Human Services: www.4woman.gov/faq/stress.htm

Section 22.2

Stress at Work and the Metabolic Syndrome

"Stress at Work and the Metabolic Syndrome," by Robert W. Griffith, M.D., February 13, 2006, http://www.healthandage.com. This article is a summary of: Chronic stress at work and the metabolic syndrome: prospective study. T. Chandola, E Brunner, M Marmot. *BMJ,* 2006; 332: 521–525. © 2006 HealthandAge Foundation. All rights reserved. Reprinted with permission.

Introduction

Previous studies have reported a link between stress at work and the metabolic syndrome.[1] This is important, as there's a known link between stress and coronary heart disease, and the metabolic syndrome is a step on the path toward coronary disease. Until now, however, such studies have been of the 'cross-sectional' type, giving a snapshot view, but not providing evidence of a cause-and-effect relationship; such evidence has to come from a prospective, or longitudinal, study, like the one reported here that has been published in the *British Medical Journal.*

What Was Done

British scientists studied over 10,000 government employees (civil servants) working in central London over a 14-year period. They were between 35 and 55 at baseline, and employed in one of 20 different civil service departments.

Enrollment was between 1985 and 1988. Postal questionnaires were completed in 1989, then 2 to 3 years after that, then 2 to 3 years later, and again 2 to 3 years later. These stages were called phase 1, 2, etc. Physical exams were done in stages 3 and 5. The necessary exams to diagnose the metabolic syndrome were done in phase 5, at the end of the study.

Work stress was measured by a self-reported Job Strain questionnaire. Job strain was considered present when job demands were registered as 'high' and decision latitude, or control over the job, was scored as 'low.' The accumulation of exposure to job stress over the study period was obtained by adding together the number of times the participant was exposed to job strain. Chronic work stress was defined as three or more instances of job strain in the five phase reports (i.e. over three quarters of the time).

Social position was also measured, using employment grades at baseline. Lifestyle measurements recorded were smoking status, daily intake of fruit and vegetables, alcohol consumption, and physical activity. A basal metabolic index (BMI) over 30 was taken as an indication of obesity (waist measurements weren't made at baseline).

What Was Found

1. Men and women from lower employment grades were more likely to have developed the metabolic syndrome.

2. Men with chronic work stress were nearly twice as likely to have developed the syndrome as those with no work stress; for women, the likelihood was over five times as great. When the sexes were combined, and adjusted for age and employment grade, those with chronic work stress were over twice as likely to develop the metabolic syndrome.

3. A health-damaging lifestyle (poor diet, smoking, heavy alcohol use, no exercise) was more likely to result in the metabolic syndrome in men than in women.

4. Excluding people with obesity at baseline from the analysis did not alter the results to a relevant extent.

What These Findings Mean

This study suggests a biological mechanism for how stress at work is linked to coronary heart disease and heart attacks. The relationship between stress and the metabolic syndrome persisted after exclusion of obese participants from the analysis, showing that pre-existing physiological changes are unlikely to explain the linkage.

The study doesn't clarify which of the remaining risk factors (insulin resistance, raised blood pressure, abnormal lipid levels) is primarily influenced by stress, but other studies indicate that all of these may be involved. And of course, it's possible that stress at work will influence any bad lifestyle habits (smoking, alcohol, no exercise) that were shown to encourage the development of the syndrome.

Other reports from this particular study indicate that those participants with the metabolic syndrome had raised cortisol and normetanephrine in their urine, which are known markers of nervous and endocrine system response to stress.

More will certainly be uncovered about the effects of stress at work. However, there's enough known to act on. While one component of job strain—high demand—is likely to persist in many (even most) jobs, the other component—control over the job, or decision latitude—can be addressed by organizations' managements. If people find their job is demanding without any opportunity for decision-making, they might be advised to look for alternative work.

Source

Chandola T, Brunner E, Marmot M. Chronic stress at work and the metabolic syndrome: prospective study. *BMJ* online: *BMJ* 2006: 386934353, doi:10.1136/bmj.38693.435301.80.

Footnote

1. The metabolic syndrome requires three of the following risk factors to be present: (a) Waist size over 40 inches (102 cm) in men, or 35 inches (88 cm) in women. (b) Serum triglyceride level over 150 mg/dL (1.7 mmol/L). (c) Serum HDL ('good') cholesterol below 40 mg/dL (1.0 mmol/L) in men, or 50 mg/dL (1.29 mmol/L) in women. (d) Blood pressure over 130/85 mm Hg (either number), or being on blood pressure medication. (e) Fasting blood sugar over 110 mg/dL (6.1 mmol/L).

Section 22.3

Therapy Helps Kids with
Type 1 Diabetes Reduce Stress

This information was provided by KidsHealth, one of the largest resources online for medically reviewed health information written for parents, kids, and teens. For more articles like this one, visit www.KidsHealth.org, or www.TeensHealth.org. © 2006 The Nemours Foundation. This information was reviewed by Steven Dowshen, M.D., January 2006.

Kids and teens who've been diagnosed with type 1 diabetes have a lot to handle—they need to eat properly, exercise regularly, test their blood sugar levels on schedule, and take the right amount of insulin. When faced with that many tasks, it's easy for teens to feel stressed. Stress can be particularly harmful for adolescents with diabetes, because it can affect hormones in the body that control blood sugar and may make it difficult for teens to stick to their diabetes management plan.

The good news is that teens with hard-to-control blood sugar levels who participate in an intense therapy program can learn to manage their diabetes better with less stress, say researchers from Wayne State University in Detroit, Michigan, and the Medical University of South Carolina in Charleston.

Researchers randomly divided 127 teens with type 1 diabetes who'd been having problems controlling their blood sugar levels into two groups. One group (the control group) received standard medical care and regularly met with diabetes specialists, nurses, social workers, dietitians, and psychologists. The teens in the other group (the intervention group) received standard care plus met with a therapist two or three times a week for about 6 months.

During the sessions (which they attended with their families), the teens had therapists help them identify problems that had been getting in the way of their blood sugar control. Over the course of the sessions, the therapists helped them overcome those obstacles with:

- **Family interventions:** The therapist taught parents to become more involved in monitoring their child's diabetes regimen.

Parents also received training in creating family routines, establishing regular mealtimes, and communicating effectively with their teens.

- **Peer interventions:** Friends learned to support the teen as he or she stuck to the diabetes plan.

- **School interventions:** The parents and therapist met with school personnel to improve communication about the teen's diabetes care needs.

- **Community interventions:** The therapist helped parents and teens find ways to make ensure care for the teens' diabetes during other activities, such as during visits to extended family members.

- **Health care system interventions:** The therapist helped the family keep health care appointments and communicate with the diabetes health care team.

At the beginning of the study and about 7 months later, the teens in both groups completed questionnaires that measured their stress due to worries about their diabetes, their interactions with family members and friends, their responsibilities for managing their diabetes, and their symptoms of high blood sugar levels and low blood sugar levels. The teens also underwent regular tests to determine how well they were controlling their blood sugar levels.

Compared with their stress levels at the beginning of the study, teens who had the intense therapy program had significantly reduced stress after treatment. In contrast, the students in the control group had more stress than they did at the start of the study. The therapy program helped reduce stress for both younger and older teens of both genders. Overall, the therapy treatment helped teens improve their blood sugar control because it helped them adhere to their diabetes management plan more effectively.

What This Means to You

According to the results of this study, an intense therapy program of this type can help teens reduce their stress levels and improve their blood sugar control by helping them follow their diabetes management plan. If your teen is having trouble following his or her diabetes management plan, talk to your child's doctor or other member of the diabetes health care team.

Source: Deborah A. Ellis, Ph.D.; Maureen A. Frey, Ph.D.; Sylvie Naar-King, Ph.D.; Thomas Templin, Ph.D.; Phillippe B. Cunningham, Ph.D.; Nedim Cakan, M.D.; *Pediatrics,* December 2005.

Chapter 23

Stress and Digestive Diseases

Chapter Contents

Section 23.1

Does Stress Cause
Irritable Bowel Syndrome?

Excerpted from the brochure "What I need to know about Irritable Bowel Syndrome" from the National Institute of Diabetes and Digestive and Kidney Diseases (NIDDK, www.niddk.nih.gov), part of the National Institutes of Health, April 2003.

What is IBS?

Irritable bowel syndrome, or IBS, is a problem that affects mainly the bowel, which is also called the large intestine. The bowel is the part of the digestive system that makes and stores stool. The word syndrome means a group of symptoms. IBS is a syndrome because it can cause several symptoms. For example, IBS causes cramping, bloating, gas, diarrhea, and constipation.

IBS is not a disease. It's a functional disorder, which means that the bowel doesn't work as it should.

With IBS, the nerves and muscles in the bowel are extra-sensitive. For example, the muscles may contract too much when you eat. These contractions can cause cramping and diarrhea during or shortly after a meal. Or the nerves can be overly sensitive to the stretching of the bowel (because of gas, for example). Cramping or pain can result.

IBS can be painful. But it does not damage the bowel or cause any other diseases.

Does stress cause IBS?

Emotional stress will not cause a person to develop IBS. But if you already have IBS, stress can trigger symptoms. In fact, the bowel can overreact to all sorts of things, including food, exercise, and hormones.

Foods that tend to cause symptoms include milk products, chocolate, alcohol, caffeine, carbonated drinks, and fatty foods. In some cases, simply eating a large meal will trigger symptoms.

Women with IBS often have more symptoms during their menstrual periods.

What are the symptoms of IBS?

The main symptoms of IBS are:

- crampy pain in the stomach area (abdomen) and
- painful diarrhea or constipation

Most people have either diarrhea or constipation, but some people have both.

Other symptoms are:

- mucus in the stool;
- swollen or bloated abdomen; and
- the feeling that you have not finished a bowel movement.

How is IBS diagnosed?

The doctor will suspect that you have IBS because of your symptoms. But the doctor may do medical tests to make sure you don't have any other diseases that could cause the symptoms.

Medical tests for IBS include:

- Physical exam
- Blood tests
- X ray of the bowel: This x-ray test is called a barium enema or lower GI (gastrointestinal) series. Barium is a thick liquid that makes the bowel show up better on the x ray. Before taking the x ray, the doctor will put barium into your bowel through the anus.
- Endoscopy: The doctor inserts a thin tube into your bowel. The tube has a camera in it, so the doctor can look at the inside of the bowel to check for problems.

What is the treatment?

IBS has no cure, but you can do things to relieve symptoms. Treatment may involve:

- diet changes;
- medicine; and
- stress relief.

You may have to try a combination of things to see which works best for you.

Diet changes: Some foods make IBS worse. Here are some foods that may cause symptoms:

- fatty foods like french fries;
- milk products like cheese or ice cream;
- chocolate;
- alcohol;
- caffeine (found in coffee and some sodas); and
- carbonated drinks like soda.

If certain foods cause symptoms, you should eat less of them or stop eating them.

To find out which foods are a problem, write down this information:

- what you eat during the day;
- what symptoms you have;
- when symptoms occur; and
- what foods always make you feel bad.

Take your notes to the doctor to see if you should stop eating certain foods.

Some foods make IBS better. Fiber reduces IBS symptoms—especially constipation—because it makes stool soft, bulky, and easier to pass. Fiber is found in bran, bread, cereal, beans, fruit, and vegetables.

- Fruits: Apples, peaches
- Vegetables: Broccoli, raw; cabbage; carrots, raw; peas
- Breads, cereals, and beans: Kidney beans; lima beans; whole-grain bread; whole-grain cereal

Add foods with fiber to your diet a little at a time to let your body get used to them. Too much fiber all at once might cause gas, which can trigger symptoms in a person with IBS.

Besides telling you to eat more foods with fiber, the doctor might also tell you to get more fiber by taking a fiber pill or drinking water mixed with a special high-fiber powder.

How much you eat matters, too. Large meals can cause cramping and diarrhea in people with IBS. If this happens to you, try eating four or five small meals a day. Or, have your usual three meals, but eat less at each meal.

Medicine: If necessary, the doctor might give you medicine to help with symptoms:

- laxatives: to treat constipation
- antispasmodics: to slow contractions in the bowel, which helps with diarrhea and pain
- antidepressants: to help those who have severe pain

You must follow your doctor's instructions when you use these medicines. Otherwise, you could become dependent on them.

Stress relief: Does stress trigger your symptoms? Learning to reduce stress can help. With less stress, you may find that you have less cramping and pain. Also, you may find it easier to manage your symptoms.

Meditation, exercise, and counseling are some things that might help. You may need to try different activities to see what works best for you.

Section 23.2

Does Stress Cause Peptic Ulcers?

Excerpted from "What I need to know about Peptic Ulcers," a publication by the National Digestive Diseases Information Clearinghouse (NDDIC), a service of the National Institute of Diabetes and Digestive and Kidney Diseases (NIDDK), October 2004. NIH Publication No. 05-5042.

What is a peptic ulcer?

A peptic ulcer is a sore in the lining of your stomach or duodenum. The duodenum is the first part of your small intestine. If peptic ulcers are found in the stomach, they're called gastric ulcers. If they're found in the duodenum, they're called duodenal ulcers. You can have more than one ulcer.

Many people have peptic ulcers. Peptic ulcers can be treated successfully. Seeing your doctor is the first step.

What are the symptoms of peptic ulcers?

A burning pain in the gut is the most common symptom. The pain:

- feels like a dull ache;
- comes and goes for a few days or weeks;
- starts 2 to 3 hours after a meal;
- comes in the middle of the night when your stomach is empty; and
- usually goes away after you eat.

Other symptoms are:

- losing weight;
- not feeling like eating;
- having pain while eating;
- feeling sick to your stomach; and
- vomiting.

Some people with peptic ulcers have mild symptoms. If you have any of these symptoms, you may have a peptic ulcer and should see your doctor.

What causes peptic ulcers?

Peptic ulcers are caused by:

- bacteria called *Helicobacter pylori*, or *H. pylori* for short;
- nonsteroidal anti-inflammatory drugs (NSAIDs) such as aspirin and ibuprofen; and
- other diseases.

Your body makes strong acids that digest food. A lining protects the inside of your stomach and duodenum from these acids. If the lining breaks down, the acids can damage the walls. Both *H. pylori* and NSAIDs weaken the lining so acid can reach the stomach or duodenal wall.

H. pylori causes almost two thirds of all ulcers. Many people have *H. pylori* infections. But not everyone who has an infection will develop a peptic ulcer.

Most other ulcers are caused by NSAIDs. Only rarely do other diseases cause ulcers.

Do stress or spicy foods cause peptic ulcers?

No, neither stress nor spicy foods cause ulcers. But they can make ulcers worse. Drinking alcohol or smoking can make ulcers worse, too.

What increases my risk of getting peptic ulcers?

You're more likely to develop a peptic ulcer if you:

- have an *H. pylori* infection;
- use NSAIDs often;
- smoke cigarettes;
- drink alcohol;
- have relatives who have peptic ulcers; and
- are 50 years old or older.

Can peptic ulcers get worse?

Peptic ulcers will get worse if they aren't treated. Call your doctor right away if you have any of these symptoms:

- sudden sharp pain that doesn't go away;
- black or bloody stools; or
- bloody vomit or vomit that looks like coffee grounds.

These could be signs that:

- the ulcer has gone through, or perforated, the stomach or duodenal wall;
- the ulcer has broken a blood vessel; or
- the ulcer has stopped food from moving from the stomach into the duodenum.

These symptoms must be treated quickly. You may need surgery.

How are peptic ulcers treated?

Peptic ulcers can be cured. Medicines for peptic ulcers are:

- proton pump inhibitors or histamine receptor blockers to stop your stomach from making acids and
- antibiotics to kill the bacteria.

Depending on your symptoms, you may take one or more of these medicines for a few weeks. They'll stop the pain and help heal your stomach or duodenum.

Ulcers take time to heal. Take your medicines even if the pain goes away. If these medicines make you feel sick or dizzy, or cause diarrhea or headaches, your doctor can change your medicines.

If NSAIDs caused your peptic ulcer, you'll need to stop taking them. If you smoke, quit. Smoking slows healing of ulcers.

Chapter 24

Stress and the Immune System

Chapter Contents

Section 24.1

What Happens When the Immune System Is under Stress?

"Stress and Disease: New Perspectives" is from the National Institute of Health (www.nih.gov) publication *Word on Health,* by Harrison Wein, Ph.D., October 2000. Reviewed by David A. Cooke, M.D., March 2007.

For thousands of years, people believed that stress made you sick. Up until the nineteenth century, the idea that the passions and emotions were intimately linked to disease held sway, and people were told by their doctors to go to spas or seaside resorts when they were ill. Gradually these ideas lost favor as more concrete causes and cures were found for illness after illness. But in the last decade, scientists like Dr. Esther Sternberg, director of the Integrative Neural Immune Program at the National Institutes of Health (NIH)'s National Institute of Mental Health (NIMH), have been rediscovering the links between the brain and the immune system.

The Immune System and the Brain

When you have an infection or something else that causes inflammation such as a burn or injury, many different kinds of cells from the immune system stream to the site. Dr. Sternberg likens them to soldiers moving into battle, each kind with its own specialized function. Some are like garbage collectors, ingesting invaders. Some make antibodies, the "bullets" to fight the infectious agents; others kill invaders directly. All these types of immune cells must coordinate their actions, and the way they do that is by sending each other signals in the form of molecules that they make in factories inside the cell.

"It turns out that these molecules have many more effects than just being the walkie-talkie communicators between different kinds of immune cells," Dr. Sternberg says. "They can also go through the bloodstream to signal the brain or activate nerves nearby that signal the brain."

These immune molecules, Dr. Sternberg explains, cause the brain to change its functions. "They can induce a whole set of behaviors that we call sickness behavior.... You lose the desire or the ability to move, you lose your appetite, you lose interest in sex." Scientists can only speculate about the purpose of these sickness behaviors, but Dr. Sternberg suggests that they might help us conserve energy when we're sick so we can better use our energy to fight disease.

These signaling molecules from the immune system can also activate the part of the brain that controls the stress response, the hypothalamus. Through a cascade of hormones released from the pituitary and adrenal glands, the hypothalamus causes blood levels of the hormone cortisol to rise. Cortisol is the major steroid hormone produced by our bodies to help us get through stressful situations. The related compound known as cortisone is widely used as an anti-inflammatory drug in creams to treat rashes and in nasal sprays to treat sinusitis and asthma. But it wasn't until very recently that scientists realized the brain also uses cortisol to suppress the immune system and tone down inflammation within the body.

Stress and the Immune System

This complete communications cycle from the immune system to the brain and back again allows the immune system to talk to the brain, and the brain to then talk back and shut down the immune response when it's no longer needed.

"When you think about this cross-talk, this two-way street," Dr. Sternberg explains, "you can begin to understand the kinds of illnesses that might result if there is either too much or too little communication in either direction."

According to Dr. Sternberg, if you're chronically stressed, the part of the brain that controls the stress response is going to be constantly pumping out a lot of stress hormones. The immune cells are being bathed in molecules which are essentially telling them to stop fighting. And so in situations of chronic stress, your immune cells are less able to respond to an invader like a bacteria or a virus.

This theory holds up in studies looking at high levels of shorter-term stress or chronic stress: in caregivers like those taking care of relatives with Alzheimer disease, medical students undergoing exam stress, Army Rangers undergoing extremely grueling physical stress, and couples with marital stress. People in these situations, Dr. Sternberg says, show a prolonged healing time, a decreased ability of their immune systems to respond to vaccination, and an increased susceptibility to viral infections like the common cold.

Some Stress Is Good

People tend to talk about stress as if it's all bad. It's not.

"Some stress is good for you," Dr. Sternberg says. "I have to get my stress response to a certain optimal level so I can perform in front of an audience when I give a talk." Otherwise, she may come across as lethargic and listless.

But while some stress is good, too much is not good. "If you're too stressed, your performance falls off," Dr. Sternberg says. "The objective should be not to get rid of stress completely because you can't get rid of stress—stress is life, life is stress. Rather, you need to be able to use your stress response optimally."

The key is to learn to move yourself to that optimal peak point so that you're not underperforming but you're also not so stressed that you're unable to perform. How much we're able to do that is the challenge, Dr. Sternberg admits. This may not be possible in all situations, or for all people, because just as with the animals Dr. Sternberg studies, some people may have a more sensitive stress response than others.

"But your goal should be to try to learn to control your stress to make it work for you," Dr. Sternberg says. "Don't just think of getting rid of your stress; think of turning it to your advantage."

Controlling the Immune Response

Problems between the brain and the immune system can go the other way, too. If for some reason you're unable to make enough of these brain stress hormones, you won't be able to turn off the immune cells once they're no longer needed.

"There has to be an exit strategy for these battles that are being fought by the immune system, and the brain provides the exit strategy through stress hormones," Dr. Sternberg says. "If your brain can't make enough of these hormones to turn the immune system off when it doesn't have to be active anymore, then it could go on unchecked and result in autoimmune diseases like rheumatoid arthritis, lupus, or other autoimmune diseases that people recognize as inflammation."

Dr. Sternberg says that there are several factors involved in these autoimmune conditions. There are many different effects that the brain and its nervous system can have on the immune system, depending on the kinds of nerve chemicals that are being made, where they're being made, what kind of nerves they come from, and whether they're in the bloodstream or not. Still, at least part of the problem in these diseases seems to involve the brain's hormonal stress response.

"So if you have too much stress hormone shutting down the immune response, you can't fight off infection and you're more susceptible to infection," Dr. Sternberg concludes. "Too little stress hormones and the immune response goes on unchecked and you could get an inflammatory disease."

Pinpointing the Problems

Why these miscommunications between the brain and the immune system come about is still largely unknown, and involves many genes and environmental factors. But by studying animals, scientists have finally been able to start understanding how the miscommunications occur.

Dr. Sternberg first started publishing work on the links between the brain and the immune system back in 1989 while studying rats with immune problems. "In many of these cases it's very hard to show the mechanism in humans," Dr. Sternberg explains, "but you can show the mechanism in animals because you can manipulate all the different parts of the system and you can begin to understand which parts affect which other parts." It has taken "a good ten years" to gather enough evidence in human studies to show that the principles her lab uncovered in rats were also relevant to human beings.

Drugs that have been tested in rats to correct brain/immune system problems have had unpredictable effects. That is because nothing happens in isolation when it comes to the brain and the immune system. Dr. Sternberg points out that our bodies are amazing machines which at every moment of the day are constantly responding to a myriad of different kinds of stimuli—chemical, psychological, and physical. "These molecules act in many different ways in different parts of the system," she says. Understanding how the brain and the immune system work together in these different diseases should help scientists develop new kinds of drugs to treat them that would never have occurred to them before.

Taking Control Now

Dr. Sternberg thinks that one of the most hopeful aspects of this science is that it tells us it's not all in our genes. A growing number of studies show that, to some degree, you can use your mind to help treat your body. Support groups, stress relief, and meditation may, by altering stress hormone levels, all help the immune system. For example, women in support groups for their breast cancer have longer life spans than women without such psychological support.

There are several components of stress to think about, including its duration, how strong it is, and how long it lasts. Every stress has some effect on the body, and you have to take into account the total additive effect on the body of all stressors when considering how to reduce stress.

Perhaps the most productive way to think about stress is in terms of control. Dr. Sternberg shows a slide of an F-14 jet flying sideways by the deck of an aircraft carrier, its wings completely vertical. "The Navy Commander who flew that jet told me that he was the only one in the photo who was not stressed, and that's because he was the one in control. The officer sitting in the seat ten feet behind him was in the exact same physical situation but was not in control. Control is a very important part of whether or not we feel stressed.

So if you can learn to feel that you're in control or actually take control of certain aspects of the situation that you're in, you can reduce your stress response. Studies show that gaining a sense of control can help patients cope with their illness, if not help the illness itself.

Until science has more solid answers, it can't hurt to participate in support groups and seek ways to relieve stress, Dr. Sternberg says. But what you need to remember is if you do these things and you're not successful in correcting whatever the underlying problem is, it's not your fault because there's a biology to the system. "You need to know the benefits of the system," she says, "but its limitations as well." In other words, try not to get too stressed about being stressed.

Stress Control

First try to identify the things in your life that cause you stress: marital problems, conflict at work, a death or illness in the family. Once you identify and understand how these stressors affect you, you can begin to figure out ways to change your environment and manage them.

If there's a problem that can be solved, set about taking control and solving it. For example, you might decide to change jobs if problems at work are making you too stressed.

But some chronic stressors can't be changed. For those, support groups, relaxation, meditation, and exercise are all tools you can use to manage your stress. If nothing you do seems to work for you, seek a health professional who can help. Also seek professional help if you find that you worry excessively about the small things in life.

Keep in mind that chronic stress can be associated with mental conditions like depression and anxiety disorders as well as physical problems. Seek professional help if you have:

- difficulty sleeping;
- changes in appetite;
- panic attacks;
- muscle tenseness and soreness;
- frequent headaches;
- gastrointestinal problems; or
- prolonged feelings of sadness or worthlessness.

Section 24.2

Stress Wears down Human Immunity over Time

"Stress affects immunity in ways related to stress type and duration, as shown by nearly 300 studies," Copyright © 2004 by the American Psychological Association. Reprinted with permission.

Psychologists have long known that stress affects our ability to fight infection, but a major new meta-analysis—a study of studies—has elucidated intriguing patterns of how stress affects human immunity, strengthening it in the short term but wearing it down over time. The report appears in the July [2004] issue of *Psychological Bulletin,* which is published by the American Psychological Association.

Major findings are three-fold. First, the overlapping findings of 293 independent studies reported in peer-reviewed scientific journals between 1960 and 2001—with some 18,941 individuals taking part in all—powerfully confirm the core fact that stress alters immunity. Second, the authors of the meta-analysis observed a distinctive pattern:

Short-term stress actually "revs up" the immune system, an adaptive response preparing for injury or infection, but long-term or chronic stress causes too much wear and tear, and the system breaks down. Third, the immune systems of people who are older or already sick are more prone to stress-related change.

Psychologists Suzanne Segerstrom, Ph.D., of the University of Kentucky, and Gregory Miller, Ph.D., of the University of British Columbia, analyzed the results of the nearly 300 studies by sorting them into different categories and statistically evaluating relationships. For example, the five stressor categories included:

- **Acute time-limited stressors:** Lab challenges such as public speaking or mental math.

- **Brief naturalistic stressors:** Real-world challenges such as academic tests.

- **Stressful event sequences:** A focal event such as loss of a spouse or major natural disaster gives rise to a series of related challenges that people know at some point will end.

- **Chronic stressors:** Pervasive demands that force people to restructure their identity or social roles, without any clear end point—such as injury resulting in permanent disability, caring for a spouse with severe dementia, or being a refugee forced from one's native country by war.

- **Distant stressors:** Traumatic experiences that occurred in the distant past yet can continue modifying the immune system because of their long-lasting emotional and cognitive consequences, such as child abuse, combat trauma, or having been a prisoner of war.

The psychologists also looked at the effects of the various stressors on different immune responses, such as natural and specific immunity. Natural immunity produces quick-acting, all-purpose cells that can attack many pathogens; they bring fever and inflammation. While they fight on the front line, the body takes a few days to mount a more efficient attack on specific invaders via the lymphocytes (T-cells and B cells) of specific immunity. Specific immunity has both cellular responses, which fight pathogens that get inside cells (such as viruses), and humoral responses, which fight pathogens that stay outside cells, such as bacteria and parasites. Scientists have identified the blood markers of these different immune responses; stress studies measure them to indicate stress response. As a result, Segerstrom and Miller were able to assess how different types of immune response correlated with different types of stress.

Write the authors, "Stressful events reliably associate with changes in the immune system and . . . characteristics of those events are important in determining the kind of change that occurs."

Acute time-limited stressors, the type that produce a "fight or flight" response, prompted the immune system to ready itself for infections resulting from bites, punctures, scrapes, or other challenges to the integrity of the skin and blood. In evolution, this response would be selected as adaptive. Brief stressors enhanced quick, energy-efficient natural immunity, to help the body meet the challenge prompting fight or flight. At the same time, certain aspects of specific immunity that consume time and energy were suppressed.

Stressful event sequences seemed to be weakly associated with different immune consequences, depending on the type of event. The data suggested different patterns for bereavement (loss) and trauma, but the authors didn't see associations strong enough to make new claims. In this regard, further study is needed.

The most chronic stressors—which change people's identities or social roles, are more beyond their control, and seem endless—were associated with the most global suppression of immunity; almost all measures of immune function dropped across the board. Duration of stress came into play: The longer the stress, the more the immune system shifted from potentially adaptive changes (such as those in the acute "fight or flight" response) to potentially detrimental changes, at first in cellular immunity and then in broader immune function. Thus, stressors that turn a person's world upside down and appear to offer no "light at the end of the tunnel" could have the greatest psychological and physiological impact.

Finally, Segerstrom and Miller found that age and disease status affected a person's vulnerability to stress-related decreases in immune function. They attribute this to how illness and age make it harder for the body to regulate itself.

The authors are satisfied that their meta-analysis confirms the value of looking at stressors and immunity in greater detail to learn the mechanisms underlying the body's response to stress. In this case, defining stressor types and examining natural vs. specific and cellular vs. humoral immune responses turned up useful information. Says Miller, "A meta-analysis lets you ask questions that are too big for any one study to answer. You see if things are consistent over the gamut of labs, methods, and people."

241

Future studies, the authors hope, will look at the role of behavior in the stress-immunity pathway. For example, optimism and coping are known to mitigate the immune response to stress. Further, they write that the most pressing question facing researchers is, "the extent to which stressor-induced changes in the immune system have meaningful implications for disease susceptibility in otherwise healthy humans." The field of psychoneuroimmunology has yet to tie together the various threads of research to determine whether immune system changes are the reason that stress makes people more likely to get sick.

Source: "Psychological Stress and the Human Immune System: A Meta-Analytic Study of 30 Years of Inquiry," Suzanne C. Segerstrom, Ph.D., University of Kentucky, and Gregory E. Miller, Ph.D., University of British Columbia; *Psychological Bulletin*, Vol. 130, No. 4.

Chapter 25

Stress, Sexuality, and the Reproductive System

Chapter Contents

Section 25.1

Does Stress Hinder Conception?

Clay, R. (2006). Does stress hinder conception? *Monitor on Psychology*, 37 (8), 46–47. Copyright © 2006 by the American Psychological Association. Reprinted with permission.

The idea that stress causes infertility is an old one. Couples struggling to conceive hear it all the time: "Just relax!" "Have a glass of wine!" "Take the pressure off by adopting a child, and you'll get pregnant in no time!"

Today's researchers, however, believe that psychological factors—while important—are secondary to biological ones. They know that the interaction between factors is complex. And while some studies support the idea that stress-reducing interventions boost pregnancy, the jury is still out.

The Impact of Stress

A 1993 study by Alice D. Domar, Ph.D., and co-authors reveals just how distressing infertility can be. The *Journal of Psychosomatic Obstetrics and Gynecology* (Vol. 14, Suppl., 45–52) article reported that infertile women's anxiety and depression levels equaled those of women with conditions such as cancer, HIV [human immunodeficiency virus], and chronic pain.

But does infertility cause stress or does stress cause infertility? Answers to that question have shifted over time, says Annette L. Stanton, Ph.D., a psychiatry professor at the University of California, Los Angeles School of Medicine.

In a 2002 article in the *Journal of Consulting and Clinical Psychology* (Vol. 70, No. 3, 751–770), Stanton and her co-authors explain that researchers under the sway of psychoanalytic theory once believed that infertility was the result of women's unconscious conflict. Now researchers have confirmed that biomedical causes account for most fertility problems, with psychological factors playing a much more limited role.

Jacky Boivin, Ph.D., a senior lecturer at the School of Psychology at Cardiff University in Wales, exemplifies that more nuanced approach.

244

Citing converging evidence from many different areas, Boivin believes stress and fertility are related. But it's not a simple causal relationship, she emphasizes. Stress can cause individuals to smoke or indulge in other fertility-harming habits, she says, or can cause them to drop out of fertility treatment prematurely. Highly stressed individuals may be ambivalent about having children and therefore avoid sex. And because of variation in people's responses to stress, a population-wide relationship between stress and infertility doesn't necessarily mean stress will impair an individual's fertility.

That complexity—and the difficulty of researching it—makes Boivin reluctant to even say there's a link between stress and fertility.

"The second you say to women that there's a connection, they think 'I'm so stressed at work, I've probably shut down my ovaries and will never get pregnant!' " she says. "Stress could disrupt fertility, but it very rarely—if ever—causes people never to conceive."

While animals shut down reproductive functioning in times of scarce resources and other stresses, Boivin explains, humans have ways of overcoming that adaptive mechanism. After all, she points out, women continue to bear children during wars, famines, and other situations far more extreme than anything modern Americans endure.

Psychological Interventions

Can treating stress improve pregnancy rates?

Domar thinks so. In a widely cited 2000 study in *Health Psychology* (Vol. 19, No. 6, 568–575), Domar and her co-authors randomly assigned 184 nondepressed women to cognitive-behavioral therapy, a support group and a control group. Those in the intervention groups not only saw significant psychological improvement but also had significantly higher pregnancy rates than the control group.

"Both intervention groups had almost triple the take-home baby rate of the control," says Domar, executive director of the Domar Center for Complementary Health Care in Waltham, Massachusetts, and an assistant professor of obstetrics/gynecology and reproductive biology at Harvard Medical School.

However, Domar and her co-authors admit that the study had some methodological problems. For one thing, many of the participants—especially those in the control group—dropped out. Some left the study because they got pregnant, others because they needed more psychological support. These and other limitations make definitive recommendations about psychological treatment impossible, the authors note.

And not all studies are as positive as Domar's, says Boivin. In a 2003 article in *Social Science and Medicine* (Vol. 57, No. 12, 2,325–2,341), Boivin reviewed the literature on psychosocial interventions for infertile patients. When it came to improving pregnancy rates, the results were mixed. Only eight of the 25 studies she analyzed examined interventions' effects on pregnancy rates, with three showing a positive effect and five showing no effect.

What the analysis did show was that interventions—especially group interventions emphasizing education about infertility and relaxation or coping training—reduced patients' anxiety, depression, and so-called infertility-specific stress. Future studies could evaluate yoga, meditation, and other such ways of achieving relaxation, adds Boivin, because what works best may vary from woman to woman.

"If people are thinking of using some kind of intervention—and you can go on the internet and find a million things claiming they'll get you pregnant—they should be motivated to use them to improve their quality of life rather than to increase their pregnancy rates," says Boivin. "That's where, chances are, it's going to work."

Rebecca A. Clay is a writer in Washington, D.C.

Section 25.2

Stress during Pregnancy: Maternal Effects

"Stress and Pregnancy," © 2006 Organization of Teratology Information Specialists (OTIS). Reprinted with permission. Member programs of OTIS are located throughout the U.S. and Canada. To find the Teratogen Information Service in your area, call OTIS toll-free at 866-626-OTIS (866-626-6847), or visit their website at www.otispregnancy.org.

Any woman who gets pregnant has a 3% to 5% chance of having a baby with a birth defect. The information below will help you to determine if stress during pregnancy increases your risk above this background risk. This information should not be used as a substitute for the medical care and advice of your health care provider.

What is stress?

Stress is the way your body reacts to something that is out of the ordinary, dangerous, unknown, or disturbing. Almost anything can cause stress and each individual responds to stressful situations in her own way. When under stress, your body makes physical and chemical changes to try to protect it.

What are some of the symptoms of stress?

- **Physical:** Chest pain, rapid heart rate, breathing problems, headaches, vision problems, teeth grinding, dizziness, fatigue, stomach problems, and muscle aches.

- **Mental:** Confusion; memory loss; nightmares; and inability to focus, make decisions, or sleep.

- **Emotional:** Feelings of anxiety, guilt, grief, denial, fear, irritability, worry, frustration, and loneliness; episodes of anger or crying.

- **Social:** Isolating yourself from others; eating too much or too little; consuming excessive alcohol; and abuse of drugs.

Why should I be concerned about stress?

While some stress can be healthy, being under excessive stress over time can be of concern for your health and well-being. Stress can increase the risk for developing conditions such as high blood pressure or depression. Stress can contribute to making existing medical problems worse. For example, if someone has diabetes and is under stress, it may be difficult to keep blood sugar levels under control.

Are these conditions a problem during pregnancy?

Having high blood pressure or depression may have an effect on your health. Sometimes medicine is needed to keep mom healthy. When the mother is healthy it improves the chances of having a healthy baby.

Can stress from a natural disaster cause my baby to have a birth defect?

No. As stressful as living through a natural disaster is, it is unlikely that this stress would cause birth defects.

247

I read that stress might cause other pregnancy problems like miscarriage. Is that true?

There are some studies that associate severe stress with an increased risk for miscarriage, preterm delivery, and low birth weight. However, these adverse outcomes may be due to other things that the person may be doing to relieve the stress such as smoking cigarettes, drinking alcohol, and abusing drugs. For now, it is unknown if stress itself increases the risk for adverse pregnancy outcomes.

Will the medicines used to treat potential health effects of stress, like high blood pressure, ulcers, or depression, hurt my baby?

Most medicines are not associated with an increased risk for birth defects. In fact, it may be more harmful to the pregnancy if some conditions are not treated. By calling toll free 866-626-6847, you can talk to a counselor about specific medication and the possible risks to a pregnancy.

Can I breastfeed my baby if I'm taking medicines used to treat things like high blood pressure, ulcers, or depression?

Most medicines get into the breast milk but at different levels and many medicines are safe to use during breastfeeding. For more information on the use specific medicines during breastfeeding call 866-626-6847.

What are ways to reduce stress from a natural disaster?

- Talk about your feelings with friends, family, and professionals and don't be afraid to ask for help.

- Follow good health habits. Don't smoke, drink alcohol, or take illegal drugs. Be sure that you maintain a healthy diet and get the rest you need. If you have been prescribed medicine, make sure you take it as directed.

- Limit watching or reading about the disaster. Reliving the event over and over again can increase the anxiety and cause more stress.

- Try to have fun. Find something you enjoy and do it. Feeling positive can be helpful.

Where can I get help?

It is very important to get help from a professional before the situation is out of control. Contact your obstetrician, pediatrician, family doctor, clinic, mental health professionals, counselors, or clergy. These individuals can help you find the resources and assistance needed to deal with stress and its effects.

References

Centers for Disease Control and Prevention. Communicating in a Crisis: Risk Communication Guideline for Public Officials. [cited 2006 March 13]. Available from URL: http://riskcommunication.samhsa.gov/index.htm

Centers for Disease Control and Prevention. Coping with a Traumatic Event: Information for the Public. [cited 2006 March 13]. Available from URL: http://www.bt.cdc.gov/masstrauma/copingpub.asp

Centers for Disease Control and Prevention. Helping Patients Cope with a Traumatic Event. [cited 2006 March 13]. Available from URL: http://www.bt.cdc.gov/masstrauma/copingpro.asp

Centers for Disease Control and Prevention. Traumatic Incident Stress: Information for Emergency Response Workers. [cited 2006 March 13]. Available from URL: http://www.cdc.gov/niosh/mining/pubs/pdfs/tisif.pdf

Hansen D, Lou HC, Olsen J. Serious life events and congenital malformations: A national study with complete follow-up. *Lancet* 2000; 356: 875–80.

McAnarney ER, Stevens-Simon C. Maternal psychological stress/depression and low birth weight. Is there a relationship? *Am J Dis Child* 1990; 144: 789–792.

Nelson DB, Grisso JA, Joffe MM, Brensinger C, Shaw L, Danter E. Does stress influence early pregnancy loss? *Ann Epidemiol* 2003; 13(4): 223–9.

Newton RW, Hunt LP. Psychological stress in pregnancy and its relations to low birth weight. *Br Med J* 1984; 288: 1191–1194.

Section 25.3

Anxiety Disorders and Pregnancy

"Anxiety Disorders and Pregnancy," © 2007 Anxiety Disorders Association of America. All Rights Reserved. Reprinted with permission. For more information visit http://www.adaa.org or call 240-485-1001.

For many women, pregnancy is a time of joy, excitement, and anticipation. For most, it is also a time of some worry. Concerns about carrying a child to term, the health of the baby, and the delivery process are common and quite natural. However, some women are plagued by persistent, excessive, and irrational anxiety and worry during, and after, pregnancy. Some may have a previous history of such excessive anxiety, while others may be experiencing it for the first time. These women may be suffering from an anxiety disorder, a serious but treatable illness.

While much has been written on the "baby blues" and postpartum depression, anxiety disorders also affect many women before, during, and after pregnancy. Read on to learn more about anxiety disorders during pregnancy and the postpartum period.

I thought women were supposed to be happy during pregnancy. Aren't there biological safeguards that protect pregnant women from anxiety and mood disorders?

No. Although pregnancy has typically been considered a time of emotional well-being, studies suggest that up to 20 percent of women suffer from anxiety or mood disorders (such as depression or bipolar disorder) during pregnancy. In fact, the childbearing years are a time when many such disorders first emerge in women.

Is there a connection between pregnancy and anxiety disorders?

Although research is limited, studies have uncovered some interesting findings. For example, some women with panic disorder experience a reduction or complete eradication of their symptoms after becoming pregnant. Conversely, some women with obsessive-compulsive disorder (OCD) suffer more severe symptoms during pregnancy or experience OCD symptoms for the first time after becoming pregnant.

Studies have found the postpartum period to be a time of increased vulnerability to reoccurring and first-time panic disorder, OCD, generalized anxiety disorder (GAD), and other disorders such as hypochondria. Among women with pregnancy-related and postpartum OCD, it is not uncommon to suffer disturbing and intrusive thoughts about harming their newborns.

Why can pregnancy change the course of a woman's anxiety disorder as described above?

It is not fully clear why pregnancy can have these effects, and much more research is needed. One likely culprit is the steadily rising hormone levels during pregnancy. The reduction in panic symptoms during this time may occur because the hormone progesterone—which has a much greater presence during pregnancy—has breakdown products that have effects similar to benzodiazepine medications like clonazepam (Klonopin) and diazepam (Valium), which are often used to treat anxiety disorders.

The hormones oxytocin and prolactin have been shown to have anti-anxiety effects in animals and may also help reduce panic during pregnancy. However, other hormonal changes during pregnancy, e.g., possible increases in androgen hormones, may contribute to the worsening of OCD symptoms that some women experience.

Although these hormone changes occur gradually during pregnancy, they reverse very suddenly after delivery. This abrupt drop likely contributes to postpartum worsening of anxiety and depression in some women.

Can a mother's mental health during pregnancy affect her baby?

There is growing evidence that suggests an untreated anxiety disorder or depression during pregnancy may contribute to poor neonatal outcomes, including preterm labor, premature delivery, low birth weight, and childhood behavioral and cognitive problems. This makes it essential for a pregnant woman to seek treatment for an anxiety disorder or depression, not just for her own health but for her baby's health. While the issue of antidepressant use to treat anxiety disorders and depression during pregnancy is a complex one, women who do decide to discontinue antidepressants should work with their treatment provider to develop an alternative plan for mental health treatment during pregnancy to prevent a relapse, which, as noted above, can have its own consequences. Nonmedication treatments include cognitive-behavioral therapy (CBT) and other methods. It is of the utmost importance for women with anxiety disorders or depression to receive some sort of treatment during this time.

Is it safe to take antidepressants during pregnancy?

The benefits of medication to the mother and risks to the baby and mother should be weighed carefully. Research on this issue is still evolving. Therefore, the decision to start, continue, or stop any medication during pregnancy should be done only in consultation with your physician.

At this time, studies have found no significant difference in the rates of miscarriages and stillbirth between women who take SSRIs [selective serotonin reuptake inhibitors], a group of antidepressants used in the treatment of anxiety disorders that include Prozac (fluoxetine), Zoloft (sertraline), Luvox (fluvoxamine), Paxil (paroxetine), Celexa (citalopram), and Lexapro (escitalopram), and those who don't. The same is true for another group of medications called tricyclic antidepressants, which include Elavil (amitriptyline) and Tofranil (imipramine).

However, some recent research has raised a few other concerns. A study published in February 2006 in the *New England Journal of Medicine* found that the babies of mothers who took SSRIs in the second half of their pregnancy were six times more likely to be born with a rare but potentially serious breathing problem called pulmonary hypertension. Although there is an increased risk for this condition, it is highly uncommon among exposed infants. Another study published in February 2006 in the *Archives of Pediatrics and Adolescent Medicine* found nearly one third of newborns whose mothers used SSRIs late in their pregnancy experienced withdrawal symptoms such as high-pitched crying, tremors, disturbed sleep, and gastrointestinal problems (a condition known as neonatal abstinence syndrome). However, these symptoms only lasted one to four days after birth and did not require medical treatment. Additionally, in 2005, the Food & Drug Administration put out a warning stating that infants exposed to Paxil during the first three months of pregnancy had an increased risk of birth defects. In 2006, a large study in the journal *Epidemiology* also found that infants exposed to SSRIs during the first trimester had an increased rate of birth defects, but the study did not determine whether some SSRIs posed more risk than others.

Antidepressants known as monoamine oxidase inhibitors (MAOIs) are generally not considered safe during pregnancy.

Because there is not a simple answer to this question, and because discontinuing treatment can have its own risks for mothers and their babies, working closely with your doctor is essential.

Is it safe to take medication while breastfeeding?

The nutritional, immunologic, and psychological benefits of breast-feeding are well documented, making breastfeeding an attractive option for many women. Women who plan to breastfeed should know that medications, including antidepressants, are secreted into the breast milk (although concentrations in the breast milk seem to vary widely). The amount of medication to which an infant is exposed depends on several factors, including dosage of medication, rate of maternal and infant drug metabolism, and frequency and timing of feedings. Scheduling feedings during certain time periods, reducing medication dosage, and using formula for some feedings can help reduce the infant's exposure to medication.

Over the past five years, data has accumulated regarding the use of antidepressants during breastfeeding. Available data on the tricyclic antidepressants fluoxetine, paroxetine, and sertraline during breastfeeding have been encouraging and suggest that significant complications related to neonatal exposure to such drugs in breast milk appear to be rare. Less information is available on the other antidepressants at this time.

The potential benefits and risks of breastfeeding by a woman taking such medications should be discussed by the patient, her physician, and her partner. Since small amounts of medication do pass into breast milk, it is important to weigh the pros and cons of each option.

Is it true that breastfeeding can have beneficial effects on anxiety?

Breastfeeding may help prevent some of the sudden hormonal transitions that occur at the end of pregnancy, since the hormones oxytocin and prolactin continue to be released. If the frequency of breastfeeding decreases gradually over time, the drop in oxytocin and prolactin for the mother will also be more gradual.

Studies have shown that women who breastfeed have reduced hormonal and nervous system reactions to acute stress. There have also been reports that breastfeeding may reduce anxiety symptoms for some women, but clearly other women continue to have anxiety. High levels of anxiety postpartum can make breastfeeding difficult because anxiety and stress suppress the release of oxytocin, a hormone needed for milk release.

Are there long-term effects on a child whose mother took medication while pregnant?

Although research suggests some medications may be used safely during pregnancy, knowledge regarding the long-term effects on a child is incomplete. At this time, few studies have thoroughly examined the impact of exposure to antidepressants during pregnancy on a child's future development and behavior.

Of the two major studies, which both looked at exposure to either tricyclic antidepressants or Prozac (fluoxetine), both found no significant differences in IQ [intelligence quotient], temperament, behavior, reactivity, mood, distractibility, or activity level between children who were and were not exposed. The authors concluded that fluoxetine and tricyclic antidepressants do not have a significant effect on cognitive development, language, or behavior.

What are nonmedication treatment approaches for an anxiety disorder?

The following are some alternatives to medication that may be appropriate for some women.

- **Behavior therapy:** The goal of behavior therapy is to modify and gain control over unwanted behavior. The individual learns to cope with difficult situations, often through controlled exposure to them.

- **Cognitive therapy:** The goal of cognitive therapy is to identify, challenge, and change unwanted, unproductive thoughts, feelings, and behaviors. The individual learns to separate unrealistic thoughts and feelings from realistic ones. As with behavior therapy, the individual is actively involved in his or her own recovery.

- **Cognitive-behavior therapy (CBT):** Many therapists use a combination of cognitive and behavior therapies. This is often referred to as CBT. With CBT, the patient learns recovery skills that are useful for a lifetime.

- **Relaxation techniques:** Relaxation techniques help individuals develop the ability to more effectively cope with the stresses that contribute to anxiety, as well as with some of the physical symptoms of anxiety. The techniques taught include breathing retraining, progressive muscle relaxation, and exercise.

- **Self-help support groups.** Support groups can be an invaluable resource for recovery and empowerment. They involve people with similar needs or experiences, and are facilitated by a consumer, layperson, or survivor.

What steps should a woman with an anxiety disorder take before becoming pregnant or after learning she is pregnant?

It is ideal for a woman who suffers from an anxiety disorder to discuss the potential of pregnancy with her doctors before becoming pregnant or as soon as possible after learning she is pregnant. Considerations you and your doctor to keep in mind when determining your treatment include:

- Severity of your illness
- History of symptoms when not on medication
- Potential effects of medications on your child
- Availability of alternative approaches to medication
- Plans for breastfeeding
- Presence of a stable support system
- Availability of child care support during postpartum period

What about postpartum depression?

Postpartum depression is a serious illness that typically emerges over the first two to three postpartum months but may occur at any point after delivery. Depression often co-occurs with an anxiety disorder. Any of these symptoms during and after pregnancy that last longer than two weeks are signs of depression and/or an anxiety disorder:

- Feeling restless or irritable

- Feeling sad, hopeless, and overwhelmed
- Crying a lot
- Having no energy or motivation
- Eating too little or too much
- Sleeping too little or too much
- Trouble focusing, remembering, or making decisions
- Feeling worthless and guilty
- Loss of interest or pleasure in activities
- Withdrawal from friends and family
- Having headaches, chest pains, heart palpitations (the heart beating fast and feeling like it is skipping beats), or hyperventilation (fast and shallow breathing)

After pregnancy, signs may also include being afraid of hurting the baby or oneself and not having any interest in the baby.

Leaving depression untreated during and after pregnancy can have serious consequences on the entire family. Women with any of the signs listed above should seek help immediately from a trained professional.

Section 25.4

Stress during Pregnancy May Increase Risk of Mental Illness in Children

Dingfelder, S. (2004). Programmed for psychopathology? *Monitor on Psychology*, 35 (2), 56–57. Copyright © 2004 by the American Psychological Association. Reprinted with permission.

Add one more apparent risk factor for mental illness to the already lengthy list: In addition to the often-studied effects of genetics and upbringing, some researchers suggest that maternal environment, the hormone-laced bath that envelops a developing embryo, may contribute to the later development of psychopathology.

In particular, stress and its effects on pregnant mothers' hormonal balance appear negatively related to the mental health of their children, according to a literature review published in the January *Psychological Bulletin* (Vol. 130, No. 1). Schizophrenia, depression, and behavioral difficulties are just a few mental health problems that children may be at increased risk for when they have stressed mothers.

Researchers at the Utrecht University Medical Center in the Netherlands reviewed 255 human and animal subject studies on the effects of maternal environment and found no single pathway responsible for increased levels of psychopathology in humans and behavioral abnormalities in animals with mothers exposed to environmental stress—from work-related stress in humans to the stress of tail-shocks in rodents.

"Exposure to maternal stress may be related to abnormalities in brain development," says primary investigator Anja Huizink, Ph.D., of Utrecht University and Erasmus Medical Center. These changes may broadly affect the later functioning of infants, says Huizink, who contends that maternal stress does not engender vulnerability to any one mental illness, a theory held by some researchers of maternal stress.

Early Theories

Unlike Huizink, some scientists have found support for the theory that prenatal stress increases vulnerability to a particular psycho-pathological outcome: schizophrenia.

One study conducted in 1998 by professor Jim van Os, M.D., Ph.D., of the Netherland's Maastricht University, investigated the connection between maternal stress caused by the German invasion of the Netherlands in May 1940 and the later psychopathology of babies born to mothers pregnant during that invasion.

Using information from the Netherlands National Psychiatric Case Register, a comprehensive record of psychiatric inpatient admissions, van Os and his colleagues tracked the mental health of more than 100,000 men and women born to mothers who were pregnant during the invasion. They found that these babies, compared with babies born in the prior or subsequent year, were more likely to later develop schizophrenia. The researchers found no significant vulnerability for affective disorders.

While stressed babies' increased incidence of schizophrenia was statistically significant, the effect was small. Overall, there was less than a 0.5 percent difference in the prevalence of the mental illness between the two groups—potentially due to the multiple genetic and environmental factors that contribute to mental illness. However, for babies exposed to stress during the first trimester, the effect proved to be more robust.

"Early effects, at least during the first or second trimester, affect the children most because that is when the development of the brain is in its most critical stages," says van Os. "You'd expect anything affecting brain development then would have long-lasting effects."

Stress Begets Fetal Distress

While the general or specific vulnerability to mental illness continues to be a hot topic, most scientists agree that maternal stress affects infants through hormonal mechanisms.

One such mechanism, discovered through animal studies, involves the hypothalamic-pituitary-adrenal (HPA) axis. Chronic activation of this system in mothers, says Huizink, may be responsible for HPA dysregulation—their offspring's difficulty controlling stress hormones. HPA dysregulation has been associated with greater emotionality and difficulty calming down after a stressful situation, explains Huizink.

Though the placenta provides embryos with some protection against mothers' increased stress hormone levels, placental levels of the stress hormone cortisol vary in direct proportion to the mother's levels of the hormone, says Huizink. In animals, increased fetal exposure to these stress hormones leads to decreased numbers of stress-hormone receptors in the hippocampus, the part of the brain responsible for mediating stress response.

Decreased sensitivity in the hippocampus may account for difficulties regulating stress responses, which have been observed in mice and primates born to stressed mothers. In a 1990 study published in *Physiology and Behavior* (Vol. 48, No. 2), Aviva Wakshlak, Ph.D., and her colleagues at Hebrew University-Hadassah Medical School in Jerusalem, found that rats born to stressed dams experienced heightened emotionality and timidity. For example, they avoided open arms of mazes and tended to defecate excessively.

In these mice, says Huizink, the stress-hormone regulatory system seems to be impaired, leading to difficulty stabilizing hormones and calming down after a danger has passed. A similar effect may be found in prenatally stressed humans, says Huizink.

"It is possible that these individuals are more sensitive to stress later in life," she says. And oversensitivity to stress, notes Huizink, is related to a variety of mental illnesses, including affective disorders.

Vivette Glover, Ph.D., who runs the Fetal and Neonatal Stress Research Group at the Imperial College of London, agrees. In a study of 7,144 mothers and babies from the Avon region of England, published in the December 2002 issue of the *Journal of the American Academy of Child and Adolescent Psychology* (Vol. 14, No. 12), Glover and her colleagues found that women who reported experiencing high levels of anxiety during pregnancy were twice as likely as nonstressed women to have children with behavioral difficulties, depression, and anxiety, which the researchers measured when the children were 4 and 7 years old.

"We were able to focus on anxiety prenatally, and not later," says Glover, who also statistically accounted for the potential confounding effects of smoking, alcohol abuse, birth weight, maternal age, and socioeconomic status—all factors that tend to correlate with maternal anxiety and may affect the developing baby directly.

However, says Huizink, while the findings of her research review converge on the idea that maternal anxiety adversely affects developing humans, precisely how this happens remains an open question. Additionally, she notes that researchers still do not know how intense maternal stress must be to adversely affect developing infants.

"There are clues we can find in animal studies," she says, "but we don't know yet if the same mechanisms apply in humans."

Further Reading

Caspi, A., Sugden, K., Moffitt, T., Taylor, A., Craig, I., Harrington, H., et al. (2003). Influence of life stress on depression: Moderation in the 5-HTT gene. *Science,* 301, 386–389.

Huizink, A., Mulder, E., & Buitelaar, J. (2004). Prenatal stress and risk for psychopathology: Specific effects or induction of general suscepti-bility? *Psychological Bulletin,* 130(1), 115–142.

O'Connor, T., Heron, J., Glover, V., & the ALSPAC Study Team. (2002). Antenatal anxiety predicts child behavioral/emotional problems in-dependently of postnatal depression. *Journal of the American Acad-emy of Child and Adolescent Psychology,* 41(12), 1470–1477.

Sagrestano, L.M., Feldman, P., Killingsworth Rini, C., Woo, G., & Dunkel-Schetter, C. (1999). Ethnicity and social support during preg-nancy. *American Journal of Community Psychology,* 27(6), 869–898.

Van Os, J., & Selton, J. (1998). Prenatal exposure to maternal stress and subsequent schizophrenia. *British Journal of Psychiatry,* 172(1), 324–326.

Section 25.5

Too Stressed for Sex: How Stress and Emotions Affect Sexuality in Later Life

Excerpted from "Sexuality in Later Life," published in *AgePages,* by the National Institute on Aging (NIA), part of the National Institutes of Health, July 2005.

People seem to want and need to be close to others. As we grow older, many of us also want to continue an active, satisfying sex life. But the aging process may cause some changes.

Normal Sexual Changes in Men and Women

Normal aging brings physical changes in both men and women. These changes sometimes affect one's ability to have and enjoy sex with another person. Some women enjoy sex more as they grow older. After menopause or a hysterectomy, they may no longer fear an unwanted pregnancy. They may feel freer to enjoy sex.

Some women do not think things like gray hair and wrinkles make them less attractive to their sexual partner. But if a woman believes that looking young or being able to give birth makes her more feminine, she may begin to worry about how desirable she is no matter what her age is. That might make sex less enjoyable for her.

A woman may notice changes in her vagina. As she ages, her vagina shortens and narrows. The walls become thinner and also a little stiffer. These changes do not mean she can't enjoy having sex. However, most women will also have less vaginal lubrication. This could affect sexual pleasure.

As men get older, impotence becomes more common. Impotence is the loss of ability to have and keep an erection hard enough for sexual intercourse. By age 65, about 15 to 25% of men have this problem at least one out of every four times they are having sex. This may happen in men with heart disease, high blood pressure, or diabetes—either because of the disease or the medicines used to treat it.

A man may find it takes longer to get an erection. His erection may not be as firm or as large as it used to be. The amount of ejaculate may be smaller. The loss of erection after orgasm may happen more quickly, or it may take longer before an erection is again possible. Some men may find they need more foreplay.

Emotional Issues and Daily Stresses: Worries That Affect Sex

Sexuality is often a delicate balance of emotional and physical issues. How you feel may affect what you are able to do. For example, men may fear that impotence will become a more common problem as they age. But, if you are too concerned with that possibility, you can cause enough stress to trigger impotence. A woman who is worried about how her looks are changing as she ages may think her partner will no longer find her attractive. This focus on youthful physical beauty may get in the way of her enjoyment of sex.

Older couples face the same daily stresses that affect people of any age. But they may also have the added concerns of age, illness, and retirement and other lifestyle changes. These worries can cause sexual difficulties. Talk openly with your doctor, or see a counselor. These health professionals can often help.

Don't blame yourself for any sexual difficulties you and your partner are having. You might want to talk with a therapist about them. If your male partner is troubled by impotence or your female partner seems less interested in sex, don't assume he or she doesn't find you attractive anymore. There can be many physical causes for sexual problems.

What Can I Do to Keep an Active Sexual Life?

There are several things you can do on your own to keep an active sexual life. Remember that sex does not have to include intercourse. Make your partner a high priority. Pay attention to his or her needs and wants. Take time to understand the changes you both are facing. Try different positions and new times, like having sex in the morning when you both may have more energy. Don't hurry—you or your partner may need to spend more time touching to become fully aroused. Masturbation is a sexual activity that some older people, especially unmarried, widowed, or divorced people and those whose partners are ill or away, may find satisfying.

Some older people, especially women, may have trouble finding a partner with whom they can share any type of intimacy. Women live longer than men, so there are more of them. In 2000 women over age

262

65 outnumbered older men by 100 to 70. Doing activities that other seniors enjoy or going places where older people gather are ways to meet new people. Some ideas include mall walking, senior centers, adult education classes at a community college, or day trips sponsored by your city or county recreation department.

If you do seem to have a problem that affects your sex life, talk to your doctor. He or she can suggest a treatment depending on the type of problem and its cause. For example, the most common sexual difficulty of older women is dyspareunia, painful intercourse caused by poor vaginal lubrication. Your doctor or a pharmacist can suggest over-the-counter, water-based vaginal lubricants to use. Or, your doctor might suggest estrogen supplements or an estrogen vaginal insert.

If impotence is the problem, it can often be managed and perhaps even reversed. There is a pill that can help. It is called sildenafil and should not be taken by men taking medicines containing nitrates, such as nitroglycerin. This pill does have possible side effects. Other available treatments include vacuum devices, self-injection of a drug (either papaverine or prostaglandin E1), or penile implants.

There is a lot you can do to continue an active sex life. Follow a healthy lifestyle—exercise, eat good food, drink plenty of fluids like water or juices, don't smoke, and avoid alcohol. Try to reduce the stress in your life. See your doctor regularly. And keep a positive outlook on life.

Chapter 26

The Relationship between Stress and Other Health Problems

Chapter Contents

Section 26.1

Chronic Stress and Periodontal Disease

"Chronic Stress, Depression and Cortisol Levels Are Potential Risk Indicators for Periodontal Disease," © 2006 American Academy of Periodontology. Reprinted with permission.

Researchers evaluated the effects that stress, depression, and cortisol may have in the accumulation of dental plaque and gingivitis in individuals 50 years and older.

Caregivers of people under psychological or physical stress, as well as those with the conditions themselves, should not overlook their oral health, according to a study printed in the *Journal of Periodontology*.

The results from the study suggest that being a caregiver to relatives with dementia, hypercortisolemia (overproduction of cortisol), or stress was associated with elevated plaque levels and increased gingival bleeding in adults aged 50 years and older.

"We found that short-term psychological stress was a risk indicator to elevated plaque levels and long-term physical stress was a risk indicator to gingivitis," said Fernando N. Hugo, DDS and Faculty of Dentistry of Piracicaba, Brazil. "These findings support the health impact of psychosocial risk factors from chronic stress, which may lead to malfunction of some biological functions."

The study indicates that the demanding task of caregiving, usually associated with increased stress, may also be a risk factor for poor oral hygiene. These findings point out that stress may contribute to a disinterest in performing oral hygiene.

"Flossing and brushing the teeth and gums had a protective effect against plaque and gingivitis," said Kenneth A. Krebs, DMD and AAP [American Academy of Periodontology] president. "That said, future research is needed to explore the relationship between stress and oral hygiene negligence."

In this study, 230 individuals were evaluated, and almost 52 percent were caregivers. Caregivers of patients with dementia were examined because they represent a well-known group suffering from the impacts of chronic stress on human health and immune functions. The results are among the first in literature to suggest that caregivers of relatives with dementia are at risk of having more plaque and gingivitis than non-caregivers.

Section 26.2

Stress and Asthma

"Stress and Asthma," © 2006 The Cleveland Clinic Foundation, 9500 Euclid Avenue, Cleveland, OH 44195, www.clevelandclinic.org. Additional information is available from the Cleveland Clinic Health Information Center, 216-444-3771, toll-free 800-223-2273 extension 43771, or at http://www.clevelandclinic.org/health.

Stress is a common asthma trigger. Stress and anxiety sometimes make you feel short of breath and may cause your asthma symptoms to become worse.

You cannot avoid stress; it is part of daily life. However, developing effective ways to manage stress and learning to relax can help you prevent shortness of breath and avoid panic.

Here are some ways to manage stress:

- **Learn to change thought patterns that produce stress:** What you think, how you think, what you expect, and what you tell yourself often determine how you feel and how well you manage rising stress levels.

- **Reduce stressors (causes of stress):** Identify the major stressors in your life: money problems, relationship problems, grief, too many deadlines, busy schedule, lack of support. If you can't resolve these stressors alone, get professional help for problems that are too difficult to deal with by yourself.

- **Try to avoid situations that trigger stress for you:** Practice effective time-management skills, such as delegating when appropriate, setting priorities, pacing yourself, and taking time out for yourself.

- **Practice relaxation exercises:** Relaxation exercises are simple to perform and combine deep breathing, releasing of muscle tension, and clearing of negative thoughts. If you practice these exercises regularly, you can use them when needed to lessen the negative effects of stress. Relaxation exercises include diaphragmatic and pursed lip breathing, imagery, repetitive phrases (repeating a phrase that triggers a physical relaxation, such as "Relax and Let Go"), and progressive muscle relaxation. Many commercial audiotapes and books that teach these exercises are available.

- **Exercise:** It's an excellent way to burn off the accumulated effects of stress.

- **Get enough sleep:** If you are not sleeping well, you will have less energy and fewer resources for coping with stress. Developing good sleep habits is very important. Here are some tips:

  - Do not go to bed until you are tired.

  - Develop specific bedtime rituals and stick to them.

  - If you have trouble sleeping, do not watch TV, read, or eat in bed.

  - Do not engage in exercise or strenuous activity immediately before bedtime.

  - Avoid caffeine.

  - Do not nap.

  - Go to bed and get up at the same time every day, including on the weekends.

- **Follow the recommended nutritional guidelines:** Junk food and refined sugars low in nutritional value and high in calories can leave you feeling out of energy and sluggish. Limiting sugar, caffeine, and alcohol can promote health and reduce stress.

- **Delegate responsibility:** Stress overload often results from having too many responsibilities. You can free up time and decrease stress by delegating responsibilities. Take a team approach and involve everyone in sharing the load. Try applying these guidelines at home or modifying them to fit your situation at work:

  - Make a list of the types of tasks involved in the job.

  - Take time to train someone to do the job or specific tasks.

  - Assign responsibility to a specific person.

  - Rotate unpleasant duties.

- Give clear, specific instructions with deadlines.
- Be appreciative; let people know you are pleased by a job well done. Allow others to do a job their own way.
- Give up being a perfectionist.

- **Seek support from your family:** The support of family and friends is very important. Social support is the single most important buffer against stress. Here are some tips you can offer to your family or friends when they ask you how they can help. Family and friends can:

  - help you remain as active and independent as possible;
  - provide emotional support;
  - help with household chores and with grocery shopping and other errands as necessary;
  - learn what they can about your condition and prescribed treatment by attending doctors' appointments with you; and
  - provide encouragement and help you follow your prescribed treatment plan.

Section 26.3

Psychological Stress and Cancer: Is There a Link?

"Psychological Stress and Cancer" is from the National Cancer Institute (NCI, www.cancer.gov), part of the National Institutes of Health, March 9, 1998. Reviewed and revised by David A. Cooke, M.D., March 2007.

The complex relationship between physical and psychological health is not well understood. Scientists know that many types of stress activate the body's endocrine (hormone) system, which in turn can cause changes in the immune system, the body's defense against infection and disease (including cancer). However, the immune system is a highly specialized network whose activity is affected not only by stress but by a number of other factors. It has not been shown that stress-induced changes in the immune system directly cause cancer.

Some studies have indicated an increased incidence of early death, including cancer death, among people who have experienced the recent loss of a spouse or other loved one. However, most cancers have been developing for many years and are diagnosed only after they have been growing in the body for a long time (from 2 to 30 years). This fact argues against an association between the death of a loved one and the triggering of cancer.

The relationship between breast cancer and stress has received particular attention. Some studies of women with breast cancer have shown significantly higher rates of this disease among those women who experienced traumatic life events and losses within several years before their diagnosis. Although studies have shown that stress factors (such as death of a spouse, social isolation, and medical school examinations) alter the way the immune system functions, they have not provided scientific evidence of a direct cause-and-effect relationship between these immune system changes and the development of cancer. One NCI-sponsored study suggests that there is no important association between stressful life events, such as the death of a loved one or divorce, and breast cancer risk. However, more research to find if there is a relationship between psychological stress and the transformation of normal cells into cancerous cells is needed.

One area that is currently being studied is the effect of stress on women already diagnosed with breast cancer. Several studies have been performed to determine whether women with breast cancer who are in support groups have better survival rates than those not in support groups. Most studies to date have not shown differences in survival, although they have found improved psychosocial status. Research in this area is continuing.

Many factors come into play when determining the relationship between stress and cancer. At present, the relationship between psychological stress and cancer occurrence or progression has not been scientifically proven. However, stress reduction is of benefit for many other health reasons.

References

"Self-Reported Stress and Risk of Breast Cancer," Felicia D. Roberts, Polly A. Newcomb, Amy Trentham-Dietz, and Barry E. Storer. *Cancer*, March 15, 1996.

"Stress and Immune Responses After Surgical Treatment for Regional Breast Cancer," Barbara L. Andersen, William B. Farrar, Deanna Golden-Kreutz, et al. *Journal of the National Cancer Institute*, January 7, 1998.

Part Three

Stress and Mental Health Disorders

Chapter 27

The Link between Stress and Depression

Chronic stress has long been shown to fuel depression, but how?

Answers are coming from scientists like those at Dalhousie University in Nova Scotia, who've found that rats repeatedly exposed to the stress hormone corticosterone show more depression-like behavior and greater signs of anxiety. Their study, which offers a rare look at sex differences, also indicates that the hormone affects males more than females. The findings appear in the December [2004] issue of *Behavioral Neuroscience* (Vol. 118, No. 6).

In the study, a team of four led by Lisa Kalynchuk, Ph.D., now at the University of Saskatchewan, studied 30 male and 30 female rats. By studying links among repeated stress, depression-like behavior and the function of the hippocampus in rats, the investigators were hunting for clues about the biological cause of depression in humans.

Kalynchuk and her co-authors cite medical evidence that depression can stem from chronic overstimulation of the body's hypothalamic-pituitary-adrenal axis, which produces stress hormones such as cortisol in humans and corticosterone in rats. For example, patients with Cushing disease have high levels of cortisol and are often depressed, and depressed people often have hippocampus-linked cognitive problems, due perhaps to smaller hippocampi.

Adelson, R. (2005). Hard-hitting hormones: The stress-depression link. *Monitor on Psychology, 36* (1), 24–26. Copyright © 2005 by the American Psychological Association. Reprinted with permission.

Thus, after the researchers injected rats with high levels of stress hormone for three weeks, they found that compared with controls, the animals showed significantly more behaviors that could be considered anxious and depressed. Voilà: The biological agent was not only unmasked, but unmasked with meticulous care.

"This is the most systematic study I've seen to date to demonstrate the stress-depression link," notes Thomas Minor, Ph.D., associate professor of behavioral neuroscience at the University of California, Los Angeles (UCLA).

Just Keep Swimming

It was important to be systematic given that, in studying the stress-hormone system and depression, it can be hard to control between-subject variation in hormone levels, the researchers say. Kalynchuk and her colleagues tried a new approach: They bypassed that system and directly injected CORT [corticosterone] for 21 days to control its levels. Each treated rat got the same supplemental dose of stress hormone to simulate in a controlled fashion what prolonged stress might do to the body. The researchers injected the control groups—half of each sex group—with salt water alone.

After three weeks of treatment, Kalynchuk and her colleagues—graduate student Andrea Gregus, undergraduate Daniel Boudreau, now a medical student, and Tara Perrot-Sinal, Ph.D.—monitored the rats for signs of anxiety and depression. The tests included:

- **Open field:** Do rats venture out into an unfamiliar open field to explore or do they hold back? Holding back is a sign of depression.

- **Resistance to capture:** How much do the rats fight being picked up? Not fighting is a sign of depression.

- **Forced swim:** When placed in a tank of water for 10 minutes, how much time do rats spend struggling, swimming or being immobile? After this, they get toweled off and dried under a heat lamp. Giving up is a sign of depression.

- **Predator odor:** Do they seem upset or run away when a collar that's been worn by a cat gets put in their cage? Showing such defensive behaviors is a sign of depression.

Sure enough, the repeated cortisone injections—which simulated three weeks of chronic stress response—increased depression-like behavior in the rats. In the forced-swim test, both male and female hormone-injected rats spent more time immobile, and they became immobile faster. In the predator-odor test, the artificially stressed rats showed more of one subset of defensive behaviors when in the presence of a cat collar.

The research team drew three main conclusions. First, exposure to repeated CORT injections produced depression-like behavior. Second, the hormonally stressed rats showed more anxiety in specific situations, such as the predator odor test, which the researchers think might be especially sensitive to anxiety in rats. Third, although the effects were generally similar in male and female rats, the hormone appeared to affect males more strongly on these tasks.

Stress Hormones and Sex Hormones

Given the greater vulnerability of male rats to stress in their study, the authors wonder whether the females' higher levels of circulating sex hormones, such as estrogen and progesterone, are "neuroprotective," supporting healthier nerve-cell life from the get-go. Prior research has linked higher sex hormones to less depression-like behavior in female rats; the inclusion of stress hormone makes this study different and an advance over previous studies, says Bruce McEwen, Ph.D., the Alfred E. Mirsky Professor and head of the Harold and Margaret Milliken Hatch Laboratory of Neuroendocrinology at Rockefeller University.

It's a welcome advance, says Tracey Shors, Ph.D., of the Center for Collaborative Neuroscience at Rutgers University. "It is my hope that these types of studies will encourage others to consider testing females when using animal models of depression," says Shors. "After all, women are much more likely to experience depression and other stress-related mental illness than men."

Although noting the limits of generalizing rat findings, author Kalynchuk says new experiments could show why female rats seem more resistant to stress-induced depression than do female humans. One obvious explanation could be that rats and humans are just plain different, and that, as she puts it, "The increased depression rate in female humans is due to an interaction between biological and psychosocial factors, which we simply cannot model in rats." The rate could also be higher, in part, because women are more likely to consult a doctor when they feel depressed, whereas men are more likely to self-medicate with alcohol or other drugs.

However, Kalynchuk also points to a possible hormonal explanation for which there's some support. It could be that, in humans, normal levels of female sex hormones could help protect against depression, but hormone fluctuations could put women at risk for problems such as postpartum depression and premenstrual dysphoric disorder. In the Dalhousie experiment, the female rats had normal levels of gonadal hormones. But, says Kalynchuk, other researchers have shown that female rats without ovaries—who have low levels of these hormones—are much more susceptible to stress.

Further experimentation, says Kalynchuk, could show whether male rats are actually more susceptible to the effects of stress than female rats with normal levels of these hormones.

Connecting the Dots

Having confirmed that the hormones released by chronic stress cause depression, researchers want to pin down the mechanism: Exactly how does CORT make us feel blue? Minor of UCLA says the study has bearing on the debate over whether CORT facilitates neurodegeneration or results in neuroprotection to produce behavioral depression.

On the one hand, Kalynchuk cites evidence that repeated stress in lab animals reduces neurogenesis—the birth of new brain cells—in the hippocampus, leading to depressive symptoms. She notes, though: "It's not clear whether a decrease in neurogenesis can cause depression or is a by-product of depression. A direct link has not yet been made."

On the other hand, Minor postulates that chronic stress hormone trips a neurological circuit breaker by causing receptors in the hippocampus and amygdala to block glucose intake, sparing these regions from neurotoxic over-excitement. This long-term coping response, he says, would drag down other responses and behaviors, causing what people experience as depression.

"Stress is when you're anxious and fatigued," says Minor. "Anxiety causes energy production, but in fatigue your energy is down, a compensatory shift." He cites accumulating evidence of depression as a metabolic problem in the brain—a view that, if confirmed, would promote regimens that help the brain build new neurons, including the traditional change of scenery, along with fresh air, exercise and regular sleep.

"In some depressed patients, the hypothalamic-pituitary-adrenal axis looks like it's being dysregulated," Minor says, noting that restoring balance to a stressed-out system—and re-regulating glucose transport to the brain—could help. Minor and his colleagues are preparing to test this hypothesis in depressed people.

Ronald Duman, Ph.D., a professor of psychiatry and pharmacology at the Yale University School of Medicine, also hopes to broaden the findings to improve treatment. The forced-swim test is, he notes, typically used to test antidepressants on rats, but their recovery is paced differently from humans. If someone could replicate the new findings with other indicators of depression, says Duman, it could lead to a better model for testing new drugs and other therapies.

For now, the Dalhousie research helps answer the "nagging question of how chronic stress gets inside the brain," says Gregory Miller, Ph.D., a psychology professor at the University of British Columbia. "To the extent that these findings generalize to the kinds of stressors and symptoms that humans experience, they'll provide valuable mechanistic insights and potentially important clinical implications."

Rachel Adelson, M.A. Rachel Adelson is an award-winning writer/editor specializing in behavioral science and neuroscience. View more information at http://www.livewirecom.com.

Chapter 28

All about Depression

In any given 1-year period, 9.5 percent of the population, or about 20.9 million American adults, suffer from a depressive illness. The economic cost for this disorder is high, but the cost in human suffering cannot be estimated. Depressive illnesses often interfere with normal functioning and cause pain and suffering not only to those who have a disorder, but also to those who care about them. Serious depression can destroy family life as well as the life of the ill person. But much of this suffering is unnecessary.

Most people with a depressive illness do not seek treatment, although the great majority, even those whose depression is extremely severe, can be helped. Thanks to years of fruitful research, there are now medications and psychosocial therapies, such as cognitive/behavioral, talk, or interpersonal therapies, that ease the pain of depression.

Unfortunately, many people do not recognize that depression is a treatable illness. If you feel that you or someone you care about is one of the many undiagnosed depressed people in this country, the information presented here may help you take the steps that may save your own or someone else's life.

From a brochure by the National Institute of Mental Health (NIMH, www .nimh.nih.gov), part of the National Institutes of Health, 2000. NIH Publication No. 00-3561. Reviewed and revised by David A. Cooke, M.D., April 2007.

What Is a Depressive Disorder?

A depressive disorder is an illness that involves the body, mood, and thoughts. It affects the way a person eats and sleeps, the way one feels about oneself, and the way one thinks about things. A depressive disorder is not the same as a passing blue mood. It is not a sign of personal weakness or a condition that can be willed or wished away. People with a depressive illness cannot merely "pull themselves together" and get better. Without treatment, symptoms can last for weeks, months, or years. Appropriate treatment, however, can help most people who suffer from depression.

Types of Depression

Depressive disorders come in different forms, just as is the case with other illnesses such as heart disease. This text briefly describes three of the most common types of depressive disorders. However, within these types there are variations in the number of symptoms, their severity, and persistence.

Major depression, also known as unipolar depression, is manifested by a combination of symptoms that interfere with the ability to work, study, sleep, eat, and enjoy once pleasurable activities. Such a disabling episode of depression may occur only once but more commonly occurs several times in a lifetime.

A less severe type of depression, dysthymia, involves long-term, chronic symptoms that do not disable, but keep one from functioning well or from feeling good. Many people with dysthymia also experience major depressive episodes at some time in their lives.

Another type of depression is bipolar disorder, also called manic-depressive illness. Not nearly as prevalent as other forms of depressive disorders, bipolar disorder is characterized by cycling mood changes: severe highs (mania) and lows (depression). Sometimes the mood switches are dramatic and rapid, occurring over days, but most often they are gradual, over weeks to months. When in the depressed cycle, an individual can have any or all of the symptoms of a depressive disorder. When in the manic cycle, the individual may be overactive, overly talkative, and have a great deal of energy. A manic individual may speak very quickly ("pressured speech") or sleep very little for days without feeling tired. Mania often affects thinking, judgment, and social behavior in ways that cause serious problems and embarrassment. For example, the individual in a manic phase may feel elated, full of grand schemes that might range from unwise business decisions to romantic sprees. Milder degrees of these symptoms are usually called hypomania. Mania, left untreated, may worsen to a psychotic state, where an individual may completely lose touch with reality. For example, a person may believe he or she is invulnerable to harm or that he or she is a religious prophet.

Symptoms of Depression and Mania

Not everyone who is depressed or manic experiences every symptom. Some people experience a few symptoms, some many. Severity of symptoms varies with individuals and also varies over time.

Depression

- Persistent sad, anxious, or "empty" mood
- Feelings of hopelessness, pessimism
- Feelings of guilt, worthlessness, helplessness
- Loss of interest or pleasure in hobbies and activities that were once enjoyed, including sex
- Decreased energy, fatigue, being "slowed down"
- Difficulty concentrating, remembering, making decisions
- Insomnia, early-morning awakening, or oversleeping
- Appetite and/or weight loss or overeating and weight gain
- Thoughts of death or suicide; suicide attempts
- Restlessness, irritability
- Persistent physical symptoms that do not respond to treatment, such as headaches, digestive disorders, and chronic pain
- Mania
- Abnormal or excessive elation
- Unusual irritability
- Decreased need for sleep
- Grandiose notions
- Increased talking
- Racing thoughts
- Increased sexual desire

- Markedly increased energy
- Poor judgment
- Inappropriate social behavior

Causes of Depression

Some types of depression run in families, suggesting that a biological vulnerability can be inherited. This seems to be the case with bipolar disorder. Studies of families in which members of each generation develop bipolar disorder found that those with the illness have a somewhat different genetic makeup than those who do not get ill. However, the reverse is not true: Not everybody with the genetic makeup that causes vulnerability to bipolar disorder will have the illness. Apparently additional factors, possibly stresses at home, work, or school, are involved in its onset.

In some families, major depression also seems to occur generation after generation. However, it can also occur in people who have no family history of depression. Whether inherited or not, major depressive disorder is often associated with changes in brain structures or brain function.

People who have low self-esteem, who consistently view themselves and the world with pessimism, or who are readily overwhelmed by stress are prone to depression. Whether this represents a psychological predisposition or an early form of the illness is not clear.

In recent years, researchers have shown that physical changes in the body can be accompanied by mental changes as well. Medical illnesses such as stroke, a heart attack, cancer, Parkinson disease, and hormonal disorders can cause depressive illness, making the sick person apathetic and unwilling to care for his or her physical needs, thus prolonging the recovery period. Also, a serious loss, difficult relationship, financial problem, or any stressful (unwelcome or even desired) change in life patterns can trigger a depressive episode. Very often, a combination of genetic, psychological, and environmental factors is involved in the onset of a depressive disorder. Later episodes of illness typically are precipitated by only mild stresses, or none at all.

Depression in Women

Women experience depression about twice as often as men.[1] Many hormonal factors may contribute to the increased rate of depression in women particularly such factors as menstrual cycle changes, pregnancy, miscarriage, postpartum period, perimenopause, and menopause. Many women also face additional stresses such as responsibilities both at work and home, single parenthood, and caring for children and for aging parents.

A recent NIMH study showed that in the case of severe premenstrual syndrome (PMS), women with a preexisting vulnerability to PMS experienced relief from mood and physical symptoms when their sex hormones were suppressed. Shortly after the hormones were reintroduced, they again developed symptoms of PMS. Women without a history of PMS reported no effects of the hormonal manipulation.[6,7]

Many women are also particularly vulnerable after the birth of a baby. The hormonal and physical changes, as well as the added responsibility of a new life, can be factors that lead to postpartum depression in some women. While transient "blues" are common in new mothers, a full-blown depressive episode is not a normal occurrence and requires active intervention. Treatment by a sympathetic physician and the family's emotional support for the new mother are prime considerations in aiding her to recover her physical and mental well-being and her ability to care for and enjoy the infant.

Depression in Men

Although men are less likely to suffer from depression than women, 6 million men in the United States are affected by the illness. Men are less likely to admit to depression, and doctors are less likely to suspect it. The rate of completed suicide in men is four times that of women, though more women attempt it. In fact, after age 70, the rate of men's suicide rises, reaching a peak after age 85.

Depression can also affect the physical health in men differently from women. A new study shows that, although depression is associated with an increased risk of coronary heart disease in both men and women, only men suffer a high death rate.[2]

Men's depression is often masked by alcohol or drugs, or by the socially acceptable habit of working excessively long hours. Depression typically shows up in men not as feeling hopeless and helpless, but as being irritable, angry, and discouraged; hence, depression may be difficult to recognize as such in men. Even if a man realizes that he is depressed, he may be less willing than a woman to seek help. Encouragement and support from concerned family members can make a difference. In the workplace, employee assistance professionals or worksite mental health programs can be of assistance in helping men understand and accept depression as a real illness that needs treatment.

Depression in the Elderly

Some people have the mistaken idea that it is normal for the elderly to feel depressed. On the contrary, most older people feel satisfied with their lives. Sometimes, though, when depression develops, it may be dismissed as a normal part of aging. Depression in the elderly, undiagnosed and untreated, causes needless suffering for the family and for the individual who could otherwise live a fruitful life. When he or she does go to the doctor, the symptoms described are usually physical, for the older person is often reluctant to discuss feelings of hopelessness, sadness, loss of interest in normally pleasurable activities, or extremely prolonged grief after a loss.

Recognizing how depressive symptoms in older people are often missed, many health care professionals are learning to identify and treat the underlying depression. They recognize that some symptoms may be side effects of medication the older person is taking for a physical problem, or they may be caused by a co-occurring illness. If a diagnosis of depression is made, treatment with medication and/or psychotherapy will help the depressed person return to a happier, more fulfilling life. Recent research suggests that brief psychotherapy (talk therapies that help a person in day-to-day relationships or in learning to counter the distorted negative thinking that commonly accompanies depression) is effective in reducing symptoms in short-term depression in older persons who are medically ill. Psychotherapy is also useful in older patients who cannot or will not take medication. Efficacy studies show that late-life depression can be treated with psychotherapy.[4]

Improved recognition and treatment of depression in late life will make those years more enjoyable and fulfilling for the depressed elderly person, the family, and caretakers.

Depression in Children

Only in the past two decades has depression in children been taken very seriously. The depressed child may pretend to be sick, refuse to go to school, cling to a parent, or worry that the parent may die. Older children may sulk, get into trouble at school, be negative, grouchy, and feel misunderstood. Because normal behaviors vary from one childhood stage to another, it can be difficult to tell whether a child is just going through a temporary "phase" or is suffering from depression. Sometimes the parents become worried about how the child's behavior has changed, or a teacher mentions that "your child doesn't seem to be himself." In such a case, if a visit to the child's pediatrician rules out physical symptoms, the doctor will probably suggest that the child be evaluated, preferably by a psychiatrist who specializes in the treatment of children. If treatment is needed, the doctor may suggest that another therapist, usually a social worker or a psychologist, provide therapy while the psychiatrist will oversee medication if it is needed. Parents should not be afraid to ask questions: What are the therapist's qualifications? What kind of therapy will the child have? Will the family as a whole participate in therapy? Will my child's therapy include an antidepressant? If so, what might the side effects be?

The National Institute of Mental Health (NIMH) has identified the use of medications for depression in children as an important area for research. The NIMH-supported Research Units on Pediatric Psychopharmacology (RUPPs) form a network of seven research sites where clinical studies on the effects of medications for mental disorders can be conducted in children and adolescents. Among the medications being studied are antidepressants, some of which have been found to be effective in treating children with depression, if properly monitored by the child's physician.[8]

Diagnostic Evaluation and Treatment

The first step to getting appropriate treatment for depression is a physical examination by a physician. Certain medications as well as some medical conditions such as a viral infection can cause the same symptoms as depression, and the physician should rule out these possibilities through examination, interview, and lab tests. If a physical cause for the depression is ruled out, a psychological evaluation should be done, by the physician or by referral to a psychiatrist or psychologist.

A good diagnostic evaluation will include a complete history of symptoms, i.e., when they started, how long they have lasted, how severe they are, whether the patient had them before and, if so, whether the symptoms were treated and what treatment was given. The doctor should ask about alcohol and drug use, and if the patient has thoughts about death or suicide. Further, a history should include questions about whether other family members have had a depressive illness and, if treated, what treatments they may have received and which were effective.

Last, a diagnostic evaluation should include a mental status examination to determine if speech or thought patterns or memory have been affected, as sometimes happens in the case of a depressive or manic-depressive illness.

Treatment choice will depend on the outcome of the evaluation. There are a variety of antidepressant medications and psychotherapies that can be used to treat depressive disorders. Some people with milder forms may do well with psychotherapy alone. People with moderate to severe depression most often benefit from antidepressants. Most do best with combined treatment: medication to gain relatively quick symptom relief and psychotherapy to learn more effective ways to deal with life's problems, including depression. Depending on the patient's diagnosis and severity of symptoms, the therapist may prescribe medication and/or one of the several forms of psychotherapy that have proven effective for depression.

Electroconvulsive therapy (ECT) is useful, particularly for individuals whose depression is severe or life threatening or who cannot take antidepressant medication.[3] ECT often is effective in cases where antidepressant medications do not provide sufficient relief of symptoms. In recent years, ECT has been much improved. A muscle relaxant is given before treatment, which is done under brief anesthesia. Electrodes are placed at precise locations on the head to deliver electrical impulses. The stimulation causes a brief (about 30 seconds) seizure within the brain. The person receiving ECT does not consciously experience the electrical stimulus. For full therapeutic benefit, at least several sessions of ECT, typically given at the rate of three per week, are required.

Medications

There are several types of antidepressant medications used to treat depressive disorders. These include newer medications chiefly the selective serotonin reuptake inhibitors (SSRIs), the tricyclics, and the monoamine oxidase inhibitors (MAOIs). The SSRIs and other newer medications that affect neurotransmitters such as dopamine or norepinephrine generally have fewer side effects than tricyclics. Sometimes the doctor will try a variety of antidepressants before finding the most effective medication or combination of medications. Sometimes the dosage must be increased to be effective. Although some improvements may be seen in the first few weeks, antidepressant medications must be taken regularly for 3 to 4 weeks (in some cases, as many as 8 weeks) before the full therapeutic effect occurs.

Patients often are tempted to stop medication too soon. They may feel better and think they no longer need the medication. Or they may think the medication isn't helping at all. It is important to keep taking medication until it has a chance to work, though side effects may appear before antidepressant activity does. Once the individual is feeling better, it is important to continue the medication for at least 4 to 9 months to prevent a recurrence of the depression. Some medications must be stopped gradually to give the body time to adjust. Never stop taking an antidepressant without consulting the doctor for instructions on how to safely discontinue the medication. For individuals with bipolar disorder or chronic major depression, medication may have to be maintained indefinitely.

Antidepressant drugs are not habit-forming. However, as is the case with any type of medication prescribed for more than a few days, antidepressants have to be carefully monitored to see if the correct dosage is being given. The doctor will check the dosage and its effectiveness regularly.

For the small number of people for whom MAO inhibitors are the best treatment, it is necessary to avoid certain foods that contain high levels of tyramine, such as many cheeses, wines, and pickles, as well as medications such as decongestants. The interaction of tyramine with MAOIs can bring on a hypertensive crisis, a sharp increase in blood pressure that can lead to a stroke. The doctor should furnish a complete list of prohibited foods that the patient should carry at all times. Other forms of antidepressants require no food restrictions.

Medications of any kind prescribed, over-the counter, or borrowed should never be mixed without consulting the doctor. One such medication that deserves particular attention is St. John's wort, an over-the-counter herbal medication that is popular for treatment of depression. While its effectiveness for depression is questionable (as discussed below), it is clear that it can cause severe and potentially fatal reactions if combined with many prescription antidepressants. Other health professionals who may prescribe a drug such as a dentist or other medical specialist should be told of the medications the patient is taking. Some drugs, although safe when taken alone can, if taken with others, cause severe and dangerous side effects. Some drugs, like alcohol or street drugs, may reduce the effectiveness of antidepressants and should be avoided. This includes wine, beer, and hard liquor. Some people who have not had a problem with alcohol use may be permitted by their doctor to use a modest amount of alcohol while taking one of the newer antidepressants.

Antianxiety drugs or sedatives are not antidepressants. They are sometimes prescribed along with antidepressants; however, they are not effective when taken alone for a depressive disorder. Stimulants, such as amphetamines, are not effective antidepressants, but they are used occasionally under close supervision in medically ill depressed patients.

Questions about any antidepressant prescribed, or problems that may be related to the medication, should be discussed with the doctor.

Lithium has for many years been the treatment of choice for bipolar disorder, as it can be effective in smoothing out the mood swings common to this disorder. Its use must be carefully monitored, as the range between an effective dose and a toxic one is small. If a person has preexisting thyroid, kidney, or heart disorders or epilepsy, lithium may not be recommended. Fortunately, other medications have been found to be of benefit in controlling mood swings. Among these are two mood-stabilizing anticonvulsants, carbamazepine (Tegretol®) and valproate (Depakote®). Both of these medications have gained wide acceptance in clinical practice, and valproate has been approved by the Food and Drug Administration for first-line treatment of acute mania. Other anticonvulsants that are being used now include lamotrigine (Lamictal®) and topiramate (Topamax®): their role in the treatment hierarchy of bipolar disorder remains under study.

Most people who have bipolar disorder take more than one medication including, along with lithium and/or an anticonvulsant, a medication for accompanying agitation, anxiety, depression, or insomnia. Finding the best possible combination of these medications is of utmost importance to the patient and requires close monitoring by the physician.

Side Effects

Antidepressants may cause mild and, usually, temporary side effects (sometimes referred to as adverse effects) in some people. Typically these are annoying, but not serious. However, any unusual reactions or side effects or those that interfere with functioning should be reported to the doctor immediately. The most common side effects of tricyclic antidepressants, and ways to deal with them, are:

- **Dry mouth:** It is helpful to drink sips of water; chew sugarless gum; and clean teeth daily.

- **Constipation:** Bran cereals, prunes, fruit, and vegetables should be in the diet.

- **Bladder problems:** Emptying the bladder may be troublesome, and the urine stream may not be as strong as usual; the doctor should be notified if there is marked difficulty or pain.

- **Sexual problems:** Sexual functioning may change; if worrisome, it should be discussed with the doctor.

- **Blurred vision:** This will pass soon and will not usually necessitate new glasses.

- **Dizziness:** Rising from the bed or chair slowly is helpful.

- **Drowsiness:** As a daytime problem this usually passes soon. A person feeling drowsy or sedated should not drive or operate heavy equipment. The more sedating antidepressants are generally taken at bedtime to help sleep and minimize daytime drowsiness.

The newer antidepressants have different types of side effects:

- **Headache:** This will usually go away.

- **Nausea:** This is also temporary, but even when it occurs, it is transient after each dose.

- **Nervousness and insomnia** (trouble falling asleep or waking often during the night): These may occur during the first few weeks; dosage reductions or time will usually resolve them.

- **Agitation** (feeling jittery): If this happens for the first time after the drug is taken and is more than transient, the doctor should be notified.

- **Sexual problems:** The doctor should be consulted if the problem is persistent or worrisome.

Herbal Therapy

In the past few years, much interest has risen in the use of herbs in the treatment of both depression and anxiety. St. John's wort (*Hypericum perforatum*), an herb used extensively in the treatment of mild to moderate depression in Europe, has recently aroused interest in the United States. St. John's wort, an attractive bushy, low-growing plant covered with yellow flowers in summer, has been used for centuries in many folk and herbal remedies. Today in Germany, *Hypericum* is used in the treatment of depression more than any other antidepressant. However, the scientific studies that have been conducted on its use have been short-term and have used several different doses.

Because of the widespread interest in St. John's wort, the National Institutes of Health (NIH) conducted a 3-year study, sponsored by three NIH components: the National Institute of Mental Health, the National Center for Complementary and Alternative Medicine, and the

Office of Dietary Supplements. The study was designed to include 336 patients with major depression of moderate severity, randomly assigned to an 8-week trial with one-third of patients receiving a uniform dose of St. John's wort, another third sertraline, a selective serotonin reuptake inhibitor (SSRI) commonly prescribed for depression, and the final third a placebo (a pill that looks exactly like the SSRI and the St. John's wort, but has no active ingredients). The study participants who responded positively were followed for an additional 18 weeks. At the end of the first phase of the study, participants were measured on two scales, one for depression and one for overall functioning. There was no significant difference in rate of response for depression, but the scale for overall functioning was better for the antidepressant than for either St. John's wort or placebo. While this study did not support the use of St. John's wort in the treatment of major depression, ongoing NIH-supported research is examining a possible role for St. John's wort in the treatment of milder forms of depression.

The Food and Drug Administration issued a Public Health Advisory on February 10, 2000. It stated that St. John's wort appears to affect an important metabolic pathway that is used by many drugs prescribed to treat conditions such as AIDS [acquired immunodeficiency syndrome], heart disease, depression, seizures, certain cancers, and rejection of transplants. Therefore, health care providers should alert their patients about these potential drug interactions.

Some other herbal supplements frequently used that have not been evaluated in large-scale clinical trials are ephedra, gingko biloba, echinacea, and ginseng. Any herbal supplement should be taken only after consultation with the doctor or other health care provider.

Psychotherapies

Many forms of psychotherapy, including some short-term (10-20 week) therapies, can help depressed individuals. Talking therapies help patients gain insight into and resolve their problems through verbal exchange with the therapist, sometimes combined with homework assignments between sessions. Behavioral therapists help patients learn how to obtain more satisfaction and rewards through their own actions and how to unlearn the behavioral patterns that contribute to or result from their depression.

Two of the short-term psychotherapies that research has shown helpful for some forms of depression are interpersonal and cognitive/behavioral therapies. Interpersonal therapists focus on the patient's disturbed personal relationships that both cause and exacerbate (or increase) the depression. Cognitive/behavioral therapists help patients change the negative styles of thinking and behaving often associated with depression.

Psychodynamic therapies, which are sometimes used to treat depressed persons, focus on resolving the patient's conflicted feelings. These therapies are often reserved until the depressive symptoms are significantly improved. In general, severe depressive illnesses, particularly those that are recurrent, will require medication (or ECT under special conditions) along with, or preceding, psychotherapy for the best outcome.

How to Help Yourself If You Are Depressed

Depressive disorders make one feel exhausted, worthless, helpless, and hopeless. Such negative thoughts and feelings make some people feel like giving up. It is important to realize that these negative views are part of the depression and typically do not accurately reflect the actual circumstances. Negative thinking fades as treatment begins to take effect. In the meantime:

- Set realistic goals in light of the depression and assume a reasonable amount of responsibility.

- Break large tasks into small ones, set some priorities, and do what you can as you can.

- Try to be with other people and to confide in someone; it is usually better than being alone and secretive.

- Participate in activities that may make you feel better.

- Mild exercise, going to a movie, a ballgame, or participating in religious, social, or other activities may help.

- Expect your mood to improve gradually, not immediately. Feeling better takes time.

- It is advisable to postpone important decisions until the depression has lifted. Before deciding to make a significant transition—change jobs, get married or divorced—discuss it with others who know you well and have a more objective view of your situation.

- People rarely snap out of a depression. But they can feel a little better day-by-day.

- Remember, positive thinking will replace the negative thinking that is part of the depression and will disappear as your depression responds to treatment.
- Let your family and friends help you.

How Family and Friends Can Help the Depressed Person

The most important thing anyone can do for the depressed person is to help him or her get an appropriate diagnosis and treatment. This may involve encouraging the individual to stay with treatment until symptoms begin to abate (several weeks), or to seek different treatment if no improvement occurs. On occasion, it may require making an appointment and accompanying the depressed person to the doctor. It may also mean monitoring whether the depressed person is taking medication. The depressed person should be encouraged to obey the doctor's orders about the use of alcoholic products while on medication. The second most important thing is to offer emotional support. This involves understanding, patience, affection, and encouragement. Engage the depressed person in conversation and listen carefully. Do not disparage feelings expressed, but point out realities and offer hope. Do not ignore remarks about suicide. Report them to the depressed person's therapist. Invite the depressed person for walks, outings, to the movies, and other activities. Be gently insistent if your invitation is refused. Encourage participation in some activities that once gave pleasure, such as hobbies, sports, religious or cultural activities, but do not push the depressed person to undertake too much too soon. The depressed person needs diversion and company, but too many demands can increase feelings of failure.

Do not accuse the depressed person of faking illness or of laziness, or expect him or her to snap out of it. Eventually, with treatment, most people do get better. Keep that in mind, and keep reassuring the depressed person that, with time and help, he or she will feel better.

Where to Get Help

If unsure where to go for help, check the Yellow Pages under "mental health," "health," "social services," "suicide prevention," "crisis intervention services," "hotlines," "hospitals," or "physicians" for phone numbers and addresses. In times of crisis, the emergency room doctor at a hospital may be able to provide temporary help for an emotional problem, and will be able to tell you where and how to get further help.

Listed below are the types of people and places that will make a referral to, or provide, diagnostic and treatment services.

- Family doctors
- Mental health specialists, such as psychiatrists, psychologists, social workers, or mental health counselors
- Health maintenance organizations
- Community mental health centers
- Hospital psychiatry departments and outpatient clinics
- University- or medical school-affiliated programs
- State hospital outpatient clinics
- Family service, social agencies, or clergy
- Private clinics and facilities
- Employee assistance programs
- Local medical and/or psychiatric societies

References

1. Blehar MD, Oren DA. Gender differences in depression. Medscape Women's Health, 1997; 2:3. Revised from: Women's increased vulnerability to mood disorders: Integrating psychobiology and epidemiology. *Depression,* 1995;3:3–12.

2. Ferketick AK, Schwartzbaum JA, Frid DJ, Moeschberger ML. Depression as an antecedent to heart disease among women and men in the NHANES I study. National Health and Nutrition Examination Survey. *Archives of Internal Medicine,* 2000; 160(9): 1261–8.

3. Frank E, Karp JF, Rush AJ (1993). Efficacy of treatments for major depression. *Psychopharmacology Bulletin,* 1993; 29:457–75.

4. Lebowitz BD, Pearson JL, Schneider LS, Reynolds CF, Alexopoulos GS, Bruce MI, Conwell Y, Katz IR, Meyers BS, Morrison MF, Mossey J, Niederehe G, Parmelee P. Diagnosis and treatment of depression in late life: consensus statement update. *Journal of the American Medical Association,* 1997; 278:1186–90.

5. Robins LN, Regier DA (Eds). *Psychiatric Disorders in America, The Epidemiologic Catchment Area Study,* 1990; New York: The Free Press.

6. Rubinow DR, Schmidt PJ, Roca CA. Estrogen-serotonin interactions: Implications for affective regulation. *Biological Psychiatry,* 1998; 44(9):839–50.

7. Schmidt PJ, Neiman LK, Danaceau MA, Adams LF, Rubinow DR. Differential behavioral effects of gonadal steroids in women with and in those without premenstrual syndrome. *Journal of the American Medical Association,* 1998; 338:209–16.

8. Vitiello B, Jensen P. Medication development and testing in children and adolescents. *Archives of General Psychiatry,* 1997; 54:871–6.

Chapter 29

The Stress-Bipolar Disorder Link

An errant enzyme linked to bipolar disorder, in the brain's prefrontal cortex, impairs cognition under stress, an animal study shows. The disturbed thinking, impaired judgment, impulsivity, and distractibility seen in mania, a destructive phase of bipolar disorder, may be traceable to overactivity of protein kinase C (PKC), suggests the study, funded by the National Institutes of Health (NIH)'s National Institute of Mental Health (NIMH) and National Institute on Aging (NIA), and the Stanley Foundation. It explains how even mild stress can worsen cognitive symptoms, as occurs in bipolar disorder, which affects 2 million Americans.

Abnormalities in the cascade of events that trigger PKC have also been implicated in schizophrenia. Amy Arnsten, Ph.D., and Shari Birnbaum, Ph.D., of Yale University, and Husseini Manji, M.D., of NIMH, and colleagues, report on their discovery in the October 29, 2004 issue of *Science*.

"Either direct or indirect activation of PKC dramatically impaired the cognitive functions of the prefrontal cortex, a higher brain region that allows us to appropriately guide our behavior, thoughts, and emotions," explained Arnsten. "PKC activation led to a reduction in memory-related cell firing, the code cells use to hold information in mind from moment-to-moment. Exposure to mild stress activated PKC

"Stress Impairs Thinking Via Mania-Linked Enzyme" is a press release from the National Institute of Mental Health (NIMH, www.nimh.nih.gov), part of the National Institutes of Health, October 29, 2004.

and resulted in prefrontal dysfunction, while inhibiting PKC protected cognitive function."

"In the future, drugs that inhibit PKC could become the preferred emergency room treatments for mania," added Manji, currently Director of NIMH's Mood and Anxiety Disorders Program, who heads a search for a fast-acting antimanic agent. "All current treatments—lithium, valproate, carbamazepine, and antipsychotics—take days, if not weeks, to work. That's because they're likely acting far upstream of where a key problem is, namely in the PKC pathway. Since PKC inhibitors could act more directly, they might quench symptoms more quickly. Patients could carry PKC inhibitors and take them preventively, as soon as they sense a manic episode coming on."

Clinical trials of a PKC inhibitor, the anti-cancer drug tamoxifen, are currently underway in bipolar disorder patients. However, these may be more important for proof-of-concept than therapeutic utility, according to Manji, who says side effects will likely rule out tamoxifen itself as a practical treatment for mania. "While there are likely other pathways involved, PKC appears to be very important for bipolar disorder," he noted.

The fact that the current antimanic drugs ultimately reduce PKC activity suggests that PKC may be a final common target of these treatments and may play a key role in bipolar disorder. Studies have also found signs of increased PKC activity in bipolar patients' blood platelets and in the brain cells of deceased patients. Susceptibility to bipolar disorder may involve variants of genes that code for a key PKC precursor and for a stress-sensitive signaling protein that normally puts the brakes on PKC activity.

The new study shows how PKC triggers cognitive symptoms in response to stress. When the stress-sensitive messenger chemical norepinephrine binds to receptors on cell membranes in the prefrontal cortex, it activates PKC through a cascade of events. The enzyme then travels out to the cell membrane, opening ion channels that heighten the cell's excitability, and stoking protein machinery that propels neurotransmitters into the synapse. PKC also moves into the cell's nucleus, where it turns on genes.

To tease out PKC's role, the researchers selectively targeted the prefrontal cortex in rats and monkeys performing working memory tasks with PKC activators, inhibitors, norepinephrine-like and stress-inducing drugs—alone and in combination. They also found that by blocking PKC, the anti-manic drugs lithium and carbamazepine protected monkeys' prefrontal cortex functioning from impairment by a norepinephrine-like drug. The researchers traced impairment to a reduction in memory-related firing of single cells in the prefrontal cortex, which was reversible by a PKC inhibitor.

Genetic and biochemical studies indicate that PKC may also be overactive in the brains of patients with schizophrenia. Antipsychotics, which are used to treat bipolar disorder as well as schizophrenia, block receptors in the brain that activate PKC.

Also participating in the study were: Dr. Peixiong Yuan, NIMH; Dr. Min Wang, Susheel Vijayraghavan, Allyson Bloom, Douglas Davis, Kevin Gobeske, Yale University; Dr. David Sweatt, Baylor College of Medicine.

Chapter 30

Understanding the Link between Stress and Anxiety Disorders

Chapter Contents

Section 30.1

What Is an Anxiety Disorder?

"What Is an Anxiety Disorder?" © 2006 Anxiety Disorders Association of America. All Rights Reserved. Reprinted with permission. For more information visit http://www.adaa.org or call 240-485-1001.

Most people experience a certain amount of anxiety and fear in their lifetimes. It is a normal part of living. For 40 million adult Americans, however, anxieties and fear are persistent and overwhelming and

Table 30.1. What's the Difference between Normal Anxiety and an Anxiety Disorder?

Normal Anxiety	Anxiety Disorder
Occasional worry about circumstantial events, a breakup, or bills, that may leave you upset	Constant, chronic, and unsubstantiated worry that causes significant distress, disturbs your life, and interferes with work
Embarrassment or self-consciousness in the face of an uncomfortable social situation	Avoidance of common social situations for fear of being judged, embarrassed, or humiliated
Random case of "nerves" or jitters, dizziness, and/or sweating over an important event like a business presentation	Repeated, random panic attacks that leave you with feelings of terror or impending doom and persistent worry about another panic attack
Realistic fear of a threatening object, place, or situation	Irrational fear or avoidance of an object, place, or situation that poses little or no threat of danger
Wanting to be sure that you are healthy and living in a safe, hazard-free environment	Performing uncontrollable, repetitive actions, such as washing your hands repeatedly or checking things over and over
Anxiety, sadness, or difficulty sleeping immediately following a traumatic event	Ongoing and recurring nightmares, flashbacks, or emotional numbing relating to a traumatic event in your life that occurred several months or years ago

302

can interfere with daily life. These people suffer from anxiety disorders, a group of psychiatric disorders that can be terrifying and crippling.

Experts believe that anxiety disorders are caused by a combination of biological and environmental factors, much like physical disorders such as heart disease or diabetes. Anxiety disorders are identified as: generalized anxiety disorder, obsessive-compulsive disorder, panic disorder, posttraumatic stress disorder, social anxiety disorder (or social phobia), and specific phobias.

Normal Anxiety or an Anxiety Disorder?

Anxiety is hardwired into all of our brains. It is part of the body's "fight or flight" response. This prepares us to act quickly in the face of danger. It is a normal response to situations of uncertainty, trouble, or feeling unprepared. However, if common everyday events bring on severe and persistent anxiety or panic that interferes with life, you may have an anxiety disorder.

Do You Relate?

If you relate to any of these anxiety disorder descriptions, talk to someone who can help as soon as possible.

Section 30.2

Anxiety Disorders:
The Most Common Psychiatric Illness

"Statistics and Facts About Anxiety Disorders," © 2006 Anxiety Disorders Association of America. All Rights Reserved. Reprinted with permission. For more information visit http://www.adaa.org or call 240-485-1001.

- Anxiety disorders are the most common mental illness in the United States, with 40 million (18.1%) of the adult U.S. population (age 18 and older) affected.

- According to "The Economic Burden of Anxiety Disorders," a study commissioned by the ADAA and based on data gathered by the association and published in the *Journal of Clinical Psychiatry*, anxiety disorders cost the United States more than $42 billion a year, almost one third of the $148 billion total mental health bill for the United States.

- More than $22.84 billion of those costs are associated with the repeated use of health care services, as those with anxiety disorders seek relief for symptoms that mimic physical illnesses.

- People with an anxiety disorder are three to five times more likely to go to the doctor and six times more likely to be hospitalized for psychiatric disorders than non-sufferers.

Note: Numbers and percentages below refer to adult U.S. population affected.

Generalized anxiety disorder: 6.8 million, 3.1%.

- Women are twice as likely to be afflicted as men.

- Very likely to be comorbid with other disorders.

Obsessive-compulsive disorder (OCD): 2.2 million, 1.0%.

- It is equally common among men and women.

- One third of afflicted adults had their first symptoms in child-hood.

- In 1990, OCD cost the United States 6% of the total $148 billion mental health bill.

Panic disorder: 6 million, 2.7%.

- Women are twice as likely to be afflicted than men.

- Has a very high comorbidity rate with major depression.

Posttraumatic stress disorder (PTSD): 7.7 million, 3.5%.

- Women are more likely to be afflicted than men.

- Rape is the most likely trigger of PTSD; 65% of men and 45.9% of women who are raped will develop the disorder.

- Childhood sexual abuse is a strong predictor of lifetime likeli-hood for developing PTSD.

Social anxiety disorder: 15 million, 6.8%.

- It is equally common among men and women.

Specific phobia: 19 million, 8.7%.

- Women are twice as likely to be afflicted as men.

Chapter 31

Types of Anxiety Disorders

Chapter Contents

Section 31.1

Panic Disorder

Excerpted from "Anxiety Disorders," a brochure by the National
Institute of Mental Health (NIMH, www.nimh.nih.gov), part of the
National Institutes of Health, June 26, 2006.

"For me, a panic attack is almost a violent experience. I feel disconnected from reality. I feel like I'm losing control in a very extreme way. My heart pounds really hard, I feel like I can't get my breath, and there's an overwhelming feeling that things are crashing in on me."

"It started 10 years ago, when I had just graduated from college and started a new job. I was sitting in a business seminar in a hotel and this thing came out of the blue. I felt like I was dying."

"In between attacks there is this dread and anxiety that it's going to happen again. I'm afraid to go back to places where I've had an attack. Unless I get help, there soon won't be any place where I can go and feel safe from panic."

Panic disorder is a real illness that can be successfully treated. It is characterized by sudden attacks of terror, usually accompanied by a pounding heart, sweatiness, weakness, faintness, or dizziness. During these attacks, people with panic disorder may flush or feel chilled; their hands may tingle or feel numb; and they may experience nausea, chest pain, or smothering sensations. Panic attacks usually produce a sense of unreality, a fear of impending doom, or a fear of losing control.

A fear of one's own unexplained physical symptoms is also a symptom of panic disorder. People having panic attacks sometimes believe they are having heart attacks, losing their minds, or on the verge of death. They can't predict when or where an attack will occur, and between episodes many worry intensely and dread the next attack.

Panic attacks can occur at any time, even during sleep. An attack usually peaks within 10 minutes, but some symptoms may last much longer. Panic disorder affects about 6 million American adults and is twice as common in women as men. Panic attacks often begin in late adolescence or early adulthood, but not everyone who experiences panic attacks will develop panic disorder. Many people have just one attack and never have another. The tendency to develop panic attacks appears to be inherited.

People who have full-blown, repeated panic attacks can become very disabled by their condition and should seek treatment before they start to avoid places or situations where panic attacks have occurred. For example, if a panic attack happened in an elevator, someone with panic disorder may develop a fear of elevators that could affect the choice of a job or an apartment, and restrict where that person can seek medical attention or enjoy entertainment.

Some people's lives become so restricted that they avoid normal activities, such as grocery shopping or driving. About one third become housebound or are able to confront a feared situation only when accompanied by a spouse or other trusted person. When the condition progresses this far, it is called agoraphobia, or fear of open spaces.

Early treatment can often prevent agoraphobia, but people with panic disorder may sometimes go from doctor to doctor for years and visit the emergency room repeatedly before someone correctly diagnoses their condition. This is unfortunate, because panic disorder is one of the most treatable of all the anxiety disorders, responding in most cases to certain kinds of medication or certain kinds of cognitive psychotherapy, which help change thinking patterns that lead to fear and anxiety.

Panic disorder is often accompanied by other serious problems, such as depression, drug abuse, or alcoholism. These conditions need to be treated separately. Symptoms of depression include feelings of sadness or hopelessness, changes in appetite or sleep patterns, low energy, and difficulty concentrating. Most people with depression can be effectively treated with antidepressant medications, certain types of psychotherapy, or a combination of the two.

Section 31.2

Obsessive-Compulsive Disorder

Excerpted from "Anxiety Disorders," a brochure by the National Institute of Mental Health (NIMH, www.nimh.nih.gov), part of the National Institutes of Health, June 26, 2006.

"I couldn't do anything without rituals. They invaded every aspect of my life. Counting really bogged me down. I would wash my hair three times as opposed to once because three was a good luck number and one wasn't. It took me longer to read because I'd count the lines in a paragraph. When I set my alarm at night, I had to set it to a number that wouldn't add up to a 'bad' number."

"I knew the rituals didn't make sense, and I was deeply ashamed of them, but I couldn't seem to overcome them until I had therapy."

"Getting dressed in the morning was tough, because I had a routine, and if I didn't follow the routine, I'd get anxious and would have to get dressed again. I always worried that if I didn't do something, my parents were going to die. I'd have these terrible thoughts of harming my parents. That was completely irrational, but the thoughts triggered more anxiety and more senseless behavior. Because of the time I spent on rituals, I was unable to do a lot of things that were important to me."

People with obsessive-compulsive disorder (OCD) have persistent, upsetting thoughts (obsessions) and use rituals (compulsions) to control the anxiety these thoughts produce. Most of the time, the rituals end up controlling them.

For example, if people are obsessed with germs or dirt, they may develop a compulsion to wash their hands over and over again. If they develop an obsession with intruders, they may lock and relock their doors many times before going to bed. Being afraid of social embarrassment may prompt people with OCD to comb their hair compulsively in front of a mirror—sometimes they get "caught" in the mirror and can't move away from it. Performing such rituals is not pleasurable. At best, it produces temporary relief from the anxiety created by obsessive thoughts.

Other common rituals are a need to repeatedly check things, touch things (especially in a particular sequence), or count things. Some

310

common obsessions include having frequent thoughts of violence and harming loved ones, persistently thinking about performing sexual acts the person dislikes, or having thoughts that are prohibited by religious beliefs. People with OCD may also be preoccupied with order and symmetry, have difficulty throwing things out (so they accumulate), or hoard unneeded items.

Healthy people also have rituals, such as checking to see if the stove is off several times before leaving the house. The difference is that people with OCD perform their rituals even though doing so interferes with daily life and they find the repetition distressing. Although most adults with OCD recognize that what they are doing is senseless, some adults and most children may not realize that their behavior is out of the ordinary.

OCD affects about 2.2 million American adults, and the problem can be accompanied by eating disorders, other anxiety disorders, or depression. It strikes men and women in roughly equal numbers and usually appears in childhood, adolescence, or early adulthood. One third of adults with OCD develop symptoms as children, and research indicates that OCD might run in families.

The course of the disease is quite varied. Symptoms may come and go, ease over time, or get worse. If OCD becomes severe, it can keep a person from working or carrying out normal responsibilities at home. People with OCD may try to help themselves by avoiding situations that trigger their obsessions, or they may use alcohol or drugs to calm themselves.

OCD usually responds well to treatment with certain medications and/or exposure-based psychotherapy, in which people face situations that cause fear or anxiety and become less sensitive (desensitized) to them. NIMH is supporting research into new treatment approaches for people whose OCD does not respond well to the usual therapies. These approaches include combination and augmentation (add-on) treatments, as well as modern techniques such as deep brain stimulation.

Section 31.3

Social Phobia (Social Anxiety Disorder)

Excerpted from "Anxiety Disorders," a brochure by the National Institute of Mental Health (NIMH, www.nimh.nih.gov), part of the National Institutes of Health, June 26, 2006.

"In any social situation, I felt fear. I would be anxious before I even left the house, and it would escalate as I got closer to a college class, a party, or whatever. I would feel sick in my stomach—it almost felt like I had the flu. My heart would pound, my palms would get sweaty, and I would get this feeling of being removed from myself and from everybody else."

"When I would walk into a room full of people, I'd turn red and it would feel like everybody's eyes were on me. I was embarrassed to stand off in a corner by myself, but I couldn't think of anything to say to anybody. It was humiliating. I felt so clumsy, I couldn't wait to get out."

Social phobia, also called social anxiety disorder, is diagnosed when people become overwhelmingly anxious and excessively self-conscious in everyday social situations. People with social phobia have an intense, persistent, and chronic fear of being watched and judged by others and of doing things that will embarrass them. They can worry for days or weeks before a dreaded situation. This fear may become so severe that it interferes with work, school, and other ordinary activities, and can make it hard to make and keep friends.

While many people with social phobia realize that their fears about being with people are excessive or unreasonable, they are unable to overcome them. Even if they manage to confront their fears and be around others, they are usually very anxious beforehand, are intensely uncomfortable throughout the encounter, and worry about how they were judged for hours afterward.

Social phobia can be limited to one situation (such as talking to people, eating or drinking, or writing on a blackboard in front of others) or may be so broad (such as in generalized social phobia) that the person experiences anxiety around almost anyone other than the family.

Physical symptoms that often accompany social phobia include blushing, profuse sweating, trembling, nausea, and difficulty talking. When these symptoms occur, people with PTSD feel as though all eyes are focused on them.

Social phobia affects about 15 million American adults. Women and men are equally likely to develop the disorder, which usually begins in childhood or early adolescence. There is some evidence that genetic factors are involved. Social phobia is often accompanied by other anxiety disorders or depression, and substance abuse may develop if people try to self-medicate their anxiety.

Social phobia can be successfully treated with certain kinds of psychotherapy or medications.

Section 31.4

Specific Phobias

Excerpted from "Anxiety Disorders," a brochure by the National Institute of Mental Health (NIMH, www.nimh.nih.gov), part of the National Institutes of Health, June 26, 2006.

"I'm scared to death of flying, and I never do it anymore. I used to start dreading a plane trip a month before I was due to leave. It was an awful feeling when that airplane door closed and I felt trapped. My heart would pound, and I would sweat bullets. When the airplane would start to ascend, it just reinforced the feeling that I couldn't get out. When I think about flying, I picture myself losing control, freaking out, and climbing the walls, but of course I never did that. I'm not afraid of crashing or hitting turbulence. It's just that feeling of being trapped. Whenever I've thought about changing jobs, I've had to think, "Would I be under pressure to fly?" These days I only go places where I can drive or take a train. My friends always point out that I couldn't get off a train traveling at high speeds either, so why don't trains bother me? I just tell them it isn't a rational fear."

A specific phobia is an intense fear of something that poses little or no actual danger. Some of the more common specific phobias are centered around closed-in places, heights, escalators, tunnels, highway driving, water, flying, dogs, and injuries involving blood. Such phobias aren't just extreme fear; they are irrational fear of a particular thing. You may be able to ski the world's tallest mountains with ease but be unable to go above the 5th floor of an office building. While adults with phobias realize that these fears are irrational, they often find that facing, or even thinking about facing, the feared object or situation brings on a panic attack or severe anxiety.

Specific phobias affect an estimated 19.2 million adult Americans and are twice as common in women as men. They usually appear in childhood or adolescence and tend to persist into adulthood. The causes of specific phobias are not well understood, but there is some evidence that the tendency to develop them may run in families.

If the feared situation or feared object is easy to avoid, people with specific phobias may not seek help; but if avoidance interferes with their careers or their personal lives, it can become disabling and treatment is usually pursued.

Specific phobias respond very well to carefully targeted psychotherapy.

Section 31.5

Generalized Anxiety Disorder

Excerpted from "Anxiety Disorders," a brochure by the National Institute of Mental Health (NIMH, www.nimh.nih.gov), part of the National Institutes of Health, June 26, 2006.

"I always thought I was just a worrier. I'd feel keyed up and unable to relax. At times it would come and go, and at times it would be constant. It could go on for days. I'd worry about what I was going to fix for a dinner party, or what would be a great present for somebody. I just couldn't let something go."

"I'd have terrible sleeping problems. There were times I'd wake up wired in the middle of the night. I had trouble concentrating, even reading the newspaper or a novel. Sometimes I'd feel a little light-headed. My heart would race or pound. And that would make me worry more. I was always imagining things were worse than they really were: when I got a stomachache, I'd think it was an ulcer."

People with generalized anxiety disorder (GAD) go through the day filled with exaggerated worry and tension, even though there is little or nothing to provoke it. They anticipate disaster and are overly concerned about health issues, money, family problems, or difficulties at work. Sometimes just the thought of getting through the day produces anxiety.

GAD is diagnosed when a person worries excessively about a variety of everyday problems for at least 6 months. People with GAD can't seem to get rid of their concerns, even though they usually realize that their anxiety is more intense than the situation warrants. They can't relax, startle easily, and have difficulty concentrating. Often they have trouble falling asleep or staying asleep. Physical symptoms that often accompany the anxiety include fatigue, headaches, muscle tension, muscle aches, difficulty swallowing, trembling, twitching, irritability, sweating, nausea, lightheadedness, having to go to the bathroom frequently, feeling out of breath, and hot flashes.

When their anxiety level is mild, people with GAD can function socially and hold down a job. Although they don't avoid certain situations as a result of their disorder, people with GAD can have difficulty carrying out the simplest daily activities if their anxiety is severe.

GAD affects about 6.8 million adult Americans and about twice as many women as men.[2] The disorder comes on gradually and can begin across the life cycle, though the risk is highest between childhood and middle age. It is diagnosed when someone spends at least 6 months worrying excessively about a number of everyday problems. There is evidence that genes play a modest role in GAD.

Other anxiety disorders, depression, or substance abuse often accompany GAD, which rarely occurs alone. GAD is commonly treated with medication or cognitive-behavioral therapy, but co-occurring conditions must also be treated using the appropriate therapies.

Chapter 32

Getting Help for Anxiety Disorders

In general, anxiety disorders are treated with medication, specific types of psychotherapy, or both. Treatment choices depend on the problem and the person's preference. Before treatment begins, a doctor must conduct a careful diagnostic evaluation to determine whether a person's symptoms are caused by an anxiety disorder or a physical problem. If an anxiety disorder is diagnosed, the type of disorder or the combination of disorders that are present must be identified, as well as any coexisting conditions, such as depression or substance abuse. Sometimes alcoholism, depression, or other coexisting conditions have such a strong effect on the individual that treating the anxiety disorder must wait until the coexisting conditions are brought under control.

People with anxiety disorders who have already received treatment should tell their current doctor about that treatment in detail. If they received medication, they should tell their doctor what medication was used, what the dosage was at the beginning of treatment, whether the dosage was increased or decreased while they were under treatment, what side effects occurred, and whether the treatment helped them become less anxious. If they received psychotherapy, they should describe the type of therapy, how often they attended sessions, and whether the therapy was useful.

Excerpted from "Anxiety Disorders," a brochure by the National Institute of Mental Health (NIMH, www.nimh.nih.gov), part of the National Institutes of Health, June 26, 2006.

Often people believe that they have "failed" at treatment or that the treatment didn't work for them when, in fact, it was not given for an adequate length of time or was administered incorrectly. Sometimes people must try several different treatments or combinations of treatment before they find the one that works for them.

Medications

Medication will not cure anxiety disorders, but it can keep them under control while the person receives psychotherapy. Medication must be prescribed by physicians, usually psychiatrists, who can either offer psychotherapy themselves or work as a team with psychologists, social workers, or counselors who provide psychotherapy. The principal medications used for anxiety disorders are antidepressants, anti-anxiety drugs, and beta-blockers to control some of the physical symptoms. With proper treatment, many people with anxiety disorders can lead normal, fulfilling lives.

Antidepressants

Antidepressants were developed to treat depression but are also effective for anxiety disorders. Although these medications begin to alter brain chemistry after the very first dose, their full effect requires a series of changes to occur; it is usually about 4 to 6 weeks before symptoms start to fade. It is important to continue taking these medications long enough to let them work.

SSRIs

Some of the newest antidepressants are called selective serotonin reuptake inhibitors, or SSRIs. SSRIs alter the levels of the neurotransmitter serotonin in the brain, which, like other neurotransmitters, helps brain cells communicate with one another.

Fluoxetine (Prozac®), sertraline (Zoloft®), escitalopram (Lexapro®), paroxetine (Paxil®), and citalopram (Celexa®) are some of the SSRIs commonly prescribed for panic disorder, OCD, PTSD, and social phobia. SSRIs are also used to treat panic disorder when it occurs in combination with OCD, social phobia, or depression. Venlafaxine (Effexor®), a drug closely related to the SSRIs, is used to treat GAD. These medications are started at low doses and gradually increased until they have a beneficial effect.

SSRIs have fewer side effects than older antidepressants, but they sometimes produce slight nausea or jitters when people first start to take them. These symptoms fade with time. Some people also experience sexual dysfunction with SSRIs, which may be helped by adjusting the dosage or switching to another SSRI.

Tricyclics

Tricyclics are older than SSRIs and work as well as SSRIs for anxiety disorders other than OCD. They are also started at low doses that are gradually increased. They sometimes cause dizziness, drowsiness, dry mouth, and weight gain, which can usually be corrected by changing the dosage or switching to another tricyclic medication.

Tricyclics include imipramine (Tofranil®), which is prescribed for panic disorder and GAD, and clomipramine (Anafranil®), which is the only tricyclic antidepressant useful for treating OCD.

MAOIs

Monoamine oxidase inhibitors (MAOIs) are the oldest class of antidepressant medications. The MAOIs most commonly prescribed for anxiety disorders are phenelzine (Nardil®), followed by tranylcypromine (Parnate®), and isocarboxazid (Marplan®), which are useful in treating panic disorder and social phobia. People who take MAOIs cannot eat a variety of foods and beverages (including cheese and red wine) that contain tyramine or take certain medications, including some types of birth control pills, pain relievers (such as Advil®, Motrin®, or Tylenol®), cold and allergy medications, and herbal supplements; these substances can interact with MAOIs to cause dangerous increases in blood pressure. The development of a new MAOI skin patch may help lessen these risks. MAOIs can also react with SSRIs to produce a serious condition called "serotonin syndrome," which can cause confusion, hallucinations, increased sweating, muscle stiffness, seizures, changes in blood pressure or heart rhythm, and other potentially life-threatening conditions.

Anti-Anxiety Drugs

High-potency benzodiazepines combat anxiety and have few side effects other than drowsiness. Because people can get used to them and may need higher and higher doses to get the same effect, benzodiazepines are generally prescribed for short periods of time, especially for people who have abused drugs or alcohol and who become dependent on medication easily. One exception to this rule is people with panic disorder, who can take benzodiazepines for up to a year without harm.

Clonazepam (Klonopin®) is used for social phobia and GAD, lorazepam (Ativan®) is helpful for panic disorder, and alprazolam (Xanax®) is useful for both panic disorder and GAD.

Some people experience withdrawal symptoms if they stop taking benzodiazepines abruptly instead of tapering off, and anxiety can return once the medication is stopped. These potential problems have led some physicians to shy away from using these drugs or to use them in inadequate doses.

Buspirone (BuSpar®), an azapirone, is a newer anti-anxiety medication used to treat GAD. Possible side effects include dizziness, headaches, and nausea. Unlike benzodiazepines, buspirone must be taken consistently for at least 2 weeks to achieve an anti-anxiety effect.

Beta-Blockers

Beta-blockers, such as propranolol (Inderal®), which is used to treat heart conditions, can prevent the physical symptoms that accompany certain anxiety disorders, particularly social phobia. When a feared situation can be predicted (such as giving a speech), a doctor may prescribe a beta-blocker to keep physical symptoms of anxiety under control.

Psychotherapy

Psychotherapy involves talking with a trained mental health professional, such as a psychiatrist, psychologist, social worker, or counselor, to discover what caused an anxiety disorder and how to deal with its symptoms.

Cognitive-Behavioral Therapy

Cognitive-behavioral therapy (CBT) is very useful in treating anxiety disorders. The cognitive part helps people change the thinking patterns that support their fears, and the behavioral part helps people change the way they react to anxiety-provoking situations.

For example, CBT can help people with panic disorder learn that their panic attacks are not really heart attacks and help people with social phobia learn how to overcome the belief that others are always watching and judging them. When people are ready to confront their fears, they are shown how to use exposure techniques to desensitize themselves to situations that trigger their anxieties.

People with OCD who fear dirt and germs are encouraged to get their hands dirty and wait increasing amounts of time before washing them.

The therapist helps the person cope with the anxiety that waiting produces; after the exercise has been repeated a number of times, the anxiety diminishes. People with social phobia may be encouraged to spend time in feared social situations without giving in to the temptation to flee and to make small social blunders and observe how people respond to them. Since the response is usually far less harsh than the person fears, these anxieties are lessened. People with PTSD may be supported through recalling their traumatic event in a safe situation, which helps reduce the fear it produces. CBT therapists also teach deep breathing and other types of exercises to relieve anxiety and encourage relaxation.

Exposure-based behavioral therapy has been used for many years to treat specific phobias. The person gradually encounters the object or situation that is feared, perhaps at first only through pictures or tapes, then later face-to-face. Often the therapist will accompany the person to a feared situation to provide support and guidance.

CBT is undertaken when people decide they are ready for it and with their permission and cooperation. To be effective, the therapy must be directed at the person's specific anxieties and must be tailored to his or her needs. There are no side effects other than the discomfort of temporarily increased anxiety.

CBT or behavioral therapy often lasts about 12 weeks. It may be conducted individually or with a group of people who have similar problems. Group therapy is particularly effective for social phobia. Often "homework" is assigned for participants to complete between sessions. There is some evidence that the benefits of CBT last longer than those of medication for people with panic disorder, and the same may be true for OCD, PTSD, and social phobia. If a disorder recurs at a later date, the same therapy can be used to treat it successfully a second time.

Medication can be combined with psychotherapy for specific anxiety disorders, and this is the best treatment approach for many people.

Taking Medications

Before taking medication for an anxiety disorder:

- Ask your doctor to tell you about the effects and side effects of the drug.

- Tell your doctor about any alternative therapies or over-the-counter medications you are using.

- Ask your doctor when and how the medication should be stopped. Some drugs can't be stopped abruptly but must be tapered off slowly under a doctor's supervision.

- Work with your doctor to determine which medication is right for you and what dosage is best.

- Be aware that some medications are effective only if they are taken regularly and that symptoms may recur if the medication is stopped.

How to Get Help for Anxiety Disorders

If you think you have an anxiety disorder, the first person you should see is your family doctor. A physician can determine whether the symptoms that alarm you are due to an anxiety disorder, another medical condition, or both.

If an anxiety disorder is diagnosed, the next step is usually seeing a mental health professional. The practitioners who are most helpful with anxiety disorders are those who have training in cognitive-behavioral therapy and/or behavioral therapy, and who are open to using medication if it is needed.

You should feel comfortable talking with the mental health professional you choose. If you do not, you should seek help elsewhere. Once you find a mental health professional with whom you are comfortable, the two of you should work as a team and make a plan to treat your anxiety disorder together.

Remember that once you start on medication, it is important not to stop taking it abruptly. Certain drugs must be tapered off under the supervision of a doctor or bad reactions can occur. Make sure you talk to the doctor who prescribed your medication before you stop taking it. If you are having trouble with side effects, it's possible that they can be eliminated by adjusting how much medication you take and when you take it.

Most insurance plans, including health maintenance organizations (HMOs), will cover treatment for anxiety disorders. Check with your insurance company and find out. If you don't have insurance, the Health and Human Services division of your county government may offer mental health care at a public mental health center that charges people according to how much they are able to pay. If you are on public assistance, you may be able to get care through your state Medicaid plan.

Many people with anxiety disorders benefit from joining a self-help or support group and sharing their problems and achievements with others. Internet chat rooms can also be useful in this regard, but any advice received over the internet should be used with caution, as internet acquaintances have usually never seen each other and false identities are common. Talking with a trusted friend or member of the clergy can also provide support, but it is not a substitute for care from a mental health professional.

Stress management techniques and meditation can help people with anxiety disorders calm themselves and may enhance the effects of therapy. There is preliminary evidence that aerobic exercise may have a calming effect. Since caffeine, certain illicit drugs, and even some over-the-counter cold medications can aggravate the symptoms of anxiety disorders, they should be avoided. Check with your physician or pharmacist before taking any additional medications.

The family is very important in the recovery of a person with an anxiety disorder. Ideally, the family should be supportive but not help perpetuate their loved one's symptoms. Family members should not trivialize the disorder or demand improvement without treatment. If your family is doing either of these things, you may want to show them this information so they can become educated allies and help you succeed in therapy.

Role of Research in Improving the Understanding and Treatment of Anxiety Disorders

NIMH supports research into the causes, diagnosis, prevention, and treatment of anxiety disorders and other mental illnesses. Scientists are looking at what role genes play in the development of these disorders and are also investigating the effects of environmental factors such as pollution, physical and psychological stress, and diet. In addition, studies are being conducted on the "natural history" (what course the illness takes without treatment) of a variety of individual anxiety disorders, combinations of anxiety disorders, and anxiety disorders that are accompanied by other mental illnesses such as depression.

Scientists currently think that, like heart disease and type 1 diabetes, mental illnesses are complex and probably result from a combination of genetic, environmental, psychological, and developmental factors. For instance, although NIMH-sponsored studies of twins and families suggest that genetics play a role in the development of some anxiety disorders, problems such as PTSD are triggered by trauma. Genetic studies may help explain why some people exposed to trauma develop PTSD and others do not.

Several parts of the brain are key actors in the production of fear and anxiety. Using brain imaging technology and neurochemical techniques, scientists have discovered that the amygdala and the hippocampus play significant roles in most anxiety disorders.

The amygdala is an almond-shaped structure deep in the brain that is believed to be a communications hub between the parts of the brain that process incoming sensory signals and the parts that interpret these signals. It can alert the rest of the brain that a threat is present and trigger a fear or anxiety response. It appears that emotional memories are stored in the central part of the amygdala and may play a role in anxiety disorders involving very distinct fears, such as fears of dogs, spiders, or flying.

The hippocampus is the part of the brain that encodes threatening events into memories. Studies have shown that the hippocampus appears to be smaller in some people who were victims of child abuse or who served in military combat. Research will determine what causes this reduction in size and what role it plays in the flashbacks, deficits in explicit memory, and fragmented memories of the traumatic event that are common in PTSD.

By learning more about how the brain creates fear and anxiety, scientists may be able to devise better treatments for anxiety disorders. For example, if specific neurotransmitters are found to play an important role in fear, drugs may be developed that will block them and decrease fear responses; if enough is learned about how the brain generates new cells throughout the lifecycle, it may be possible to stimulate the growth of new neurons in the hippocampus in people with PTSD.

Current research at NIMH on anxiety disorders includes studies that address how well medication and behavioral therapies work in the treatment of OCD, and the safety and effectiveness of medications for children and adolescents who have a combination of anxiety disorders and attention deficit hyperactivity disorder.

Chapter 33

Tobacco Addiction and Stress

Smokers often talk about the magic of cigarettes for managing stress. Many smokers report that smoking provides a sense of well-being and reduces stress. While this may be true from a psychological standpoint, the nicotine in cigarette smoke is actually a stimulant that increases smokers' physiological stress. What's more, the carbon monoxide in cigarette smoke adds to physiological stress by robbing the body of needed oxygen.

So why would smokers say that cigarettes calm them down? The answer may lie in the whipsaw effect of nicotine dependency (Parrott, 1999). Smokers' bodies and minds become used to certain levels of nicotine. In between cigarettes, plasma nicotine levels drop and smokers notice increased edginess and cravings. In short, they experience withdrawal. When smokers light up, the withdrawal symptoms abate and they feel calm. Ironically, at the same time, the nicotine is actually adding to their bodies' overall stress levels. This is the cruel paradox. What feels to smokers like stress relief is, in truth, a buildup of stress. Moreover, the back-and-forth experience of withdrawal and relief can be quite stressful in itself.

"Stress and Smoking: A Cruel Paradox," by Gary Tedeschi, Ph.D., *Helpline Wire,* the Newsletter of the California Smoker's Helpline, Fall 2003/Winter 2004. © 2003 Regents of the University of California. For additional information, visit www.CaliforniaSmokersHelpline.org

The benefits of smoking for stress management seem very real to smokers. Few realize that they are adding to their stress by smoking. When asked how smoking helps with stress, many clients say smoking takes them away from it for a few minutes so they can regroup and ease back into the situation. Some say smoking helps them concentrate, so they can figure out what to do. Others note the calming effect of the smoking ritual: taking out a cigarette, lighting it, and deeply inhaling and exhaling. Most admit, however, that although they feel more relaxed after smoking, the source of the stress remains. While smoking offers momentary relief, it does not solve the problem.

Clients' perception of smoking as a stress reliever may be one reason that pharmacotherapy for smoking cessation does not work for everyone. Pharmacotherapy, such as nicotine replacement therapy (NRT), has become the quitting method of choice in recent years, due in part to the growing focus on the physical aspect of quitting. If clients can find a way to curb the tension of physical withdrawal, they have won a good part of the battle. Yet, even curbing withdrawal is not the whole battle. Clients also must change the way they view their smoking.

Many clients have come to trust smoking as a reliable way of dealing with stress. This trust is an example of positive expectancy (Bandura, 1997). To aid clients in quitting, counselors work with two types of positive expectancy: specific and general. Often smokers cannot imagine doing anything else but smoking to help them with stress. Viewing cigarettes as the only choice for coping is an example of specific positive expectancy. Counselors guide clients toward finding other approaches to stress management. A number of healthy strategies can also provide the desired effect (or close to it): deep breathing, drinking water, exercising, calling a friend, meditating, taking a hot shower, etc. Viewing several options as viable is an example of general positive expectancy. Smokers can succeed at quitting if they shift their positive expectancy from specific to general. That is, they must come to trust that several things besides smoking can help them manage stress.

Many smokers find it daunting to face stress without their cigarettes. Because the immediate stress relief is so reinforcing, it's hard for smokers to imagine that the very thing they do to reduce stress actually creates more of it. Once they grasp this paradox, they begin to see their smoking in a new way. This crucial change in perspective makes it easier for smokers to replace smoking with new, healthy behaviors and to develop confidence that quitting will actually reduce their stress level over the long term.

References

Bandura, A., (1997). *Self-efficacy: The Exercise of Control,* W.H. Freeman & Company: New York, NY.

Parrott, A.C. (1999). Does cigarette smoking cause stress? *American Psychologist,* 54(10), 817–820.

Gary Tedeschi, Ph.D. is a licensed psychologist and Clinical Director of the California Smokers' Helpline.

Chapter 34

Alcohol Use, Addiction, and Stress

Chapter Contents

Section 34.1

Alcohol and Stress

Excerpted from text published in *Alcohol Alert* No. 32-1996, a publication of the National Institute on Alcohol Abuse and Alcoholism (NIAAA), April 1996. For a complete list of references, see www.niaaa.nih.gov. Reviewed by David A. Cooke, M.D., April 2007.

The term "stress" often is used to describe the subjective feeling of pressure or tension. However, when scientists refer to stress, they mean the many objective physiological processes that are initiated in response to a stressor. As this text explains, the stress response is a complex process; the association between drinking and stress is more complicated still. Because both drinking behavior and an individual's response to stress are determined by multiple genetic and environmental factors, studying the link between alcohol consumption and stress may further our understanding of drinking behavior.

The Stress Response

The maintenance of the body's relatively steady internal state, or homeostasis, is essential for survival. The body's delicate balance of biochemical and physiological function is constantly challenged by a wide variety of stressors, including illness, injury, and exposure to extreme temperatures; by psychological factors, such as depression and fear; and by sexual activity and some forms of novelty-seeking. In response to stress, or even perceived stress, the body mobilizes an extensive array of physiological and behavioral changes in a process of continual adaptation, with the goal of maintaining homeostasis and coping with the stress.

The stress response is a highly complex, integrated network involving the central nervous system, the adrenal system, and the cardiovascular system. When homeostasis is threatened, the hypothalamus gland, at the base of the brain, initiates the stress response by secreting corticotropin releasing factor (CRF). CRF coordinates the stress response by triggering an integrated series of physiological and behavioral reactions. CRF is transported in blood within the brain and in seconds triggers the pituitary gland to release adrenocorticotropin hormone (ACTH), also referred to as corticotropin. ACTH then triggers secretion of glucocorticoid hormones (i.e., "steroids") by the adrenal glands, located at the top of the kidneys. Glucocorticoid hormones play a key role in the stress response and its termination.

Activation of the stress response affects smooth muscle, fat, the gastrointestinal tract, the kidneys, and many other organs and the body functions that they control. The stress response affects the body's regulation of temperature; appetite and satiety; arousal, vigilance, and attention; mood; and more. Physical adaptation to stress allows the body to redirect oxygen and nutrients to the stressed body site, where they are needed most.

Both the perception of what is stressful and the physiological response to stress vary considerably among individuals. These differences are based on genetic factors and environmental influences that can be traced back to infancy.

Stress is usually thought of as harmful; but when the stress response is acute and transient, homeostasis is maintained and no adverse effects result. Under chronic stress, however, when the body either fails to compensate or when it overcompensates, damage can occur. Such damage may include suppression of growth, immune system dysfunction, and cell damage resulting in impaired learning and memory.

Does Stress Influence Drinking?

Human research to clarify the connection between alcohol and stress usually has been conducted using either population surveys based on subject self-reports or experimental studies. In many but not all of these studies, individuals report that they drink in response to stress and do so for a variety of reasons. Studies indicate that people drink as a means of coping with economic stress, job stress, and marital problems, often in the absence of social support, and that the more severe and chronic the stressor, the greater the alcohol consumption. However, whether an individual will drink in response to stress appears to depend on many factors, including possible genetic determinants of drinking in response to stress, an individual's usual drinking behavior, one's expectations regarding the effect of alcohol on stress, the intensity and type of stressor, the individual's sense of control over the stressor, the range of one's responses to cope with the perceived stress, and the availability of social support to buffer the effects of stress. Some researchers have found that high levels of stress may influence drinking when alternative resources are lacking, when alcohol is accessible, and when the individual believes that alcohol will help to reduce the stress.

Numerous studies have found that stress increases alcohol consumption in animals and that individual animals may differ in the amount of alcohol they consume in response to stress. Such differences may be related in part to an animal's experiencing chronic stress early in life: Prolonged stress in infancy may permanently alter the hormonal stress response and subsequent reactions to new stressors, including alcohol consumption. For example, monkeys who were reared by peers, a circumstance regarded as a stressor compared to mother-rearing, consumed twice as much alcohol as monkeys who were mother-reared. According to research, adult rats handled for the first 3 weeks of life demonstrate markedly reduced hormonal responses to a variety of stressors compared with rats not handled during this time. In humans, researchers reported an association between certain types of alcoholism and adverse early childhood experiences.

Animal studies reporting a positive correlation between stress and alcohol consumption suggest that drinking may take place in response to chronic stress perceived as unavoidable. For instance, rats chronically exposed to unavoidable shock learn to be helpless or passive when faced with any new stressor—including shock that is avoidable—and to demonstrate increased alcohol preference compared with rats that received only avoidable shock. The rats exposed to unavoidable shock exhibit the hormonal changes indicative of the stress response, including increased levels of corticosteroid hormones.

Whether humans drink in response to uncontrollable stress is less clear. In a review investigating the connection between alcohol consumption and stress, researchers noted several studies in which researchers sampled individuals from areas affected by natural disaster. One study found that alcohol consumption increased by 30 percent in the 2 years following a flood at Buffalo Creek, West Virginia. Similarly, there was evidence of increased drinking in the towns surrounding Mount St. Helens following eruption of the volcano. Following the nuclear plant accident at Three Mile Island, however, alcohol consumption was infrequently used by those sampled as a means of coping with the resulting stress.

In both humans and animals, drinking appears to follow stress. Some human research, however, shows that drinking may take place in anticipation of or during times of stress.

Does Drinking Reduce or Induce Stress?

Some studies have reported that acute exposure to low doses of alcohol may reduce the response to a stressor in animals and humans. For example, low doses of alcohol reduced the stress response in rats subjected to strenuous activity in a running wheel. In humans, a low dose of alcohol improved performance of a complex mental problem-solving task under stressful conditions. However, in some individuals, at certain doses, alcohol may induce rather than reduce the body's stress response.

Much research demonstrates that alcohol actually induces the stress response by stimulating hormone release by the hypothalamus, pituitary, and adrenal glands. This finding has been demonstrated in animal studies. In one study with rats, the administration of alcohol initiated the physiological stress response, measured by increased levels of corticosterone. In addition to stimulating the hormonal stress response, chronic exposure to alcohol also results in an increase in adrenaline.

Stress, Alcoholism, and Relapse

Stress may be linked to social drinking, and the physiological response to stress is different in actively drinking alcoholics compared with nonalcoholics. Researchers have found that animals preferring alcohol over water have a different physiological response to stress than animals that do not prefer alcohol. Nonetheless, a clear association between stress, drinking behavior, and the development of alcoholism in humans has yet to be established.

There may, however, in the already established alcoholic, be a clearer connection between stress and relapse: Among abstinent alcoholics, personally threatening, severe, and chronic life stressors may lead to alcohol relapse. Researchers studied a group of men who completed inpatient alcoholism treatment and later experienced severe and prolonged psychosocial stress prior to and independent of any alcohol use. The researchers found that subjects who relapsed experienced twice as much severe and prolonged stress before their return to drinking as those who remained abstinent. In this study, severe psychosocial stress was related to relapse in alcoholic males who expected alcohol to reduce their stress. Those most vulnerable to stress-related relapse scored low on measures of coping skills, self-efficacy, and social support. Stress-related relapse was greatest among those who had less confidence in their ability to resist drinking and among those who relied on drinkers for social support. Although many factors can influence a return to drinking, researchers noted that stress may exert its greatest influence on the initial consumption of alcohol after a period of abstinence.

Section 34.2

Study Links Receptor to Stress-Induced Alcohol Relapse

From the National Institute on Alcohol Abuse and Alcoholism (NIAAA), part of the National Institutes of Health, October 2, 2006.

Relapse to uncontrolled drinking after periods of sobriety is a defining characteristic of alcoholism and is often triggered by stress. A study in rats reports that a specific receptor for a stress-response transmitter may play an important role in stress-induced relapse. The study, a collaboration between scientists at the National Institute on Alcohol Abuse and Alcoholism (NIAAA), part of the National Institutes of Health (NIH), and at Camerino University, Italy, appears in the *Proceedings of the National Academy of Sciences* on October 2, 2006.

"This finding helps untangle the complex interplay of genetic and environmental factors that influence relapse," says NIAAA Director T.-K. Li, M.D. "It also points to potential approaches for treating individuals at risk for relapse."

Anita C. Hansson, Ph.D., a fellow in NIAAA's Laboratory of Clinical and Translational Studies, and other NIAAA scientists worked with Camerino University scientists to examine stress-induced relapse in rats that were bred to have a greater-than-normal preference for alcohol.

"These animals provide an excellent model for identifying genes involved in stress-mediated relapse," says Dr. Hansson. "Not only do they voluntarily consume large amounts of alcohol they also display anxiety and depression-like traits, characteristics that are common among human alcoholics and which indicate a maladaptive response to stress."

A series of behavioral experiments confirmed that the alcohol-preferring rats were more sensitive to stressful situations. For example, they explored a new environment significantly less than did the normal rats, and also remained immobile longer than normal rats did in the novel environment. Each group of rats then learned that, by pressing a bar, they gained access to as much alcohol as they cared to drink. Under these conditions, the alcohol-preferring rats consume more than twice the amount of regular rats, and do so in order to obtain the intoxicating effects of alcohol. This behavior was extinguished, or unlearned, by a 15-day period during which bar-pressing yielded no alcohol, thus allowing the alcohol-preferring rats to achieve a state of sobriety.

Investigators then assessed whether a stressful stimulus—mild electric foot shock—would induce the rats to again seek alcohol by resuming the bar-pressing behavior. Alcohol-seeking was reinstated in the alcohol-preferring rats by foot shocks of much lower intensity than normal rats required.

"The resumption of alcohol-seeking by alcohol-preferring rats under these conditions is analogous to stress-induced relapse to drinking by human alcoholics," says NIAAA Clinical Director Markus Heilig, M.D., Ph.D., a senior author of the paper.

To determine if a particular gene or genes might underlie the stress-induced drinking of the alcohol-preferring rats, the researchers compared gene expression patterns in the brains of rats from each group. They focused on several families of known stress-related genes, including those associated with corticotropin-releasing hormone (CRH), which influences behavioral responses to stress through a number of different receptors. They found that alcohol-preferring rats had higher expression levels of Crhr1, a gene encoding the corticotropin-releasing hormone receptor 1 (CRH-R1). Subsequent experiments showed that antalarmin, a compound that blocks CRH-R1, suppressed alcohol drinking and completely blocked stress-induced reinstatement of drinking in alcohol-preferring rats, but had no effect on normal rats. Dr. Heilig notes that NIAAA and other NIH institutes have begun to develop antalarmin for human use.

"Our findings demonstrate that the Crhr1 genotype and its expression interact with environmental stress to reinstate alcohol-seeking behavior in this animal model of excessive drinking," says Dr. Hansson. She and her colleagues conclude that their data "provide a functional validation for antagonism at CRH-R1 receptors as a mechanism for novel treatments aimed at relapse prevention in susceptible individuals."

The National Institute on Alcohol Abuse and Alcoholism, part of the National Institutes of Health, is the primary U.S. agency for conducting and supporting research on the causes, consequences, prevention, and treatment of alcohol abuse, alcoholism, and alcohol problems and disseminates research findings to general, professional, and academic audiences. Additional alcohol research information and publications are available at www.niaaa.nih.gov.

Chapter 35

Drug Addiction and Stress

Chapter Contents

Section 35.1

The Relationship between Drug Use and Stress

"Studies Link Stress and Drug Addiction," is by Steven Stocker, from *NIDA Notes*, a publication of the National Institute of Drug Abuse (NIDA, www.drugabuse.gov), part of the National Institutes of Health. Volume 14, Number 1, April 1999. Reviewed by David A. Cooke, M.D., April 2007.

Drug-addicted patients who are trying to remain off drugs can often resist the cravings brought on by seeing reminders of their former drug life, NIDA-funded researcher Dr. Mary Jeanne Kreek of Rockefeller University in New York City has noted. "For 6 months or so, they can walk past the street corner where they used to buy drugs and not succumb to their urges. But then all of a sudden they relapse," she says. "When we ask them why they relapse, almost always they tell us something like, 'Well, things weren't going well at my job,' or 'My wife left me.' Sometimes, the problem is as small as 'My public assistance check was delayed,' or 'The traffic was too heavy.'"

Anecdotes such as these are common in the drug abuse treatment community. These anecdotes plus animal studies on this subject point toward an important role for stress in drug abuse relapse. In addition, the fact that addicts often relapse apparently in response to what most people would consider mild stressors suggests that addicts may be more sensitive than nonaddicts to stress.

This hypersensitivity may exist before drug abusers start taking drugs and may contribute to their initial drug use, or it could result from the effects of chronic drug abuse on the brain, or its existence could be due to a combination of both, Dr. Kreek has proposed. She has demonstrated that the nervous system of an addict is hypersensitive to chemically induced stress, which suggests that the nervous system also may be hypersensitive to emotional stress.

How the Body Copes with Stress

The body reacts to stress by secreting two types of chemical messengers—hormones in the blood and neurotransmitters in the brain.

Scientists think that some of the neurotransmitters may be the same or similar chemicals as the hormones but acting in a different capacity.

Some of the hormones travel throughout the body, altering the metabolism of food so that the brain and muscles have sufficient stores of metabolic fuel for activities, such as fighting or fleeing, that help the person cope with the source of the stress. In the brain, the neurotransmitters trigger emotions, such as aggression or anxiety, that prompt the person to undertake those activities.

Normally, stress hormones are released in small amounts throughout the day, but when the body is under stress the level of these hormones increases dramatically. The release of stress hormones begins in the brain. First, a hormone called corticotropin-releasing factor (CRF) is released from the brain into the blood, which carries the CRF to the pituitary gland, located directly underneath the brain. There, CRF stimulates the release of another hormone, adrenocorticotropin (ACTH), which, in turn, triggers the release of other hormones—principally cortisol—from the adrenal glands. Cortisol travels throughout the body, helping it to cope with stress. If the stressor is mild, when the cortisol reaches the brain and pituitary gland it inhibits the further release of CRF and ACTH, which return to their normal levels. But if the stressor is intense, signals in the brain for more CRF release outweigh the inhibitory signal from cortisol, and the stress-hormone cycle continues.

Researchers speculate that CRF and ACTH may be among the chemicals that serve dual purposes as hormones and neurotransmitters. The researchers posit that if, indeed, these chemicals also act as neurotransmitters, they may be involved in producing the emotional responses to stress.

The stress hormone cycle is controlled by a number of stimulatory chemicals in addition to CRF and ACTH and inhibitory chemicals in addition to cortisol both in the brain and in the blood. Among the chemicals that inhibit the cycle are neurotransmitters called opioid peptides, which are chemically similar to opiate drugs such as heroin and morphine. Dr. Kreek has found evidence that opioid peptides also may inhibit the release of CRF and other stress-related neurotransmitters in the brain, thereby inhibiting stressful emotions.

How Addiction Changes the Body's Response to Stress

Heroin and morphine inhibit the stress-hormone cycle and presumably the release of stress-related neurotransmitters just as the natural opioid peptides do. Thus, when people take heroin or morphine, the drugs add to the inhibition already being provided by the opioid peptides. This may be a major reason that some people start taking heroin or morphine in the first place, suggests Dr. Kreek. "Every one of us has things in life that really bother us," she says. "Most people are able to cope with these hassles, but some people find it very difficult to do so. In trying opiate drugs for the first time, some people who have difficulty coping with stressful emotions might find that these drugs blunt those emotions, an effect that they might find rewarding. This could be a major factor in their continued use of these drugs."

When the effects of opiate drugs wear off, the addict goes into withdrawal. Research has shown that, during withdrawal, the level of stress hormones rises in the blood and stress-related neurotransmitters are released in the brain. These chemicals trigger emotions that the addict perceives as highly unpleasant, which drive the addict to take more opiate drugs. Because the effects of heroin or morphine last only 4 to 6 hours, opiate addicts often experience withdrawal three or four times a day. This constant switching on and off of the stress systems of the body heightens whatever hypersensitivity these systems may have had before the person started taking drugs, Dr. Kreek says. "The result is that these stress chemicals are on a sort of hair-trigger release. They surge at the slightest provocation," she says.

Studies have suggested that cocaine similarly heightens the body's sensitivity to stress, although in a different way. When a cocaine addict takes cocaine, the stress systems are activated, much like when an opiate addict goes into withdrawal, but the person perceives this as part of the cocaine rush because cocaine is also stimulating the parts of the brain that are involved in feeling pleasure. When cocaine's effects wear off and the addict goes into withdrawal, the stress systems are again activated—again, much like when an opiate addict goes into withdrawal. This time, the cocaine addict perceives the activation as unpleasant because the cocaine is no longer stimulating the pleasure circuits in the brain. Because cocaine switches on the stress systems both when it is active and during withdrawal, these systems rapidly become hypersensitive, Dr. Kreek theorizes.

Evidence for the Link between Stress and Addiction

This theory about stress and drug addiction is derived in part from studies conducted by Dr. Kreek's group in which addicts were given a test agent called metyrapone. This chemical blocks the production of cortisol in the adrenal glands, which lowers the level of cortisol in the blood. As a result, cortisol is no longer inhibiting the release of CRF from the brain and ACTH from the pituitary. The brain and pituitary then start producing more of these chemicals.

Physicians use metyrapone to test whether a person's stress system is operating normally. When metyrapone is given to nonaddicted people, the ACTH level in the blood increases. However, when Dr. Kreek and her colleagues administered metyrapone to active heroin addicts, the ACTH level hardly rose at all. When the scientists gave metyrapone to heroin addicts who were abstaining from heroin use and who were not taking methadone, the synthetic opioid medication that suppresses cravings for opiate drugs, the ACTH level in the majority of the addicts increased about twice as high as in nonaddicts. Finally, when the scientists gave metyrapone to heroin addicts maintained for at least 3 months on methadone, the ACTH level rose the same as in nonaddicts.

Addicts on heroin under-react because all the excess opioid molecules in the brain greatly inhibit the brain's stress system, Dr. Kreek explains. Addicts who are heroin-free and methadone-free overreact because the constant on-off of daily heroin use has made the stress system hypersensitive, she says, and heroin addicts who are on methadone react normally because methadone stabilizes this stress system. Methadone acts at the same sites in the brain as heroin, but methadone stays active for about 24 hours while the effects of heroin are felt for only 4 to 6 hours. Because methadone is long-acting, the heroin addict is no longer going into withdrawal three or four times a day. Without the constant activation involved in these withdrawals, the brain's stress system normalizes.

Recently, Dr. Kreek's group reported that a majority of cocaine addicts who are abstaining from cocaine use overreact in the metyrapone test, just like the heroin addicts who are abstaining from heroin and not taking methadone. As with heroin addicts, this overreaction in cocaine addicts reflects hypersensitivity of the stress system caused by chronic cocaine abuse.

"We think that addicts may react to emotional stress in the same way that their stress-hormone system reacts to the metyrapone test," says Dr. Kreek. At the slightest provocation, CRF and other stress-related neurotransmitters pour out into the brain, producing unpleasant emotions that make the addict want to take drugs again, she suggests. Since life is filled with little provocations, addicts in withdrawal are constantly having their stress system activated, she concludes.

Sources

Kreek, M.J., and Koob, G.F. Drug dependence: Stress and dysregulation of brain reward pathways. *Drug and Alcohol Dependence* 51:23–47, 1998.

Kreek, M.J., et al. ACTH, cortisol, and b-endorphin response to metyrapone testing during chronic methadone maintenance treatment in humans. *Neuropeptides* 5:277–278, 1984.

Schluger, J.H., et al. Abnormal metyrapone tests during cocaine abstinence. In: L.S. Harris, ed. Problems of Drug Dependence, 1997: Proceedings of the 59th Annual Scientific Meeting, College on Problems of Drug Dependence, Inc. *NIDA Research Monograph Series, Number 178*. NIH Publication No. 98-4305. Pittsburgh, PA: Superintendent of Documents, U.S. Government Printing Office, p. 105, 1998.

Schluger, J.H., et al. Nalmefene causes greater hypothalamic-pituitary-adrenal axis activation than naloxone in normal volunteers: Implications for the treatment of alcoholism. *Alcoholism: Clinical and Experimental Research* 22(7):1430–1436, 1998.

Section 35.2

Opiate Drugs Increase Vulnerability to Stress

Copyright © 2005 by the American Psychological Association.
Reprinted with permission.

A 2005 study has found that opiate drugs such as morphine leave animals more vulnerable to stress. This means that stress and opiates are in a vicious cycle: Not only does stress trigger drug use, but in return the drug leaves animals more vulnerable to stress. The study, conducted at the University of New South Wales, helps to explain why people who use opiates such as heroin have very high rates of anxiety problems, including posttraumatic stress disorder, even after they stop using. That emotional fragility can also make them more likely to start using again.

The study appears in the journal *Behavioral Neuroscience,* which is published by the American Psychological Association (APA). Understanding how opiate users respond to and cope with stress may lead to better treatment and help prevent relapses. Co-author Gavan McNally, Ph.D., notes that heroin is the most commonly used illicit opiate, followed perhaps by morphine. In medical settings, pethidine, fentanyl, morphine, and codeine are typically used.

McNally and his colleagues conducted four experiments with rats, injecting them with either morphine or saline solution every day for 10 days. Then, either one or seven days after the final injection, they gently restrained each rat for 30 minutes as a form of stress.

The team then measured the rats' biological responses to the restraint stress. They also studied behaviors that reflect anxiety, checking the rats' levels of social interaction and general activity. The researchers tested anxiety responses for three different dose levels and different durations of exposure (0, 1, 5 or 10 days).

In the absence of stress, the opiate-treated rats were exactly the same as the control rats. Only when the animals were exposed to a stressor were there marked differences in nervous-system and behavioral responses. For example, in terms of anxiety, the impact of stress was twice as great for the morphine-treated rats as for the saline-treated rats. Whereas stress reduced social interaction by about 31 percent in the saline-treated animals, it reduced social interaction by 68 percent in the morphine-treated animals.

Thus, exposure to morphine left those rats significantly more anxious in response to stress. This effect was sensitive to both dose and duration: The longer the duration or the higher the dose of morphine, the greater the difference in anxiety between morphine- and saline-treated rats.

The authors say this is the first important evidence that opiate use increases subsequent vulnerability to stress—a tough knot to untie given that stress leads to drug use. The results also were first to show that the vulnerability could last at least a week, evidence that the altered response was independent of any recent effect of the opiate or of opiate withdrawal.

McNally points out that brief exposure to opiates, of five or fewer days, was not enough to change vulnerability to stress. He says, "It appears the development of opiate dependence is the critical variable, and there are marked individual differences in humans in the development of dependence. A few days of codeine to relieve postoperative pain are unlikely to lead to the development of dependence."

Because rodent nervous systems are so like ours, animal models allow neuroscientists to study the behavioral and brain mechanisms for drug addiction. McNally says, "Our goal is the translation of these findings in the clinical domain. Our data suggest that implementing treatments that are designed to reduce vulnerability to stress—such as cognitive-behavioral therapy, pharmacological approaches, or both—in opiate addicts may be therapeutically useful."

As for why opiate exposure raises vulnerability to stress, the authors speculate that opiates may, by altering the expression of specific anxiety-related genes, prime the nervous system in a lasting way to be more vulnerable to stress. McNally notes the paradox that drugs used to escape from stress instead may heighten its impact.

Source: Increased Vulnerability to Stress Following Opiate Exposures: Behavioral and Autonomic Correlates; Kate E. Blatchford, BPsychol, Keri Diamond, BPsychol, Frederick Westbrook, DPhil, and Gavan P. McNally, PhD; University of New South Wales; *Behavioral Neuroscience,* Vol. 119, No. 4.

Part Four

Stress after Trauma, Loss, or Disaster

Chapter 36

Trauma, Loss, and Traumatic Grief

Few things in life are as painful as the death of a loved one. Grief is simultaneously a universal and very personal response to loss that, even in the best of circumstances, can dominate one's emotional life for many months and, frequently, many years. Ideally, the anguish of acute grief is gradually transformed over time into a way of remembering and honoring the loved one that is less emotionally painful and disruptive. Over time, the loved one can be remembered without being flooded with the pervasive heartache of acute grief.

But sometimes grief becomes complicated, and bereaved survivors remain shaken and acutely distressed for months or years after the loss. They may find it difficult to get through the day, to connect with others, to have hopes for the future; in short, grief-stricken people may find it exceptionally hard to move on with their lives. In many instances, these complications and additional problems indicate or impede adjustment to the death. Professional help may remedy this so that grief no longer presents an insurmountable obstacle to adaptation to life in the aftermath of the loss.

Sudden shocking losses can be particularly difficult. These include: (1) deaths that occur without warning, providing no opportunity to anticipate, prepare, or say goodbye; (2) the death of one's child (some evidence it's worse with young children than adult children); (3) deaths that occur as the result of violence or of violent harm to the body; (4) a death in which the body is never recovered; (5) multiple losses/deaths

"Trauma, Loss and Traumatic Grief," © 2005 International Society for Traumatic Stress Studies. All rights reserved. Reprinted with permission.

of more than one person; and (6) deaths that occur as a result of the willful misconduct of others, carelessness, or negligence. Causes of such losses include disease, accidents, suicide, homicide, war, and terrorism.

What is the difference between normal grief and complications of grief?

Grieving reactions can vary a great deal from person to person and from culture to culture. Grief is not a single emotion, but usually involves a wide range of intense emotions. There is an overwhelming sense of loss with strong feelings of yearning or longing for the loved one. Survivors may feel a profound sense of emptiness and a sense that a part of them has died. Some may feel confused or unsure of who they are without the deceased and wonder what exactly they should be doing. They often speak of generalized pain or heaviness in their chest. They may feel depressed and hopeless about the future. Things that were once important may not seem to matter so much any more. In addition, they may cry easily, lose interest in eating, or experience stomach upset, headaches, and feelings of restlessness.

It can take a significant amount of time to accept the reality of a death. Survivors may know intellectually that their loved one is dead, but find themselves expecting the loved one to walk through the door or call on the telephone. It can be particularly hard to part with the loved one's possessions. The death of a loved one may provoke existential, spiritual, or identity crises that challenge one's faith or one's assumptions about life's meaning. Current research on grief and loss teaches us to respect an individual's way of coping with a loss, while at the same time looking for signs and symptoms of potentially serious complications that could be alleviated. For example, plans to commit suicide, a persistent inability to function for weeks to months after the death, abuse of alcohol and drugs, or symptoms of severe major depression or posttraumatic stress disorder should all be addressed professionally and immediately, even if the person is grief-stricken.

Although grief resembles major depression in many ways, a skilled clinician can determine whether a bereaved person is suffering with depression. It is a mistake to assume that a bereaved person with major depressive symptoms is just having a "normal" reaction, since depression is a serious but treatable disorder. When the death is particularly shocking in some way, there also can be symptoms of posttraumatic stress disorder (PTSD). There are four groups of symptoms that indicate PTSD: (1) re-experiencing of the traumatic event as indicated by painful, intrusive thoughts or nightmares about the death;

(2) avoidance or emotional numbing, as indicated by marked efforts to stay away from activities, places, or things related to the loved one's death; (3) feeling detached from others and an inability to feel positive emotions; and (4) increased persistent anxiety and physiologic arousal, as indicated by difficulty sleeping, irritability, difficulty concentrating, and a tendency to become startled easily. Although many of these symptoms also are common in normal grief, if all four clusters are present it is likely that the person is also experiencing PTSD.

Survivor guilt is common among bereaved persons, but may be excessive and unreasonable in those with major depression or traumatic grief. Survivors may blame themselves for the death or for not protecting their loved one somehow.

After loss, how long will the feelings last?

Because survivors of the death of a loved one must often come to terms with not only the death itself, but the manner of the death (e.g., if it were violent or painful) as well as all the day-to-day consequences of being without the person (e.g., financial, social), it can take many months for the most painful feelings and thoughts to diminish. It is common for survivors to agonize about what their loved ones experienced during their final moments of life. If other persons were directly or indirectly responsible for the death, the survivor must grapple with the realization that others can and will commit malevolent acts. This awareness can provoke intense reactions including powerful rage toward those perceived to be responsible. If the loved one's actions led to the death (for example by suicide or drug overdose), anger at him or her is a common feeling as is feeling abandoned by the deceased.

It also may take longer to deal with the loss if the survivor (1) has previously experienced psychological problems, such as major depression or separation anxiety; (2) was very dependent (e.g., practically, financially, as well as emotionally) on the person who died; (3) has experienced previous trauma or traumatic loss, especially if it is similar in some way to this loss ; (4) has few friends or relatives who are supportive; or (5) is simultaneously coping with other serious concerns, such as dislocation, major health problems, psychosocial stresses, or other losses. Other factors which contribute to greater difficulty in recovery include loss of parent before age 16, physical/sexual abuse, or serious neglect as a child.

As the initial shock of the death diminishes, there may be intervals when the survivor is able to focus on other issues and not feel the pain of the loss so intensely. Gradually, these intervals will become longer, and there will be good days and bad days. However, people can experience setbacks during the process. On a relatively good day, the bereaved person may encounter a reminder of the loved one, and this may cause the reemergence of painful feelings of loss. People often have difficulty dealing with occasions such as holidays, birthdays, the anniversary date of the death, or other times that have meaning.

Recent research suggests that if after about six months the acute grief reaction has not shifted into a set of feelings that is easier to bear, the bereaved person should consider taking extra steps to facilitate this process.

What can survivors do to help themselves?

Because physical health may be affected by grief, it is important for survivors to try to maintain adequate nutrition, sleep, and exercise. It's especially important for individuals with any chronic health problems, such as heart disease, to stay in contact with a physician, if at all possible, to ensure proper monitoring of their condition. Survivors often are preoccupied by their grief and may be prone to other sorts of mishaps, such as accidents, so extra caution is important. Similarly, it may be more difficult if survivors must make major decisions during the first several months after a loss, since life changes may bring on additional stress.

Most experts recommend that survivors confide in someone about the loss and find a support system. This can be a friend, a member of the clergy or another person who has experienced similar loss. It may take some time to identify friends who can be good listeners. Not everyone knows what to say or do to be helpful. Some survivors withdraw from social contact to avoid hearing hurtful comments. This is unfortunate, because the bereaved person loses the opportunity to heal with the help of others.

Through the grieving process, the many memories that come to mind of the loved one may at times seem like more than the survivor can bear. It can be helpful for survivors to learn ways to calm themselves. These might include such things as taking a walk, being with people, or participating in a distracting activity. Some survivors find it useful to write or to read.

When is it a good idea to seek professional help?

If the intensity of grief is unremitting after about six months or more, or if there are also symptoms of posttraumatic stress disorder or major depression, or if these reactions interfere with other parts of normal life such as being able to care for one's children or hold a job, asking for support from a professional can be helpful. In addition, any of the following experiences suggest that professional help may be needed:

- Continuing to experience intense yearning for the deceased that does not diminish over time
- Struggling with substantial feelings of guilt or uncontrolled rage
- Becoming severely depressed and feeling hopeless about the future
- Harboring persistent suicidal thoughts
- Abusing alcohol or other drugs or increasing tobacco use

How can treatment help?

No matter how long someone has been suffering from the impact of a sudden traumatic loss, comforting and effective treatments are available. It is important for survivors of sudden traumatic loss to select a therapist who is experienced in treating both trauma and bereavement. A variety of individual psychotherapies and support groups are available. Medication and psychotherapy may be effective with symptoms of both depression and PTSD. In addition, temporary medication may be useful for those who initially experience intense anxiety or the inability to sleep at all. A family doctor, clergy person, local mental health association, state psychiatric, psychological, or social work association, or health insurer may be helpful in providing a referral to a counselor or therapist with experience in treating sudden traumatic loss.

Chapter 37

Common Reactions to Trauma

Following a traumatic event, people typically describe feeling things like relief to be alive, followed by stress, fear, and anger. They also often find they are unable to stop thinking about what happened. Having stress reactions is what happens to most people and has nothing to do with personal weakness. Many will also exhibit high levels of arousal. For most, if the following symptoms occur, they will slowly decrease over time.

Remember that most trauma survivors (including veterans, children, disaster rescue or relief workers) experience common stress reactions. Understanding what is happening when you or someone you know reacts to a traumatic event will help you be less fearful and better able to handle things. These reactions may last for several days or even a few weeks and may include:

- feeling hopeless about the future and detached or unconcerned about others;
- having trouble concentrating and making decisions;
- feeling jumpy and startling easily at sudden noise;
- on guard and constantly alert;
- having disturbing dreams/memories or flashbacks; or
- work or school problems.

From the National Center for Posttraumatic Stress Disorder (www.ncptsd.va .gov), part of the U.S. Department of Veterans Affairs, July 2006.

You may also experience more physical reactions such as:

- stomach upset or trouble eating;

- trouble sleeping and exhaustion;

- pounding heart, rapid breathing, edginess;

- severe headache if thinking of the event or sweating;

- failure to engage in exercise, diet, safe sex, or regular health care;

- excess smoking, alcohol, drugs, or food; or

- worsening of chronic medical problems.

Or have more emotional troubles such as:

- feeling nervous, helpless, fearful, or sad;

- feeling shock, numb, or an inability to experience love or joy;

- avoiding people, places, and things related to the event;

- being irritable or having outbursts of anger;

- becoming easily upset or agitated;

- self-blame or negative views of oneself or the world;

- distrust of others, conflict, or being over-controlling;

- withdrawal or feeling rejected or abandoned; or

- loss of intimacy or feeling detached.

Use your personal support systems, family, and friends when you are ready to talk. Recovery is an ongoing gradual process. It doesn't happen through suddenly being "cured" and it doesn't mean that you will forget what happened. For most, fear, anxiety, remembering, efforts to avoid reminders, and arousal symptoms, if present, will gradually decrease over time. Most people will recover from trauma naturally. If your emotional reactions are getting in the way of your relationships, work, or other important activities, you may want to talk to a counselor or your doctor. Good treatments are available.

Common Problems That Can Occur

Posttraumatic stress disorder (PTSD): PTSD is a condition that can develop after someone has experienced a life-threatening situation. People with PTSD often can't stop thinking about what happened to them. They may try to avoid people and places that remind them of the trauma and may work hard to push thoughts of the even out of their head. Feeling numb is another common reaction. Finally, people find that they have trouble relaxing. They startle easily and are often on guard.

Depression: Depression involves feeling down or sad more days than not, and losing interest in activities that used to be enjoyable or fun. You may feel low in energy and be overly tired. People may feel hopelessness or despair or feel that things will never get better. Depression may be especially likely when a person experiences losses such as the death of close friends. This sometimes leads a depressed person to think about hurting or killing him or herself. Because of this, it is important to get help.

Self-blame, guilt, and shame: Sometimes in trying to make sense of a traumatic event, people take too much responsibility for bad things that happened, for what they did or did not do, or for surviving when others didn't. Remember, we all tend to be our own worst critics and that guilt, shame, and self-blame are usually unjustified.

Suicidal thoughts: Trauma and personal loss can lead depressed people to think about hurting or killing themselves. If you think someone you know may be feeling suicidal, you should directly ask them. You will **not** put the idea in their head. If they have a plan to hurt themselves and the means to do it and cannot make a contract with you to stay safe, try to get them to a counselor or call 911 immediately. You can also call the National Suicide Prevention Lifeline (www.suicidepreventionlifeline.org) at 800-273-TALK (8255).

Anger or aggressive behavior: Trauma can be connected with anger in many ways. After a trauma people often feel that the situation was unfair or unjust. They can't comprehend why the event has happened and why it has happened to them. These thoughts can result in intense anger. Although anger is a natural and healthy emotion, intense feelings of anger and aggressive behavior can cause relationship and job problems and loss of friendships. If people become violent when angry, this can just make the situation worse as people can become injured and there may be legal consequences.

Alcohol/drug abuse: Drinking or "self-medicating" with drugs is a common way many cope with upsetting events to numb themselves and to try to deal with the difficult thoughts, feelings, and memories related to the trauma. While this may offer a quick solution, it can actually lead to more problems. If someone close begins to lose control of drinking or drug use, it is important to assist them in getting appropriate care.

Recovery

Immediately following a trauma, almost everyone will find themselves unable to stop thinking about what happened. Many will also exhibit high levels of arousal. For most, fear, anxiety, remembering, efforts to avoid reminders, and arousal symptoms, if present, will gradually decrease over time. Use your personal support systems, family and friends, when you are ready to talk. Recovery is an ongoing gradual process. It doesn't happen through suddenly being "cured" and it doesn't mean that you will forget what happened. But, most people will recover from trauma naturally over time. If your emotional reactions are getting in the way of your relationships, work, or other important activities you may want to talk to a counselor or your doctor. Good treatments are available.

Chapter 38

Stress after Loss: The Effects of Traumatic Experiences

When people find themselves suddenly in danger, sometimes they are overcome with feelings of fear, helplessness, or horror. These events are called traumatic experiences. Some common traumatic experiences include being physically attacked, being in a serious accident, being in combat, being sexually assaulted, and being in a fire or a disaster like a hurricane or a tornado. After traumatic experiences, people may have problems that they didn't have before the event. If these problems are severe and the survivor does not get help for them, they can begin to cause problems in the survivor's family.

How Do Traumatic Experiences Affect People?

People who go through traumatic experiences often have symptoms and problems afterward. How serious the symptoms and problems are depends on many things including a person's life experiences before the trauma, a person's own natural ability to cope with stress, how serious the trauma was, and what kind of help and support a person gets from family, friends, and professionals immediately following the trauma.

Excerpted from "Effects of Traumatic Experiences," a fact sheet from the National Center for Posttraumatic Stress Disorder (NCPTSD, www.ncptsd.va .gov), part of the U.S. Department of Veterans Affairs, July 2006. By Eve B. Carlson, Ph.D. and Joseph Ruzek, Ph.D.

Because most trauma survivors are not familiar with how trauma affects people, they often have trouble understanding what is happening to them. They may think the trauma is their fault, that they are going crazy, or that there is something wrong with them because other people who experienced the trauma don't appear to have the same problems. Survivors may turn to drugs or alcohol to make themselves feel better. They may turn away from friends and family who don't seem to understand. They may not know what to do to get better.

What Do Trauma Survivors Need to Know?

- Traumas happen to many competent, healthy, strong, good people. No one can completely protect him- or herself from traumatic experiences.

- Many people have long-lasting problems following exposure to trauma. Up to 8% of individuals will have PTSD at some time in their lives.

- People who react to traumas are not going crazy. They are experiencing symptoms and problems that are connected with having been in a traumatic situation.

- Having symptoms after a traumatic event is not a sign of personal weakness. Many psychologically well-adjusted and physically healthy people develop PTSD. Probably everyone would develop PTSD if they were exposed to a severe enough trauma.

- When a person understands trauma symptoms better, he or she can become less fearful of them and better able to manage them.

- By recognizing the effects of trauma and knowing more about symptoms, a person is better able to decide about getting treatment.

What Are the Common Effects of Trauma?

During a trauma, survivors often become overwhelmed with fear. Soon after the traumatic experience, they may re-experience the trauma mentally and physically. Because this can be uncomfortable and sometimes painful, survivors tend to avoid reminders of the trauma. These symptoms create a problem that is called posttraumatic stress disorder (PTSD). PTSD is a specific set of problems resulting from a traumatic experience and is recognized by medical and mental-health professionals.

Re-Experiencing Symptoms

Trauma survivors commonly re-experience their traumas. This means that the survivor experiences again the same mental, emotional, and physical experiences that occurred during or just after the trauma. These include thinking about the trauma, seeing images of the event, feeling agitated, and having physical sensations like those that occurred during the trauma. Trauma survivors find themselves feeling as if they are in danger, experiencing panic sensations, wanting to escape, getting angry, and thinking about attacking or harming someone else. Because they are anxious and physically agitated, they may have trouble sleeping and concentrating. The survivor usually can't control these symptoms or stop them from happening. Mentally re-experiencing the trauma can include:

- upsetting memories such as images or thoughts about the trauma;

- feeling as if the trauma is happening again (flashbacks);

- bad dreams and nightmares;

- getting upset when reminded about the trauma (by something the person sees, hears, feels, smells, or tastes);

- anxiety or fear or feeling in danger again;

- anger or aggressive feelings and feeling the need to defend oneself;

- trouble controlling emotions because reminders lead to sudden anxiety, anger, or upset; or

- trouble concentrating or thinking clearly.

People also can have physical reactions to trauma reminders such as:

- trouble falling or staying asleep;

- feeling agitated and constantly on the lookout for danger;

- getting very startled by loud noises or something or someone coming up on you from behind when you don't expect it;

- feeling shaky and sweaty; or

- having your heart pound or having trouble breathing.

Because trauma survivors have these upsetting feelings when they feel stress or are reminded of their trauma, they often act as if they are in danger again. They might get overly concerned about staying safe in situations that are not truly dangerous. For example, a person living in a safe neighborhood might still feel that he has to have an alarm system, double locks on the door, a locked fence, and a guard dog. Because traumatized people often feel like they are in danger even when they are not, they may be overly aggressive and lash out to protect themselves when there is no need. For example, a person who was attacked might be quick to yell at or hit someone who seems to be threatening.

Re-experiencing symptoms are a sign that the body and mind are actively struggling to cope with the traumatic experience. These symptoms are automatic, learned responses to trauma reminders. The trauma has become associated with many things so that when the person experiences these things, he or she is reminded of the trauma and feels that he or she is in danger again. It is also possible that re-experiencing symptoms are actually a part of the mind's attempt to make sense of what has happened.

Avoidance Symptoms

Because thinking about the trauma and feeling as if you are in danger is upsetting, people who have been through traumas often try to avoid reminders of the trauma. Sometimes survivors are aware that they are avoiding reminders, but other times survivors do not realize that their behavior is motivated by the need to avoid reminders of the trauma.

Ways of avoiding thoughts, feelings, and sensations associated with the trauma can include:

- actively avoiding trauma-related thoughts and memories;
- avoiding conversations and staying away from places, activities, or people that might remind you of the trauma;
- trouble remembering important parts of what happened during the trauma;
- shutting down emotionally or feeling emotionally numb;
- trouble having loving feelings or feeling any strong emotions;
- finding that things around you seem strange or unreal;
- feeling strange;

- feeling disconnected from the world around you and things that happen to you;
- avoiding situations that might make you have a strong emotional reaction;
- feeling weird physical sensations;
- feeling physically numb;
- not feeling pain or other sensations; or
- losing interest in things you used to enjoy doing.

Trying to avoid thinking about the trauma and avoiding treatment for trauma-related problems may keep a person from feeling upset in the short term, but avoiding treatment means that in the long term, trauma symptoms will persist.

What Are Common Secondary and Associated Posttraumatic Symptoms?

Secondary symptoms are problems that arise because of the post-traumatic re-experiencing and avoidance symptoms. For example, because a person wants to avoid talking about a traumatic event, she might cut off from friends, which would eventually cause her to feel lonely and depressed. As time passes after a traumatic experience, more secondary symptoms may develop. Over time, secondary symptoms can become more troubling and disabling than the original re-experiencing and avoidance symptoms.

Associated symptoms don't come directly from being overwhelmed with fear; they occur because of other things that were going on at the time of the trauma. For example, a person who is psychologically traumatized in a car accident might also be physically injured and then get depressed because he can't work or leave the house.

All of the following problems can be secondary or associated trauma symptoms.

Depression can develop when a person has losses connected with the trauma or when a person avoids other people and becomes isolated.

Despair and hopelessness can result when a person is afraid that he or she will never feel better again.

Survivors may lose **important beliefs** when a traumatic event makes them lose faith that the world is a good and safe place.

Aggressive behavior toward oneself or others can result from frustration over the inability to control PTSD symptoms (feeling that

PTSD symptoms run your life). People may also become aggressive when other things that happened at the time of trauma make the person angry (the unfairness of the situation). Some people are aggressive because they grew up with people who lashed out and they were never taught other ways to cope with angry feelings. Because angry feelings may keep others at a distance, they may stop a person from having positive connections and getting help. Anger and aggression can cause job problems, marital and relationship problems, and loss of friendships.

Self-blame, guilt, and shame can arise when PTSD symptoms make it hard to fulfill current responsibilities. They can also occur when people fall into the common trap of second-guessing what they did or didn't do at the time of a trauma. Many people, in trying to make sense of their experience, blame themselves. This is usually completely unwarranted and fails to hold accountable those who may have actually been responsible for the event. Self-blame causes a lot of distress and can prevent a person from reaching out for help. Sometimes society also blames the victim of a trauma. Unfortunately, this may reinforce the survivor's hesitation to seek help.

People who have experienced traumas may have **problems in relationships with others** because they often have a hard time feeling close to people or trusting people. This is especially likely to happen when the trauma was caused or worsened by other people (as opposed to an accident or natural disaster).

Trauma survivors may **feel detached or disconnected from others** because they have difficulty feeling or expressing positive feelings. After traumas, people can become overwhelmed by their problems or become numb and stop putting energy into their relationships with friends and family.

Survivors may get into **arguments and fights with other people** because of the angry or aggressive feelings that are common after a trauma. Also, a person's constant avoidance of social situations (such as family gatherings) may create hurt feelings or animosity in the survivor's relationships.

Less interest or participation in things the person used to like to do may result from depression following a trauma. When a person spends less time doing fun things and being with people, he or she has fewer chances to feel good and have pleasant interactions.

Social isolation can happen because of social withdrawal and a lack of trust in others. This often leads to the loss of support, friendships, and intimacy, and it increases fears and worries.

Survivors may have **problems with identity** when PTSD symptoms change important aspects of a person's life such as relationships or whether the person can do his or her work well. A person may also question his or her identity because of the way he or she acted during a trauma. For instance, a person who thinks of himself as unselfish might think he acted selfishly by saving himself during a disaster. This might make him question whether he really is who he thought he was.

Feeling permanently damaged can result when trauma symptoms don't go away and a person doesn't believe they will get better.

Survivors may develop **problems with self-esteem** because PTSD symptoms make it hard for a person to feel good about him- or herself. Sometimes, because of how they behaved at the time of the trauma, survivors feel that they are bad, worthless, stupid, incompetent, evil, etc.

Physical health symptoms and problems can happen because of long periods of physical agitation or arousal from anxiety. Trauma survivors may also avoid medical care because it reminds them of their trauma and causes anxiety, and this may lead to poorer health. For example, a rape survivor may not visit a gynecologist and an injured motor vehicle accident survivor may avoid doctors because they remind him or her that a trauma occurred. Habits used to cope with posttraumatic stress, like alcohol use, can also cause health problems. In addition, other things that happened at the time of the trauma may cause health problems (for example, an injury).

Survivors may turn to **alcohol and drug abuse** when they want to avoid the bad feelings that come with PTSD symptoms. Many people use alcohol and drugs as a way to try to cope with upsetting trauma symptoms, but it actually leads to more problems.

Remember

Although individuals with PTSD may feel overwhelmed by their symptoms, it is important for them to remember that there are other, positive aspects of their lives. There are helpful mental-health and medical resources available, and survivors have their strengths, interests, commitments, relationships with others, past experiences that were not traumatic, desires, and hopes for the future.

Treatments are available for individuals with PTSD and associated trauma-related symptoms.

Understanding the effects of trauma on relationships can also be an important step for family members or friends.

Chapter 39

Mass Disasters, Trauma, and Loss

Disasters occur commonly and affect individuals as well as their communities. They may be human-made, caused by deliberate intention, as with terrorism, civil unrest, and war experiences, or caused by people through mishap or neglect, such as a work accident or an apartment fire. In addition, disasters may be caused by nature, including earthquakes, floods, wildfires, hurricanes, or tornadoes.

Often large numbers of people are affected and they share their experience of trauma and traumatic loss. Many losses may occur after a disaster, including loss of loved ones, coworkers, neighbors, and pets, and loss of homes, workplaces, schools, houses of worship, possessions, and communities. Survivors may also lose their routine way of living and working, going to school, and being with others. Some may lose their confidence in the future.

Some disasters, such as terrorism, continue over a long period. These may create an ongoing insecurity and exposure to danger or threat of danger, which may make it more difficult for some people to function in their lives.

After a disaster, it is normal to experience a number of stress reactions that may continue for a significant period. And after the sudden, traumatic loss caused by disasters, it is normal for grieving and mourning to be uneven, more intensely felt, and extended over time. In all disasters, the experience of safety, security, and predictability in the world is challenged, and a sense of uncertainty becomes a part of life.

"Mass Disasters, Trauma, and Loss," © 2005 International Society for Traumatic Stress Studies. All rights reserved. Reprinted with permission.

What can I expect after experiencing a disaster?

Most child, adolescent, adult, and older adult survivors experience some of the following normal stress responses to varying degrees. They may last for many months after the disaster has ended, and even longer. Normal stress reactions include:

- **emotional (feeling) reactions:** feelings of shock, disbelief, anxiety, fear, grief, anger, resentment, guilt, shame, helplessness, hopelessness, betrayal, depression, emotional numbness (difficulty having feelings, including those of love and intimacy, or taking interest and pleasure in day-to-day activities);

- **cognitive (thinking) reactions:** confusion, disorientation, indecisiveness, worry, shortened attention span, difficulty concentrating, memory loss, unwanted memories, repeated imagery, self-blame;

- **physical (bodily) reactions:** tension, fatigue, edginess, difficulty sleeping, nightmares, being startled easily, racing heartbeat, nausea, aches and pains, worsening health conditions, change in appetite, change in sex drive;

- **interpersonal reactions:** neediness; dependency; distrust; irritability; conflict; withdrawal; isolation; feeling rejected or abandoned; being distant, judgmental, or over-controlling in friendships, marriages, family, or other relationships; and

- **spiritual (meaning) reactions:** wondering why, why me, where was God; feeling as if life is not worth living, loss of hope.

What factors increase the risk of lasting vulnerability?

During or after massive disasters, many survivors may be directly exposed to or witness things that may make them particularly vulnerable to serious stress reactions.

Disaster stress may revive memories or experiences of earlier trauma, as well as possibly intensifying pre-existing social, economic, spiritual, psychological, or medical problems. While trauma reactions can become lasting problems, the shared experience of disasters and people's resiliency can provide support. Being aware of risk factors is important. They include:

- loss of family, neighborhood, or community;
- life-threatening danger or physical harm (especially to children);

- exposure to horrible death, bodily injury, or bodies;

- extreme environmental or human violence or destruction;

- loss of home or valued possessions;

- loss of communication with or support from important people in one's life;

- intense emotional demands;

- extreme fatigue, weather exposure, hunger, or sleep deprivation;

- extended exposure to danger, loss, emotional/physical strain; or

- exposure to toxic contamination (such as gas, fumes, chemicals, radioactivity, or biological agents).

Studies show that some individuals are more vulnerable to serious stress reactions and lasting difficulty, including those whose histories include:

- other traumatic experiences (such as severe accidents, abuse, assault, combat, immigrant and refugee experiences, rescue work);

- chronic medical illness or psychological problems;

- chronic poverty, homelessness, unemployment, or discrimination; or

- recent or earlier major life stressors or emotional strain (such as divorce or job loss).

What can survivors do to reduce vulnerability to serious emotional reactions and to achieve the best recovery from disaster stress?

Observations by mental health specialists who assist survivors in the wake of disaster suggest that the following steps help to reduce stress symptoms and to promote post-disaster readjustment:

- **Protect:** Find a safe haven that provides shelter, food and water, sanitation, privacy, and opportunities to sit quietly, relax, and sleep, at least briefly.

- **Direct:** Begin working on immediate personal and family priorities to help you and your loved ones preserve or regain a sense of hope, purpose, and self-esteem.

- **Connect:** Maintain or re-establish communication with family, peers, and counselors in order to talk about the experiences. Survivors may want to find opportunities to "tell their stories" to others who express interest and concern and, when they are able, to listen to others as they tell theirs, in order to release the stress a little bit at a time and try to create meaning.

- **Select:** Identify key resources such as Federal Emergency Management Agency (FEMA), the Red Cross, the Salvation Army, local and state health departments for cleanup, health, housing, and basic emergency assistance. Identify local cultural or community supports to help maintain or reestablish normal activities such as attending religious services.

Taking every day one at a time is essential in disaster's wake. Each day is a new opportunity to take steps toward recovery. People affected by disasters should try to:

- focus on what's most important to themselves and their families today;

- try to learn and understand what they and their loved ones are experiencing, to help remember what's important;

- understand personally what these experiences mean as a part of their lives, so that they will feel able to go on with their lives and even grow personally;

- take good care of themselves physically, including exercising regularly, eating well, and getting enough sleep, to reduce stress and prevent physical illness; and

- work together with others in their communities to improve conditions, reach out to persons who are marginalized or isolated, and otherwise promote recovery.

How would I decide I need professional help?

Most disaster survivors experience many normal responses and for some, their personal resources and capacities may grow and their relationships may strengthen. However, many survivors experience reactions during and after disasters that concern them, often when the disaster was caused by human action or included horror or loss of life. Some problematic responses are as follows:

- intrusive re-experiencing (terrifying memories, nightmares, or flashbacks)

- unsafe attempts to avoid disturbing memories (such as through substance use or alcohol)

- ongoing emotional numbing (unable to feel emotion, as if empty)

- extended hyperarousal (panic attacks, rage, extreme irritability, intense agitation, exaggerated startle response)

- severe anxiety (paralyzing worry, extreme helplessness)

- severe depression (loss of energy, interest, self-worth, or motivation)

- loss of meaning and hope

- sustained anger or rage

- dissociation (feeling unreal or outside oneself, as in a dream; having "blank" periods of time one cannot remember)

If after the end of a disaster, these normal experiences do not slowly improve, if they worsen with time, or if they cause difficulties in relationships or work, it is helpful to find professional support. People who wish to consider therapy should select a trained mental health professional who is knowledgeable about trauma as well as natural- and human-caused disasters. A family doctor, clergy person, local mental health association, state psychiatric, psychological, or social work association, or health insurer may be helpful in providing a referral to a counselor or therapist.

Chapter 40

Severe Stress Reactions after Disaster

Chapter Contents

Section 40.1

Managing Grief after a Disaster

Excerpted from "Managing Grief after Disaster," by Katherine Shear, Ph.D., from the National Center for Posttraumatic Stress Disorder (NCPTSD, www.ncptsd.va.gov), part of the U.S. Department of Veterans Affairs, 2007.

The Experience of Grief

Grief is the process by which we adjust to the loss of a close relationship. Therefore, grief is an inevitable companion to love and attachment. The lives of those we love are interwoven with our own in thousands of small and large ways. One's immediate family, in particular, contributes to a sense of comfort, security, and happiness and reinforces behavior. Endocrine function can become entrained by cues from another person. When this happens, losing that person requires a period of physiological adjustment. In all cases, loss of a loved one engenders feelings of loneliness, sadness, and vulnerability. The death of someone close also makes one's own death imaginable, thus evoking fear of dying. When a person experiences the death of someone close, that person is confronted by mortality and undergoes a certain degree of acute separation distress. Sometimes, there is also guilt about being alive when the other person has died, or there is guilt about not being able to save the person or make his or her life or dying easier.

While grief is not the same for every person, there are certain commonalities. During the initial phase, the bereaved person is preoccupied with the deceased, preoccupied with feelings of yearning and longing, and with searching for him or her. While grieving, most people withdraw from the world and turn inward, often reviewing the course of the relationship, including positive and negative thoughts and feelings. People often also review the meaning the relationship had in their lives. Grief entails a host of painful emotions that can sometimes be very strong and persistent. Strong feelings of sadness and loneliness almost always occur following the death of a close friend or family member. Fear and anxiety are also common. Difficult feelings of resentment, anger, and guilt can occur. Experiencing any or all of these emotions following the loss of a friend or family member is perfectly normal.

As the transition to life without a friend or family member progresses, the intensity of grief subsides. The bereaved person accepts the death and begins to take some comfort in positive memories, establishing a permanent sense of connection to the person who died. It becomes possible to reengage in activities and relationships while still having memories of and maintaining a sense of closeness to the deceased. The period over which this adjustment occurs is variable, depending on the circumstances of the death, the characteristics of the bereaved, and the nature of the relationship. In some circumstances, intense grief persists for many months or even years. Intrusive images and disturbing ideas inhibit the healing process, and there is a sense that the death is unacceptable and unfair. For some who have difficulty coping with the death, grief sometimes seems to be all that is left of the relationship. Also, a decrease in the intensity of the grief may feel like a betrayal of the person who died. Some people also have persistent feelings of guilt. When a death is sudden, violent, and untimely, the bereaved will most likely also face other difficulties. The condition in which unmanageably intense and/or persistent grief symptoms occur is called traumatic grief. Work is under way to establish diagnostic criteria and to develop treatments for this condition. Traumatic grief may predispose a person to other psychiatric, medical, and behavioral problems that can complicate bereavement. These are generally treatable conditions and need to be recognized by professionals and by the bereaved individuals themselves.

Complications of Bereavement

Bereavement is a risk factor for a range of mental and physical health problems. Among these are the following:

- Prolonged grief or traumatic grief
- Onset or recurrence of major depressive disorder
- Onset or recurrence of panic disorder or other anxiety disorders
- Possible increased vulnerability to posttraumatic stress disorder (PTSD)
- Alcohol and other substance abuse
- Smoking, poor nutrition, low levels of exercise

- Suicidal ideation
- Onset or worsening of health problems, especially cardiovascular and immunologic dysfunction

Traumatic Grief

Grief will inevitably disrupt mental functioning following the death of a loved one. While it should be emphasized that grief itself is a normal process of adapting emotionally and cognitively to the loss or absence of a loved one, sometimes the intensity of a person's grief may be overwhelming or last longer than is healthy. This may occur for a variety of reasons. The relationship between the deceased and the bereaved might have been very close or complicated; the circumstances of the death may be sudden or traumatic, as in accident, disaster, or illness; or the grieving person may not have good coping skills or the social support that would help the grieving process. In situations like these, it may be helpful to seek professional help or counseling in order to resolve the grief.

When grief goes on longer than is healthy or when it is overwhelming, a diagnosis of traumatic grief might be appropriate. It may be helpful to draw an analogy to a physical illness. An illness is not a characteristic of a person; it is a state a person is in at a given time. Many illnesses are very treatable. Another analogy is to an acute injury. People are more or less vulnerable to disability from an injury, but some types of injury are so severe that they always cause impairment. Using such an analogy, it is possible to see that following an accident or disaster or the sudden death of a very close person, it is entirely normal to experience traumatic grief, just as it is quite normal to develop tuberculosis upon exposure to a virulent organism, and it is normal to be unable to walk on a broken leg. It is also clear that it is a good idea to diagnose and treat these conditions. No one would tell a person with pneumonia "pull yourself together" or "get on with it" or expect a person with a deep cut or a broken bone to heal him- or herself. Although labels can be hurtful if misused, they can also be helpful. An ill person needs to have a "sick role" and to receive treatment. An ill person benefits from support and assistance from family and friends, as well as from treatment by a trained professional.

Symptoms of traumatic grief:

- Preoccupation with the deceased
- Pain in the same area as the deceased
- Memories that are upsetting

- Avoidance of reminders of the death
- Feeling that death is unacceptable
- Feeling life is empty
- Longing for the person
- Hearing the voice of the person who died
- Being drawn to places and things associated with the deceased
- Seeing the person who died
- Anger about the death
- Feeling it is unfair to live when this person died
- Disbelief about the death
- Bitterness about the death
- Feeling stunned or dazed
- Envy of others
- Difficulty trusting others
- Feeling lonely most of the time
- Difficulty caring about others

Risk Factors for Complications of Bereavement

Risk factors are those aspects of a situation that tend to increase vulnerability to complications and that may slow recovery. Existing studies suggest that risk factors relate to the characteristics of an individual, the nature of the relationship to the deceased, the circumstances of the death, and the social context within which recovery takes place. Some risk factors relate to the larger situation in which the bereaved finds him- or herself, and some risk factors relate to the bereaved individual's specific history and makeup. While both kinds of risk factors raise the distress level of the bereaved person, it is useful for clinicians to be particularly aware of the bereaved's individual situation.

The following risk factors have been identified.

Demographic Factors

- **Socioeconomic status:** Lower socioeconomic status is related to a poorer health status in general. Bereavement appears to affect people similarly, regardless of socioeconomic status.

- **Age:** Bereavement appears to be somewhat more stressful for younger individuals than it is for older individuals, with the exception of elderly people. The disparity between how older individuals are affected and how elderly people are affected may be because the stress experienced by elderly people is related to preexisting health problems.

- **Gender:** There is some evidence that men, especially widowers, have more bereavement-related health problems than women, especially when dealing specifically with the loss of a spouse. Although both men and women are deeply affected by the loss of close family members and friends, the death of a child may be more difficult for mothers than for fathers. Women may also recognize the effects of bereavement more readily than men, and men and women may cope differently.

- **Individual characteristics:** Overall, individuals who are defined as "neurotic" have been shown to have more health problems. Low internal locus of control is generally associated with more depression. This is not specific for bereavement. On the other hand, high internal locus of control does not act as a buffer for bereavement-related distress. Anecdotal evidence suggests that a belief in life after death may be protective. However, when this was examined in a study, a protective effect was not found. Guilt or self-blame about the death may contribute to traumatic grief.

- **Relationship quality:** Relationship quality may affect men and women differently when it comes to difficulty with bereavement. A good marriage may be associated with more bereavement-related problems in women, while the opposite may be true for men. In general, data does not support clinical lore that implies that bereavement problems occur because of ambivalence or problems in a relationship. It is very clear that in some instances an especially positive relationship may be associated with very difficult bereavement reactions.

Circumstances of the Death

Not surprisingly, sudden death is associated with more symptoms of bereavement difficulty in the first 6 months after the loss. In some studies this difference was not present in later interviews, while in other studies it was. A low score on a measure of internal locus of control signified a greater likelihood for difficulty for younger bereaved spouses. In some studies, there is evidence of continuing distress from the loss for many years following a sudden, violent loss. Experiencing multiple losses or witnessing the death (especially a factor for children who witness a death) has been found to correlate with levels of grief intensity. Feelings of helplessness and powerlessness, survivor guilt, threat to one's own life, confrontation with the massive and shocking deaths and mutilations of others, and a violation of one's assumptive world of safety and meaning are traumatic factors that may impact a person's ability to resolve grief. It is clear that many of those bereaved by the WTC [World Trade Center] disaster may experience treatable psychiatric difficulties for a long period of time. It is important for professionals to be vigilant about this possibility.

Social Context

Both perceived and received social support are related to lower symptoms of depression in the general population, but there does not appear to be a specific relationship between social support and bereavement outcome. However, it is important to note that bereaved individuals often perceive that others lack empathy and that others are hostile about the bereaved's continued symptoms. This perception is likely related to a poorer outcome but has not been specifically studied. In general, however, social support and positive family functioning, along with the opportunity to express grief, may help to mitigate the negative effects of bereavement.

Treatment of Bereaved Individuals

Grief support groups and grief counseling are widespread and undoubtedly highly variable. Little information is available related to support group and counseling outcome. There is specific controversy regarding the importance of confronting the death (also called "grief work") in the early phase of grief. In one study, investigators developed a measure to assess the extent to which individuals confronted or avoided their loss and used scores on this instrument to predict outcomes at later times. They found that low scores for widows did not influence outcome, but low scores for widowers predicted poorer outcome. There is some evidence that the occurrence of symptoms of major depression in the first month following the death predicts a worse course later, especially for suicidally bereaved individuals.

It goes without saying that the loss of a close relationship permanently affects the bereaved person. It is not reasonable to think that one can recover from such a loss or resolve the loss. Such a loss is permanent and has permanent effects on the bereaved. Still, it is possible and important that the bereaved person will eventually have comforting memories of the deceased and feel interested in and able to engage in life. Grief experts provide a list of reasonable expectations we can have for the bereaved. A person who has lost someone should eventually have (1) the ability to give energy to everyday life, (2) psychological comfort, or freedom from pain and distress, (3) the ability to experience satisfaction and gratification in life, (4) hopefulness for the future, and (5) the ability to function adequately in a range of social roles.

Section 40.2

Which Individuals Are at Risk for Severe Stress Responses?

From "Mental Health Reactions after Disaster: A Fact Sheet for Providers," from the National Center for Posttraumatic Stress Disorder (NCPTSD, www.ncptsd.va.gov), part of the U.S. Department of Veterans Affairs, 2007.

In the immediate aftermath of a disaster, almost everyone will find themselves unable to stop thinking about what happened. These are called intrusion or re-experiencing symptoms. They will also exhibit high levels of arousal. For most, fear, anxiety, re-experiencing, efforts to avoid reminders, and arousal symptoms, if present, will gradually decrease over time. The expected psychological outcome is recovery, not psychopathology.

What are common stress reactions in the wake of disaster?

Practitioners should remember that most disaster survivors (including children and disaster rescue or relief workers) experience common stress reactions after a traumatic event. These reactions may last for several days or even a few weeks.

Common reactions after disaster include:

- **Emotional reactions:** Shock; fear; grief; anger; guilt; shame; feeling helpless; feeling numb, sadness.

- **Cognitive reactions:** Confusion, indecisiveness, worry, shortened attention span, trouble concentrating.

- **Physical reactions:** Tension, fatigue, edginess, insomnia, bodily aches or pain, startling easily, racing heartbeat, nausea, change in appetite, change in sex drive.

- **Interpersonal reactions:** Distrust, conflict, withdrawal, work or school problems, irritability, loss of intimacy, feeling rejected or abandoned.

What are some more severe reactions to a disaster?

Because stress reactions are so pervasive after a major disaster, it can be difficult to know when a stress reaction is more severe and may require clinical intervention. The following are severe stress symptoms that indicate increased risk for acute stress disorder or posttraumatic stress disorder (PTSD). Even more important than the symptoms listed below is the individual's functional capacity. Symptomatic individuals who can continue to function effectively at work or at home are at much lower risk for developing psychiatric problems that those who are functionally incapacitated.

Severe reactions after disaster include:

- **Intrusive re-experiencing:** Terrifying memories, nightmares, or flashbacks.

- **Extreme emotional numbing:** Completely unable to feel emotion, as if empty.

- **Extreme attempts to avoid disturbing memories:** Such as through substance use.

- **Hyperarousal:** Panic attacks, rage, extreme irritability, intense agitation, violence.

- **Severe anxiety:** Debilitating worry, extreme helplessness, compulsions or obsessions.

- **Severe depression:** Loss of the ability to feel hope, pleasure, or interest; feeling worthless, suicidal ideation or intent.

- **Dissociation:** Fragmented thoughts, spaced out, unaware of surroundings, amnesia.

Which individuals are at risk for severe stress responses?

Some individuals have a higher than typical risk for severe stress symptoms and lasting PTSD, including those with a history of the following risk factors.

- **Trauma and stress:** Severe exposure to the disaster, especially injury, threat to life, and extreme loss. Living in a highly disrupted or traumatized community. High secondary stress.

- **Survivor characteristics:** Female gender, being age 40 and 60, being an ethnic minority, low socioeconomic status, and pre-disaster psychiatric history.

- **Family context:** In an adult survivor, having children in the home. If female, the presence of a spouse. If a child, the presence of parental distress. A significantly distressed family member, interpersonal conflict, or lack of support in the home.

- **Resource context:** Lacking belief in one's ability to cope or few, weak, or deteriorating social resources.

Chapter 41

Posttraumatic Stress Disorder: Chronic Stress after Trauma

Posttraumatic stress disorder (PTSD) is an anxiety disorder that can occur following the experience or witnessing of a traumatic event. A traumatic event is a life-threatening event such as military combat, natural disasters, terrorist incidents, serious accidents, or physical or sexual assault in adult or childhood. Most survivors of trauma return to normal given a little time. However, some people will have stress reactions that do not go away on their own, or may even get worse over time. These individuals may develop PTSD.

People with PTSD experience three different kinds of symptoms. The first set of symptoms involves reliving the trauma in some way such as becoming upset when confronted with a traumatic reminder or thinking about the trauma when you are trying to do something else. The second set of symptoms involves either staying away from places or people that remind you of the trauma, isolating from other people, or feeling numb. The third set of symptoms includes things such as feeling on guard, irritable, or startling easily.

In addition to the symptoms described above, we now know that there are clear biological changes that are associated with PTSD. PTSD is complicated by the fact that people with PTSD often may develop additional disorders such as depression, substance abuse, problems of memory and cognition, and other problems of physical and

"What Is Posttraumatic Stress Disorder (PTSD)?" is from the National Center for Posttraumatic Stress Disorder (www.ncptsd.va.gov), part of the U.S. Department of Veterans Affairs, July 2006.

mental health. These problems may lead to impairment of the person's ability to function in social or family life, including occupational instability, marital problems, and family problems.

PTSD can be treated with psychotherapy (talk therapy) and medicines such as antidepressants. Early treatment is important and may help reduce long-term symptoms. Unfortunately, many people do not know that they have PTSD or do not seek treatment. This information will help you to better understand PTSD and how it can be treated.

How does PTSD develop?

PTSD develops in response to a traumatic event. About 60% of men and 50% of women experience a traumatic event in their lifetime. Most people who are exposed to a traumatic event will have some of the symptoms of PTSD in the days and weeks after the event. For some people these symptoms are more severe and long lasting. The reasons why some people develop PTSD are still being studied. There are biological, psychological, and social factors that affect the development of PTSD.

What are the symptoms of PTSD?

Although PTSD symptoms can begin right after a traumatic event, PTSD is not diagnosed unless the symptoms last for at least one month, and either cause significant distress or interfere with work or home life. In order to be diagnosed with PTSD, a person must have three different types of symptoms: re-experiencing symptoms, avoidance and numbing symptoms, and arousal symptoms.

Re-experiencing symptoms: Re-experiencing symptoms are symptoms that involve reliving the traumatic event. There are a number of ways in which people may relive a trauma. They may have upsetting memories of the traumatic event. These memories can come back when they are not expecting them. At other times the memories may be triggered by a traumatic reminder such as when a combat veteran hears a car backfire, a motor vehicle accident victim drives by a car accident, or a rape victim sees a news report of a recent sexual assault. These memories can cause both emotional and physical reactions. Sometimes these memories can feel so real it is as if the event is actually happening again. This is called a flashback. Reliving the event may cause intense feelings of fear, helplessness, and horror similar to the feelings they had when the event took place.

Avoidance and numbing symptoms: Avoidance symptoms are efforts people make to avoid the traumatic event. Individuals with PTSD may try to avoid situations that trigger memories of the traumatic event. They may avoid going near places where the trauma occurred or seeing TV programs or news reports about similar events. They may avoid other sights, sounds, smells, or people that are reminders of the traumatic event. Some people find that they try and distract themselves as one way to avoid thinking about the traumatic event.

Numbing symptoms are another way to avoid the traumatic event. Individuals with PTSD may find it difficult to be in touch with their feelings or express emotions toward other people. For example, they may feel emotionally "numb" and may isolate from others. They may be less interested in activities you once enjoyed. Some people forget, or are unable to talk about, important parts of the event. Some think that they will have a shortened life span or will not reach personal goals such as having a career or family.

Arousal symptoms: People with PTSD may feel constantly alert after the traumatic event. This is known as increased emotional arousal, and it can cause difficulty sleeping, outbursts of anger or irritability, and difficulty concentrating. They may find that they are constantly on guard and on the lookout for signs of danger. They may also find that they get startled.

What other problems do people with PTSD experience?

It is very common for other conditions to occur along with PTSD, such as depression, anxiety, or substance abuse. More than half of men with PTSD also have problems with alcohol. The next most common co-occurring problems in men are depression, followed by conduct disorder, and then problems with drugs. In women, the most common co-occurring problem is depression. Just under half of women with PTSD also experience depression. The next most common co-occurring problems in women are specific fears, social anxiety, and then problems with alcohol.

People with PTSD often have problems functioning. In general, people with PTSD have more unemployment, divorce or separation, spouse abuse, and chance of being fired than people without PTSD. Vietnam veterans with PTSD were found to have many problems with family and other interpersonal relationships, problems with employment, and increased incidents of violence.

People with PTSD also may experience a wide variety of physical symptoms. This is a common occurrence in people who have depression and other anxiety disorders. Some evidence suggests that PTSD may be associated with increased likelihood of developing medical disorders. Research is ongoing, and it is too soon to draw firm conclusions about which disorders are associated with PTSD.

Chapter 42

Coping with Traumatic Stress Reactions

The Importance of Active Coping

When people take direct action to cope with their stress reactions and trauma-related problems, they put themselves in a position of power. Active coping makes you begin to feel less helpless.

- Active coping means recognizing and accepting the impact of trauma on your life and taking direct action to improve things.

- Active coping occurs even when there is no crisis; coping is an attitude and a habit that must be strengthened.

Understanding the Recovery Process

Knowing how recovery happens puts you in more control of the recovery process.

- Recovery is an ongoing, daily, gradual process. It is not a matter of suddenly being cured.

- Some amount of continued reaction to the traumatic event(s) is normal and reflects a normal body and mind. Healing doesn't mean forgetting traumatic experiences or having no emotional pain when thinking about them.

From the National Center for Posttraumatic Stress Disorder (NCPTSD, www .ncptsd.va.gov), part of the U.S. Department of Veterans Affairs, July 2006.

- Healing may mean fewer symptoms, symptoms that are less disturbing, greater confidence in your ability to cope with your memories and reactions, or an improved ability to manage your emotions.

Coping with Traumatic Stress Reactions: Behaviors That Don't Help

These are behaviors you should not use to cope.

- Using drugs and alcohol to reduce anxiety, relax, stop thinking about experiences, or go to sleep. Alcohol and drug use cause more problems than they cure.

- Keeping away from other people. Social isolation means loss of support, friendship, and closeness with others, and more time to worry or feel hopeless and alone.

- Dropping out of pleasurable or recreational activities. This leads to fewer opportunities to feel good and feel a sense of achievement.

- Using anger to control others. Anger helps keep other people away. Anger may keep bad emotions away temporarily, but it also keeps away positive connections and help from loved ones.

- Trying to constantly avoid people, places, or thoughts that are reminders of the traumatic event. Avoiding thoughts about the trauma or treatment doesn't keep away distress, and it prevents you from making progress on coping with stress reactions.

- Working all the time to try to avoid distressing memories of the trauma (the workaholic).

Coping with Traumatic Stress Reactions: Behaviors That Can Help

There are many ways you can cope with posttraumatic stress. Here are some things you can do if you have any of the following symptoms.

Unwanted Distressing Memories, Images, or Thoughts

- Remind yourself that they are just that: memories.

- Remind yourself that it's natural to have some memories of the traumatic event(s).

- Talk about them to someone you trust.

- Remember that, although reminders of trauma can feel overwhelming, they often lessen with time.

Sudden Feelings of Anxiety or Panic

These are a common part of traumatic stress reactions and include sensations of your heart pounding and feeling lightheaded or spacey (usually caused by rapid breathing). If this happens, remember that:

- These reactions are not dangerous. If you had them while exercising, they probably would not worry you.

- It is the addition of inaccurate frightening thoughts (e.g., I'm going to die, I'm having a heart attack, I will lose control) that makes them especially upsetting.

- Slowing down your breathing may help.

- The sensations will pass soon and you can go about your business after they decrease.

Each time you think in these positive ways about your arousal/anxious reactions, you will be working toward making them happen less frequently. Practice will make it easier to cope.

Feeling Like the Trauma Is Happening Again (Flashbacks)

- Keep your eyes open. Look around you and notice where you are.

- Talk to yourself. Remind yourself where you are, what year you're in, and that you are safe. The trauma happened in the past, and you are in the present.

- Get up and move around. Have a drink of water and wash your hands.

- Call someone you trust and tell them what is happening.

- Remind yourself that this is a common traumatic stress reaction.

- Tell your counselor or doctor about the flashback(s).

Trauma-Related Dreams and Nightmares

If you awaken from a nightmare in a panic, remind yourself that you are reacting to a dream and that's why you are anxious/aroused, not because there is real danger now.

- Consider getting up out of bed, regrouping, and orienting yourself.

- Engage in a pleasant, calming activity (e.g., listen to soothing music).

- Talk to someone if possible.

- Talk to your doctor about your nightmares; certain medications can be helpful.

Difficulty Falling or Staying Asleep

- Keep to a regular bedtime schedule.

- Avoid strenuous exercise for the few hours just before going to bed.

- Avoid using your sleeping area for anything other than sleeping or sexual intimacies.

- Avoid alcohol, tobacco, and caffeine. These harm your ability to sleep.

- Do not lie in bed thinking or worrying. Get up and enjoy something soothing or pleasant; read a calming book, drink a glass of warm milk, or do a quiet hobby.

Irritability, Anger, and Rage

- Take a time out to cool off or think things over. Walk away from the situation.

- Get in the habit of exercising daily. Exercise reduces body tension and helps get the anger out in a positive and productive way.

- Remember that staying angry doesn't work. It actually increases your stress and can cause health problems.

- Talk to your counselor or doctor about your anger. Take classes in anger management.

- If you blow up at family members or friends, find time as soon as you can to talk to them about it. Let them know how you feel and what you are doing to cope with your reactions.

Difficulty Concentrating

- Slow down. Give yourself time to focus on what it is you need to learn or do.

- Write things down. Making to-do lists may be helpful.

- Break tasks down into small doable chunks.

- Plan a realistic number of events or tasks for each day.

- You may be depressed; many people who are depressed have trouble concentrating. Again, this is something you can discuss with your counselor, doctor, or someone close to you.

Having Difficulty Feeling or Expressing Positive Emotions

- Remember that this is a common reaction to trauma, that you are not doing this on purpose, and that you should not feel guilty for something you do not want to happen and cannot control.

- Make sure to regularly participate in activities that you enjoy or used to enjoy. Sometimes, these activities can rekindle feelings of pleasure.

- Take steps to communicate your caring to loved ones in little ways: write a card, leave a small gift, or phone someone and say hello.

A Final Word

Experiment with these ways of coping to find which ones are helpful to you. Practice them; like other skills, they work better with practice. Talk to your counselor or doctor about them. Reach out to people that can help, such as your family and your community. You're not alone.

Chapter 43

Helping Children and Adolescents with Traumatic Stress

Chapter Contents

Section 43.1

Posttraumatic Stress Disorder and the Family

From the National Center for Posttraumatic Stress Disorder (NCPTSD, www.ncptsd.va.gov), part of the U.S. Department of Veterans Affairs, 2007. By Eve B. Carlson, Ph.D. and Joseph Ruzek, Ph.D.

How Does PTSD Affect Family Members?

Because the symptoms of PTSD and other trauma reactions change how a trauma survivor feels and acts, traumatic experiences that happen to one member of a family can affect everyone else in the family. When trauma reactions are severe and go on for some time without treatment, they can cause major problems in a family. This information will describe family members' reactions to the traumatic event and to the survivor's symptoms and behaviors.

It's no wonder that family members react to the fact that their loved one has gone through a trauma. It's upsetting when someone you care about goes through a terrible ordeal. And it's no wonder that people react to the way a traumatized family member feels and acts. Trauma symptoms can make a family member hard to get along with or cause him or her to withdraw from the rest of the family. It can be very difficult for everyone when these changes occur. Just as people have different reactions to traumatic experiences, families also react differently when a loved one is traumatized. In the section that follows, many different types of reactions are described. A family may experience many of these reactions, or only a few. All of the reactions described, however, are common in families who have had to deal with trauma.

Sympathy

One of the first reactions many family members have is sympathy for their loved one. People feel very sorry that someone they care about has had to suffer through a terrifying experience. And they feel sorry when the person continues to suffer from symptoms of PTSD and other trauma responses. It can be helpful for the person who has experienced the trauma to know that his or her family members sympathize with him or her, especially just after the traumatic event occurs.

Sympathy from family members can have a negative effect, though. When family members' sympathy leads them to "baby" a trauma survivor and have low expectations of him or her, it may send a message that the family doesn't believe the trauma survivor is strong enough to overcome the ordeal. For example, if a wife has so much sympathy for her husband that she doesn't expect him to work after a traumatic experience, the husband may think that she doesn't have any confidence in his ability to recover and go back to work.

Depression

One source of depression for family members can be the traumatic event itself. All traumas involve events where people suddenly find themselves in danger. When this happens in a situation or place where people are used to feeling safe, just knowing the event happened could cause a person to lose faith in the safety and predictability of life. For example, if a woman gets mugged in the parking lot of a neighborhood shopping center, her family may find they feel depressed by the idea that they are not really as safe as they thought they were, even in their own neighborhood.

It can also be very depressing when a traumatic event threatens a person's ideals about the world. For instance, if a man gets traumatized in combat by seeing someone tortured, it can be very depressing to know that people are capable of doing such cruel things to each other. Before the man was faced with that event, he may have been able to believe that people are basically good and kind.

Depression is also common among family members when the traumatized person acts in a way that causes feelings of pain or loss. There may be changes in family life when a member has PTSD or other symptoms after trauma. The traumatized person may feel too anxious to go out on family outings as he or she did in the past. The traumatized person may not be able to work because of PTSD symptoms. As a result, the family income may decrease and the family may be unable to buy things and do things the way they did before the traumatic event. A husband may feel unloved or abandoned when—because of her depression—his traumatized wife withdraws emotionally and avoids being intimate or sexual. Children whose father can't be in crowds because of combat trauma may feel hurt that their father won't come to see them play sports. When PTSD lasts for a long time, family members can begin to lose hope that their loved one or their family will ever get "back to normal."

Fear and Worry

Knowing that something terrible can happen "out of the blue" can make people very fearful. This is especially true when a family member feels unsafe and often reminds others about possible dangers. Very often, trauma survivors feel "on edge" and become preoccupied with trying to stay safe. They may want to get a guard dog, or put up security lights, or have weapons in the house in order to protect themselves and their family members. When one person in a family is very worried about safety, it can make everyone else feel unsafe too. However, something that helps one person feel safe—like a loaded weapon under the bed—may make another person feel unsafe.

Family members can also experience fear when the trauma survivor is angry or aggressive. As described above, trauma survivors can become angry and aggressive automatically if they feel they are in danger. Trauma survivors may also become angry and aggressive because they are frustrated that they have trauma symptoms, or because they learned to be aggressive as a way to protect themselves in the trauma situation. No matter what the reason for the anger and aggression, it naturally makes family members fearful.

Many trauma symptoms can cause family members to worry. A wife might worry that her traumatized husband who becomes angry and violent at the least provocation will be injured in a fight or get in trouble with the police. A daughter may worry that her mother will make herself ill by drinking heavily as a result of a traumatic event. A man's inability to keep a job because of trauma-related problems may cause his family to worry constantly about money and the future.

Avoidance

Just as trauma survivors are often afraid to address what happened to them, family members are frequently fearful of examining the traumatic event as well. Family members may want to avoid talking about the trauma or trauma-related problems, even with friends. People who have experienced trauma hope that if they don't talk about the problem, it will go away. People also don't wish to talk about the trauma with others because they are afraid that others won't understand or will judge them. Sometimes, if the traumatic event is one associated with shame, such as rape, family members may avoid talking about the event and its effects because of social "rules" that tell us it is inappropriate to talk about such things. Family members may also not discuss the trauma with others because they fear it will bring their loved one more shame.

Family members may avoid the things that the trauma survivor avoids because they want to spare the survivor further pain, or because they are afraid of his or her reaction. For example, the wife of a combat veteran who is anxious about going out in public may not make plans for family outings or vacations because she is afraid to upset her husband. Though she doesn't know what she can do to "fix" the problem, she does know that if the family goes to a public event, the husband will be anxious and irritable the whole time.

Guilt and Shame

Family members can feel guilt or shame after a traumatic event for a number of reasons. A family member may experience these feelings if he or she feels responsible for the trauma. For instance, a husband whose wife is assaulted may feel guilt or shame because he was unable to protect her from the attack. A wife may feel responsible for her husband's car accident if she thinks she could have prevented it if she had gotten the car's brakes fixed. A family member may feel guilt and shame if he or she feels responsible for the trauma survivor's happiness or general well-being, but sees no improvement no matter how hard he or she tries to help. Sometimes, after years of trauma-related problems in a family, a family member may learn about post-traumatic stress disorder and realize that this is the source of their family problems. The family member may then feel guilty that he or she was unsupportive during the years.

Anger

Anger is a very common problem in families that have survived a trauma. Family members may feel angry about the trauma and its effect on their lives. They may be angry at whomever they believe is responsible for the traumatic event (this includes being angry at God). They can also feel anger toward the trauma survivor. Family members may feel that the survivor should just "forget about it" and get on with life. They may be angry when their loved one continues to "dwell" on the trauma. A wife may be mad because her husband can't keep a job or because he drinks too much or won't go with her to social events or avoids being intimate with her or doesn't take care of the kids. Family members may also feel angry and irritable in response to the anger and irritability the trauma survivor directs at them.

Negative Feelings

Sometimes family members have surprisingly negative feelings about the traumatized family member. They may believe the trauma survivor no longer exhibits the qualities that they loved and admired. A person who was outgoing before a trauma may become withdrawn. A person who was fun-loving and easygoing before a trauma may become ill-tempered. It may be hard to feel good toward a person who seems to have changed in many ways. Family members may also respond negatively to behaviors that develop following a trauma. For instance, family members may be disgusted by a woman's over-drinking in response to a trauma.

Family members may also have negative feelings about the survivor that are directly related to the traumatic event. For example, a wife may no longer respect her husband if she feels he didn't behave bravely during a traumatic event. A husband whose wife was raped may feel disgusted about what happened and wonder if she could have done something to prevent the assault. A son may feel ashamed that his father didn't fight back when he was beaten during a robbery. Sometimes people have these negative feelings even when they know that their assessment of the situation is unfair.

Drug and Alcohol Abuse

Drug and alcohol abuse can become a problem for the families of trauma survivors. Family members may try to escape from bad feelings by using drugs or drinking. A child or spouse may spend time drinking with friends to avoid having to go home and face an angry parent or spouse. On the other hand, spouses sometimes abuse drugs or alcohol to keep their loved ones "company" when they're drinking or using drugs to avoid trauma-related feelings.

Sleep Problems

Sleep can become a problem for family members, especially when it is a problem for the trauma survivor. When the trauma survivor stays up late to avoid going to sleep, can't get to sleep, tosses and turns in his or her sleep, or has nightmares, it is difficult for family members to sleep well. Often family members are also unable to sleep well because they are depressed and/or they are worried about the survivor.

Health Problems

Family members of trauma survivors can develop health problems for a number of reasons. Bad habits, such as drinking, smoking, and not exercising, may worsen as a result of coping with a loved one's trauma responses. In addition, many illnesses can be caused by trauma-related stress if it goes on for an extended period of time. When family members constantly feel anxious, worried, angry, or depressed, they are more likely to develop stomach problems, bowel problems, headaches, muscle pain, and other health problems.

What Can Families Do to Care for Themselves and the Survivor?

Trauma survivors and their families often don't know what to do to care for themselves. First, it is important to continue to learn more about trauma and its effects. Some books are listed below that may be helpful. For veterans, educational classes may be available through a local VA Medical Center or VA Readjustment Counseling Service Vet Center.

Treatment for PTSD is available in most communities through psychologists and social workers in private practice. Insurance may help pay for this treatment. Community mental-health centers and private mental-health clinics (such as those run by charitable or church organizations) may also provide treatment, sometimes at low or reduced fees. To find phone numbers for mental-health professionals, you can look in the yellow pages of your local phone book under "Mental Health Services" and "Therapists."

Veterans can receive treatment at a local VA Medical Center or VA Readjustment Counseling Service Vet Center 1-800-905-4675. Insurance may help pay for treatment at a VA center, and treatment for some veterans is provided at no cost (when their PTSD is determined to be service-related). To find phone numbers for local VA Medical Center or VA Readjustment Counseling Service Vet Centers, you can look in the "Government Pages" of your local phone book under "Veterans Affairs". In that section, look under "Medical Care" for a VA Medical Center phone number and under "Vet Center" for the Readjustment Counseling Service Vet Center phone number.

Family members of a traumatized person should find out as much as they can about PTSD and get help for themselves, even if their loved one doesn't seek treatment. Family members can encourage the survivor to inquire about education and counseling, but they should not pressure or try to force their loved one to get help. Classes or treatment may also be useful for stress and anger management, addiction, couples communication, or parenting.

While in the process of getting help, if family members feel comfortable, they should let their loved one know that they are willing to listen if the survivor would like to talk about his or her trauma. But the family should stop if anyone gets too upset or overwhelmed. If everyone is able, it is also important to talk about how the trauma is affecting the family and what can be done about it.

Suggested Readings

Allen, J. G. (1995). *Coping with Trauma: A Guide to Self-Understanding*. Washington, DC: American Psychiatric Press.

Mason, P. (1990). Recovering *from the War: A Woman's Guide to Helping Your Vietnam Vet, Your Family, and Yourself.*

Matsakis, A. (1996). *Vietnam Wives: Facing the Challenges of Life with Veterans Suffering Post Traumatic Stress* (Sidran Press, 1996, ISBN 1-886968-00-4).

Section 43.2

Helping Children Heal after a Traumatic Event

Excerpted from "Helping Children and Adolescents Cope with Violence and Disasters," a fact sheet by the National Institute of Mental Health (NIMH, www.nimh.nih.gov), part of the National Institutes of Health, 2001. NIH Publication No. 01-3518. Reviewed by David A. Cooke, M.D., April 2007.

Helping young people avoid or overcome emotional problems in the wake of violence or disaster is one of the most important challenges a parent, teacher, or mental health professional can face. The National Institute of Mental Health and other federal agencies are working to address the issue of assisting children and adolescents who have been victims of or witnesses to violent and/or catastrophic events. The purpose of this text is to tell what is known about the impact of violence and disasters on children and adolescents and suggest steps to minimize long-term emotional harm.

In the aftermath of the terrorist attacks on New York City and Washington, D.C., both adults and children struggled with the emotional impact of such large-scale damage and losses of life. Other major acts of violence that have been felt across the country include the 1995 bombing of the Alfred P. Murrah Federal Building in Oklahoma City and the 1999 shootings at Columbine High School in Littleton, Colorado. While these disastrous events have caught the nation's attention, they are only a fraction of the many tragic episodes that affect children's lives. Each year many children and adolescents sustain injuries from violence, lose friends or family members, or are adversely affected by witnessing a violent or catastrophic event. Each situation is unique, whether it centers upon a plane crash where many people are killed, automobile accidents involving friends or family members, or natural disasters such as the Northridge, California Earthquake (1994) or Hurricane Floyd (1999) where deaths occur and homes are lost—but these events have similarities as well and cause similar reactions in children. Even in the course of everyday life, exposure to violence in the home or on the streets can lead to emotional harm.

Research has shown that both adults and children who experience catastrophic events show a wide range of reactions. Some suffer only worries and bad memories that fade with emotional support and the passage of time. Others are more deeply affected and experience long-term problems. Research on posttraumatic stress disorder (PTSD) shows that some soldiers, survivors of criminal victimization, torture and other violence, and survivors of natural and manmade catastrophes suffer long-term effects from their experiences. Children who have witnessed violence in their families, schools, or communities are also vulnerable to serious long-term problems. Their emotional reactions, including fear, depression, withdrawal, or anger, can occur immediately or some time after the tragic event. Youngsters who have experienced a catastrophic event often need support from parents and teachers to avoid long-term emotional harm. Most will recover in a short time, but the few who develop PTSD or other persistent problems need treatment.

Trauma: What Is It?

"Trauma" has both a medical and a psychiatric definition. Medically, "trauma" refers to a serious or critical bodily injury, wound, or shock. This definition is often associated with trauma medicine practiced in emergency rooms and represents a popular view of the term. Psychiatrically, "trauma" has assumed a different meaning and refers to an experience that is emotionally painful, distressful, or shocking, which often results in lasting mental and physical effects.

Psychiatric trauma, or emotional harm, is essentially a normal response to an extreme event. It involves the creation of emotional memories about the distressful event that are stored in structures deep within the brain. In general, it is believed that the more direct the exposure to the traumatic event, the higher the risk for emotional harm. Thus in a school shooting, for example, the student who is injured probably will be most severely affected emotionally; and the student who sees a classmate shot, even killed, is likely to be more emotionally affected than the student who was in another part of the school when the violence occurred. But even secondhand exposure to violence can be traumatic. For this reason, all children and adolescents exposed to violence or a disaster, even if only through graphic media reports, should be watched for signs of emotional distress.

How Children and Adolescents React to Trauma

Reactions to trauma may appear immediately after the traumatic event or days and even weeks later. Loss of trust in adults and fear of the event occurring again are responses seen in many children and adolescents who have been exposed to traumatic events. Other reactions vary according to age:

For children 5 years of age and younger, typical reactions can include a fear of being separated from the parent, crying, whimpering, screaming, immobility and/or aimless motion, trembling, frightened facial expressions and excessive clinging. Parents may also notice children returning to behaviors exhibited at earlier ages (these are called regressive behaviors), such as thumb-sucking, bedwetting, and fear of darkness. Children in this age bracket tend to be strongly affected by the parents' reactions to the traumatic event.

Children 6 to 11 years old may show extreme withdrawal, disruptive behavior, and/or inability to pay attention. Regressive behaviors, nightmares, sleep problems, irrational fears, irritability, refusal to attend school, outbursts of anger, and fighting are also common in traumatized children of this age. Also the child may complain of stomachaches or other bodily symptoms that have no medical basis. Schoolwork often suffers. Depression, anxiety, feelings of guilt, and emotional numbing or "flatness" are often present as well.

Adolescents 12 to 17 years old may exhibit responses similar to those of adults, including flashbacks, nightmares, emotional numbing, avoidance of any reminders of the traumatic event, depression, substance abuse, problems with peers, and anti-social behavior. Also common are withdrawal and isolation, physical complaints, suicidal thoughts, school avoidance, academic decline, sleep disturbances, and confusion. The adolescent may feel extreme guilt over his or her failure to prevent injury or loss of life and may harbor revenge fantasies that interfere with recovery from the trauma.

Some youngsters are more vulnerable to trauma than others, for reasons scientists don't fully understand. It has been shown that the impact of a traumatic event is likely to be greatest in the child or adolescent who previously has been the victim of child abuse or some other form of trauma or who already had a mental health problem. And the youngster who lacks family support is more at risk for a poor recovery.

Helping the Child or Adolescent Trauma Survivor

Early intervention to help children and adolescents who have suffered trauma from violence or a disaster is critical. Parents, teachers, and mental health professionals can do a great deal to help these youngsters recover. Help should begin at the scene of the traumatic event.

According to the National Center for Posttraumatic Stress Disorder of the Department of Veterans Affairs, workers in charge of a disaster scene should:

- Find ways to protect children from further harm and from further exposure to traumatic stimuli. If possible, create a safe haven for them. Protect children from onlookers and the media covering the story.

- When possible, direct children who are able to walk away from the site of violence or destruction, away from severely injured survivors, and away from continuing danger. Kind but firm direction is needed.

- Identify children in acute distress and stay with them until initial stabilization occurs. Acute distress includes panic (marked by trembling, agitation, rambling speech, becoming mute, or erratic behavior) and intense grief (signs include loud crying, rage, or immobility).

- Use a supportive and compassionate verbal or non-verbal exchange (such as a hug, if appropriate) with the child to help him or her feel safe. However brief the exchange, or however temporary, such reassurances are important to children.

After violence or a disaster occurs, the family is the first-line resource for helping. Among the things that parents and other caring adults can do are:

- Explain the episode of violence or disaster as well as you are able.

- Encourage the children to express their feelings and listen without passing judgment. Help younger children learn to use words that express their feelings. However, do not force discussion of the traumatic event.

- Let children and adolescents know that it is normal to feel upset after something bad happens.

- Allow time for the youngsters to experience and talk about their feelings. At home, however, a gradual return to routine can be reassuring to the child.

- If your children are fearful, reassure them that you love them and will take care of them. Stay together as a family as much as possible.

- If behavior at bedtime is a problem, give the child extra time and reassurance. Let him or her sleep with a light on or in your room for a limited time if necessary.

- Reassure children and adolescents that the traumatic event was not their fault.

- Do not criticize regressive behavior or shame the child with words like "babyish."

- Allow children to cry or be sad. Don't expect them to be brave or tough.

- Encourage children and adolescents to feel in control. Let them make some decisions about meals, what to wear, etc.

- Take care of yourself so you can take care of the children.

When violence or disaster affects a whole school or community, teachers and school administrators can play a major role in the healing process. Some of the things educators can do are:

- If possible, give yourself a bit of time to come to terms with the event before you attempt to reassure the children. This may not be possible in the case of a violent episode that occurs at school, but sometimes in a natural disaster there will be several days before schools reopen and teachers can take the time to prepare themselves emotionally.

- Don't try to rush back to ordinary school routines too soon. Give the children or adolescents time to talk over the traumatic event and express their feelings about it.

- Respect the preferences of children who do not want to participate in class discussions about the traumatic event. Do not force discussion or repeatedly bring up the catastrophic event; doing so may re-traumatize children.

- Hold in-school sessions with entire classes, with smaller groups of students, or with individual students. These sessions can be very useful in letting students know that their fears and concerns are normal reactions. Many counties and school districts have teams that will go into schools to hold such sessions after a disaster or episode of violence. Involve mental health professionals in these activities if possible.

- Offer art and play therapy for young children in school.

- Be sensitive to cultural differences among the children. In some cultures, for example, it is not acceptable to express negative emotions. Also, the child who is reluctant to make eye contact with a teacher may not be depressed, but may simply be exhibiting behavior appropriate to his or her culture.

- Encourage children to develop coping and problem-solving skills and age-appropriate methods for managing anxiety.

- Hold meetings for parents to discuss the traumatic event, their children's response to it, and how they and you can help. Involve mental health professionals in these meetings if possible.

Most children and adolescents, if given support such as that described above, will recover almost completely from the fear and anxiety caused by a traumatic experience within a few weeks. However, some children and adolescents will need more help perhaps over a longer period of time in order to heal. Grief over the loss of a loved one, teacher, friend, or pet may take months to resolve, and may be reawakened by reminders such as media reports or the anniversary of the death.

In the immediate aftermath of a traumatic event, and in the weeks following, it is important to identify the youngsters who are in need of more intensive support and therapy because of profound grief or some other extreme emotion. Children and adolescents who may require the help of a mental health professional include those who show avoidance behavior, such as resisting or refusing to go places that remind them of the place where the traumatic event occurred, and emotional numbing, a diminished emotional response or lack of feeling toward the event. Youngsters who have more common reactions including re-experiencing the trauma, or reliving it in the form of nightmares and disturbing recollections during the day, and hyperarousal, including sleep disturbances and a tendency to be easily startled, may respond well to supportive reassurance from parents and teachers.

Posttraumatic Stress Disorder

As mentioned earlier, some children and adolescents will have prolonged problems after a traumatic event. These potentially chronic conditions include depression and prolonged grief. Another serious and potentially long-lasting problem is posttraumatic stress disorder (PTSD). This condition is diagnosed when the following symptoms have been present for longer than one month:

- Re-experiencing the event through play or in trauma-specific nightmares or flashbacks, or distress over events that resemble or symbolize the trauma.

- Routine avoidance of reminders of the event or a general lack of responsiveness (e.g., diminished interests or a sense of having a foreshortened future).

- Increased sleep disturbances, irritability, poor concentration, startle reaction, and regressive behavior.

Rates of PTSD identified in child and adult survivors of violence and disasters vary widely. For example, estimates range from 2 percent after a natural disaster (tornado), 28 percent after an episode of terrorism (mass shooting), and 29 percent after a plane crash.

The disorder may arise weeks or months after the traumatic event. PTSD may resolve without treatment, but some form of therapy by a mental health professional is often required in order for healing to occur. Fortunately, it is more common for traumatized individuals to have some of the symptoms of PTSD than to develop the full-blown disorder.

As noted above, people differ in their vulnerability to PTSD, and the source of this difference is not known in its entirety. Researchers have identified factors that interact to influence vulnerability to developing PTSD. These factors include:

- characteristics of the trauma exposure itself (e.g., proximity to trauma, severity, and duration),

- characteristics of the individual (e.g., prior trauma exposures, family history/prior psychiatric illness, gender—women are at greatest risk for many of the most common assaultive traumas), and

- post-trauma factors (e.g., availability of social support, emergence of avoidance/numbing, hyperarousal and re-experiencing symptoms).

Research has shown that PTSD clearly alters a number of fundamental brain mechanisms. Abnormal levels of brain chemicals that affect coping behavior, learning, and memory have been detected among people with the disorder. In addition, recent imaging studies have discovered altered metabolism and blood flow in the brain as well as structural brain changes in people with PTSD.

Treatment of PTSD

People with PTSD are treated with specialized forms of psychotherapy and sometimes with medications or a combination of the two. One of the forms of psychotherapy shown to be effective is cognitive behavioral therapy, or CBT. In CBT, the patient is taught methods of overcoming anxiety or depression and modifying undesirable behaviors such as avoidance of reminders of the traumatic event. The therapist helps the patient examine and re-evaluate beliefs that are interfering with healing, such as the belief that the traumatic event will happen again. Children who undergo CBT are taught to avoid "catastrophizing." For example, they are reassured that dark clouds do not necessarily mean another hurricane, that the fact that someone is angry doesn't necessarily mean that another shooting is imminent, etc. Play therapy and art therapy also can help younger children to remember the traumatic event safely and express their feelings about it. Other forms of psychotherapy that have been found to help persons with PTSD include group and exposure therapy. A reasonable period of time for treatment of PTSD is 6 to 12 weeks with occasional follow-up sessions, but treatment may be longer depending on a patient's particular circumstances. Research has shown that support from family and friends can be an important part of recovery.

There has been a good deal of research on the use of medications for adults with PTSD, including research on the formation of emotionally charged memories and medications that may help block the development of symptoms. Medications appear to be useful in reducing overwhelming symptoms of arousal (such as sleep disturbances and an exaggerated startle reflex), intrusive thoughts, and avoidance; reducing accompanying conditions such as depression and panic; and improving impulse control and related behavioral problems. Research is just beginning on the use of medications to treat PTSD in children and adolescents.

There is accumulating empirical evidence that trauma/grief-focused psychotherapy and selected pharmacologic interventions can be effective in alleviating PTSD symptoms and in addressing co-occurring depression. However, more medication treatment research is needed.

A mental health professional with special expertise in the area of child and adolescent trauma is the best person to help a youngster with PTSD. Organizations on the accompanying resource list may help you to find such a specialist in your geographical area.

What Are Scientists Learning about Trauma in Children and Adolescents?

The National Institute of Mental Health (NIMH), a part of the federal government's National Institutes of Health, supports research on the brain and a wide range of mental disorders, including PTSD and related conditions. The Department of Veterans Affairs also conducts research in this area with adults and their family members.

Recent research findings include:

- Some studies show that counseling children very soon after a catastrophic event may reduce some of the symptoms of PTSD. A study of trauma/grief-focused psychotherapy among early adolescents exposed to an earthquake found that brief psychotherapy was effective in alleviating PTSD symptoms and preventing the worsening of co-occurring depression.

- Parents' responses to a violent event or disaster strongly influence their children's ability to recover. This is particularly true for mothers of young children. If the mother is depressed or highly anxious, she may need to get emotional support or counseling in order to be able to help her child.

- Either being exposed to violence within the home for an extended period of time or exposure to a one-time event like an attack by a dog can cause PTSD in a child.

- Community violence can have a profound effect on teachers as well as students. One study of Head Start teachers who lived through the 1992 Los Angeles riots showed that 7 percent had severe posttraumatic stress symptoms, and 29 percent had moderate symptoms. Children also were acutely affected by the violence and anxiety around them. They were more aggressive and noisy and less likely to be obedient or get along with each other.

- Research has demonstrated that PTSD after exposure to a variety of traumatic events (family violence, child abuse, disasters, and community violence) is often accompanied by depression. Depression must be treated along with PTSD, and early treatment is best.

- Inner-city children experience the greatest exposure to violence. A study of young adolescent boys from inner-city Chicago showed that 68 percent had seen someone beaten up and 22.5 percent

407

had seen someone shot or killed. Youngsters who had been exposed to community violence were more likely to exhibit aggressive behavior or depression within the following year.

NIMH-supported scientists are continuing to conduct research into the impact of violence and disaster on children and adolescents. For example, one study will follow 6,000 Chicago children from 80 different neighborhoods over a period of several years.

It will examine the emotional, social, and academic effects of exposure to violence. In some of the children, the researchers will look at the role of stress hormones in a child or adolescent's response to traumatic experiences. Another study will deal specifically with the victims of school violence, attempting to determine what places children at risk for victimization at school and what factors protect them.

It is particularly important to conduct research to discover which individual, family, school, and community interventions work best for children and adolescents exposed to violence or disaster, and to find out whether a well-intended but ill-designed intervention could set the youngsters back by keeping the trauma alive in their minds. Through research, NIMH hopes to gain knowledge to lessen the suffering that violence and disasters impose on children and adolescents and their families.

Section 43.3

Tips on Helping Children Cope with Fear and Anxiety

"How Families Can Help Children Cope with Fear and Anxiety" is from the Substance Abuse and Mental Health Services Administration (SAMHSA, www.samhsa.gov), June 2002.

Whether tragic events touch your family personally or are brought into your home via newspapers and television, you can help children cope with the anxiety that violence, death, and disasters can cause.

Listening and talking to children about their concerns can reassure them that they will be safe. Start by encouraging them to discuss how they have been affected by what is happening around them. Even young children may have specific questions about tragedies. Children react to stress at their own developmental level.

Here are some pointers for parents and other caregivers:

- **Encourage children to ask questions:** Listen to what they say. Provide comfort and assurance that address their specific fears. It's okay to admit you can't answer all of their questions.

- **Talk on their level:** Communicate with your children in a way they can understand. Don't get too technical or complicated.

- **Find out what frightens them:** Encourage your children to talk about fears they may have. They may worry that someone will harm them at school or that someone will try to hurt you.

- **Focus on the positive:** Reinforce the fact that most people are kind and caring. Remind your child of the heroic actions taken by ordinary people to help victims of tragedy.

- **Pay attention:** Your children's play and drawings may give you a glimpse into their questions or concerns. Ask them to tell you what is going on in the game or the picture. It's an opportunity to clarify any misconceptions, answer questions, and give reassurance.

- **Develop a plan:** Establish a family emergency plan for the future, such as a meeting place where everyone should gather if something unexpected happens in your family or neighborhood. It can help you and your children feel safer.

If you are concerned about your child's reaction to stress or trauma, call your physician or a community mental health center.

Section 43.4

Age-Specific Interventions for Your Traumatized Child or Adolescent

From "Age-specific Interventions at Home for Children in Trauma: From Preschool to Adolescence," a fact sheet from the Substance Abuse and Mental Health Services Administration (SAMHSA, www.samhsa.gov), October 2002.

Children are just as affected as adults are by a disaster or traumatic event. Some may be affected even more, but no one realizes it. Without intending to, we, as parents, may send our children a message that it is not all right to talk about the experience. This may cause confusion, self-doubt, and feelings of helplessness for a child. Children need to hear that it is normal to feel frightened during and after a disaster or traumatic event. When you acknowledge and normalize these feelings for your children, it will help them make peace with their experience and move on. Following exposure to a disaster or traumatic event, children are likely to show signs of stress. Signs include sadness and anxiety, outbursts and tantrums, aggressive behavior, a return to earlier behavior that was outgrown, stomachaches and headaches, and an ongoing desire to stay home from school or away from friends. These reactions are normal and usually do not last long. Whether your child is a preschooler, adolescent, or somewhere in between, you can help your child by following these suggestions.

Preschooler

- Stick to regular family routines.

- Make an extra effort to provide comfort and reassurance.
- Avoid unnecessary separations.
- Permit a child to sleep in the parents' room temporarily.
- Encourage expression of feelings and emotions through play, drawing, puppet shows, and storytelling.
- Limit media exposure.
- Develop a safety plan for future incidents.

Elementary-Age Children

- Provide extra attention and consideration.
- Set gentle but firm limits for acting out behavior.
- Listen to a child's repeated telling of his or her trauma experience.
- Encourage expression of thoughts and feelings through conversation and play.
- Provide home chores and rehabilitation activities that are structured, but not too demanding.
- Rehearse safety measures for future incidents.
- Point out kind deeds and the ways in which people helped each other during the disaster or traumatic event.

Preadolescents and Adolescents

- Provide extra attention and consideration.
- Be there to listen to your children, but don't force them to talk about feelings and emotions.
- Encourage discussion of trauma experiences among peers.
- Promote involvement with community recovery work.
- Urge participation in physical activities.
- Encourage resumption of regular social and recreational activities.
- Rehearse family safety measures for future incidents.
- It is important to remember that you do not have to "fix" how your child feels.

- Instead, focus on helping your child understand and deal with his or her experiences.

- Healing is an evolving state for most children, but some may need professional help.

- If signs of stress do not subside after a few weeks, or if they get worse, consider consulting a mental health professional who has special training in working with children. In time and with help, your children will learn that life does go on.

Chapter 44

Posttraumatic Stress Disorder and the Risk of Suicide

This information explores the relationship between posttraumatic stress disorder (PTSD) and suicide. It also addresses important questions about understanding and coping with suicide. This information is not intended to replace mental health assistance obtained from a professional.

Does PTSD Increase an Individual's Suicide Risk?

A large body of research indicates that there is a correlation between PTSD and suicide. There is evidence that traumatic events such as sexual abuse, combat trauma, rape, and domestic violence generally increase a person's suicide risk. Considerable debate exists, however, about the reason for this increase. Whereas some studies suggest that suicide risk is higher due to the symptoms of PTSD, others claim that suicide risk is higher in these individuals because of related psychiatric conditions. Some studies that point to PTSD as the cause of suicide suggest that high levels of intrusive memories can predict the relative risk of suicide. High levels of arousal symptoms and low levels of avoidance have also been shown to predict suicide risk. In contrast, other researchers have found that conditions that co-occur with PTSD, such as depression, may be more predictive of suicide. Furthermore, some cognitive styles of coping, such as using suppression to

"PTSD and Suicide," is a fact sheet by William Hudenko, Ph.D., from the National Center for PTSD (www.ncptsd.va.gov), part of the U.S. Department of Veterans Affairs, April 2007.

deal with stress, may be additionally predictive of suicide risk in individuals with PTSD.

Given the high rate of PTSD in veterans, considerable research has examined the relationship between PTSD and suicide in this population. Multiple factors contribute to suicide risk in veterans. Some of the most common factors are listed below:

- male gender
- alcohol abuse
- family history of suicide
- older age
- poor social-environmental support (exemplified by homelessness and unmarried status)
- possession of firearms
- the presence of medical and psychiatric conditions (including combat-related PTSD) associated with suicide

Currently there is debate about the exact influence of combat-related trauma on suicide risk. For those veterans who have PTSD as a result of combat trauma, however, it appears that the highest relative suicide risk is in veterans who were wounded multiple times or hospitalized for a wound. This suggests that the intensity of the combat trauma, and the number of times it occurred, may influence suicide risk in veterans with PTSD. Other research on veterans with combat-related PTSD suggests that the most significant predictor of both suicide attempts and preoccupation with suicide is combat-related guilt. Many veterans experience highly intrusive thoughts and extreme guilt about acts committed during times of war. These thoughts can often overpower the emotional coping capacities of veterans.

Reasons for Suicide

Individuals who have lost someone to suicide often question why that person chose to end his or her life. Unfortunately, there is no easy answer to this question. Suicide often appears to be related to environmental stresses or traumatic events, but it is also the case that some individuals commit suicide without any identifiable reason. Although survivors will always feel devastation and confusion when a loved one commits suicide, available research may help survivors better understand some common reasons for suicide.

Specific reasons for suicide are as diverse as the individuals who commit it. Nevertheless, there are some common causal factors that appear to be related to suicide. For example, more than 90% of suicide victims have a significant psychiatric illness at the time of their death. These illnesses are often both undiagnosed and untreated. The two most common psychiatric conditions associated with suicide are mood disorders and substance abuse. When an individual has both a mood disorder and a substance abuse issue, the risk of suicide is much higher. This is especially the case for adolescents and young adults. This research suggests that the presence of mental illness is a primary contributor to the cause of suicide. For individuals who suffer from clinical depression specifically, of utmost concern are those who exhibit open aggression, anxiety, or agitation, as these factors significantly increase the risk of suicide.

Some researchers suggest that suicide can be understood as a type of coping mechanism for individuals who feel overwhelmed and trapped by their situations. For these people, suicide is seen as a way of dealing with extremely strong negative emotions through escape. This conceptualization of suicide is exemplified by the relation between suicide rates and media coverage, particularly in the young. Research reveals that the magnitude of increase in suicides following a suicide story is proportional to the amount, duration, and prominence of media coverage. These data suggest that suicide is more likely to occur when it is no longer perceived as "taboo" and instead is seen as a viable coping method for stress. This hypothesis of suicide as a coping device is further supported by evidence that a family history of suicide greatly increases an individual's suicide risk, regardless of the presence of mental illness.

When trying to understand suicide, some helpful questions to consider are:

- Did the individual ever receive treatment for depression or another mental disorder?

- Did the individual have a problem with substance abuse?

- Did the individual have a history of suicide attempts?

- Did the individual have a family history of suicide attempts?

Suicide as a Traumatic Event

A considerable amount of research examines exposure to suicide as a traumatic event. Studies show that trauma from exposure to suicide can contribute to PTSD. In particular, adults and adolescents are more likely to develop PTSD as a result of exposure to suicide if one or more of the following conditions are true: if they witness the suicide, if they are very connected with the person who dies, or if they have a history of psychiatric illness. However, relative to other traumatic events, there appears to be nothing unique about developing PTSD as a consequence of exposure to suicide. Studies do show, however, that traumatic grief is more likely to arise after exposure to traumatic death such as suicide. Traumatic grief refers to a syndrome in which individuals experience functional impairment, a decline in physical health, and suicidal ideation. These symptoms occur independent of other conditions such as depression and anxiety.

What Can I Do?

I Am Suicidal

Everyone feels down occasionally. Feeling suicidal, however, is not normal. If you have thoughts about hurting yourself, it is important to seek professional help. Many people who experience suicidal thoughts also struggle with a mood disorder or substance abuse problem. If you think you may have one of these conditions, there are many places to seek help. For conditions such as PTSD, depression, or substance abuse, helpful treatments include medication from a primary care physician or psychiatrist, and therapy from a mental health provider such as a psychologist. To locate a mental health provider near you, call your doctor's office or ask a friend for a recommendation. The following link may also be a helpful way to locate a mental health professional: http://www.mentalhealth.samhsa.gov/databases. If you work for a large company or organization, call the human resources office to find out if they provide mental health services or make referrals. If you are ever considering suicide and feel unsafe, you may call the following hotline (available 24 hours a day) to speak with someone who can help: 800-273-TALK (800-273-8255) (en Español 888-628-9454).

If you do not struggle with a psychiatric illness, you may need to learn additional coping strategies for high levels of stress. There are many therapeutic treatments that could be helpful in this situation. Consider using one of the methods mentioned above to locate a mental health professional near you.

Someone I Know Is Suicidal

It is likely that sometime during your life you will be exposed to a family member, peer, or coworker who is feeling suicidal. When someone discloses information about feeling suicidal, the information can be overwhelming, anxiety provoking, and frightening. This is particularly true if the disclosure is made in confidence and you feel pressure not to share the information with others. If someone you know is thinking about suicide, the issue should be taken very seriously. Individuals who contemplate suicide may not necessarily take action, but evaluating the risk can be complicated and should be done by a qualified mental health professional.

Helping a suicidal individual can be a difficult process. The person's age will influence your first course of action. If your acquaintance is an adult, try to be supportive and listen to his or her concerns. Next, encourage that person to seek treatment immediately. Help the person with this process by remaining calm and providing information about mental health options in the area. Call 800-273-TALK (800-273-8255) or visit http://www.mentalhealth.samhsa.gov/databases to obtain referral information.

Often the most difficult part of obtaining treatment is the initial call to a mental health professional. It is usually easier for a suicidal individual to accept professional help if they have assistance with this part of the process. The decision to seek treatment is typically voluntary for adults. Their ability to maintain safety will determine the treatment options. Options include outpatient therapy, medication management, and inpatient treatment. Inpatient hospital visits are typically only prescribed when an individual is no longer safe without supervision. Sometimes involuntary hospital admission is necessary. However, because of federal laws protecting adult civil rights, this course of action in uncommon. Involuntary admission only occurs when an individual demonstrates unsafe behavior. If you feel that your acquaintance may hurt him- or herself or others, contact your local police department for assistance.

If the person with suicidal thoughts is a minor (under the age of 18), it is important to contact the minor's parent or legal guardian. If the caregiver is unwilling or unable to take action, contact a mental health professional or law enforcement agent for assistance. United States federal law states that individuals under the age of 18 are not able to make mental health treatment decisions. Therefore, it is important that responsible adults see that minors receive the appropriate services. Treatment options for children and adolescents are similar to those outlined for adults. Unlike adults, however, minors may receive inpatient hospitalization without their consent if it is deemed necessary by their parents or the legal system.

While helping a suicidal person can be a difficult process, remember that the assistance you provide could save someone's life.

Someone I Know Has Committed Suicide

It is always difficult to cope when an acquaintance commits suicide. Overcoming the suicide will be particularly challenging if you were emotionally close to the victim, if you witnessed the event, or if you have a prior history of psychiatric illness. Additional factors that complicate the grieving process include low socioeconomic status and low social support. Grieving the loss of a loved one is a natural process. It may take several months to feel "normal" again after your acquaintance commits suicide. Due to the traumatic nature of suicide, you may experience traumatic grief as part of the healing process. If you experience pronounced levels of grief several months after the suicide, contact a mental health professional for assistance. Lastly, many people experience intense guilt following the suicide of an acquaintance. This feeling is often related to thoughts about being unable to prevent the suicide. Suicide is never your fault. It is a complicated and difficult phenomenon to understand, with many contributing factors. To gain a better understanding of suicide or the grieving process, consider finding a mental health provider at http://www.mentalhealth.samhsa.gov/databases.

References

1. Amir, M., Kaplan, Z., Efroni, R., & Kotler, M. (1999). Suicide risk and coping styles in posttraumatic stress disorder patients. *Psychotherapy and Psychosomatics,* 68(2), 76–81.

2. Andress, V. R., & Corey, D. M. (1978). Survivor-victims: Who discovers or witnesses suicide? *Psychological Reports,* 42(3, Pt 1), 759–764.

3. Barraclough, B., & Hughes, J. (1987). *Suicide: Clinical and epidemiological studies.* New York, NY: Croom Helm.

4. Ben-Ya'acov, Y., & Amir, M. (2004). Posttraumatic symptoms and suicide risk. *Personality and Individual Differences,* 36, 1257–1264.

5. Brent, D. A., Perper, J. A., Moritz, G., Allman, C., Friend, A., Roth, C., et al. (1993a). Psychiatric risk factors for adolescent suicide: A case-control study. *Journal of the American Academy of Child and Adolescent Psychiatry,* 32(3), 521–529.

6. Brent, D. A., Perper, J. A., Moritz, G., Friend, A., Schweers, J., Allman, C., et al. (1993b). Adolescent witnesses to a peer suicide.

Journal of the American Academy of Child and Adolescent Psychiatry, 32(6), 1184–1188.

7. Brent, D. A., Perper, J. A., Moritz, G., Liotus, L., Richardson, D., Canobbio, R., et al. (1995). Posttraumatic stress disorder in peers of adolescent suicide victims: Predisposing factors and phenomenology. *Journal of the American Academy of Child and Adolescent Psychiatry,* 34(2), 209–215.

8. Bullman, T. A., & Kang, H. K. (1995). A study of suicide among Vietnam veterans. *Federal Practitioner,* 12(3), 9–13.

9. Conwell, Y., Duberstein, P. R., Cox, C., Herrmann, J. H., Forbes, N. T., Caine, E. D. (1996). Relationship of age and axis I diagnoses in victims of completed suicide: A psychological autopsy study. *American Journal of Psychiatry,* 153(8), 1001–1008.

10. Dyregrov, K., Nordanger, D., & Dyregrov, A. (2003). Predictors of psychosocial distress after suicide, SIDS and accidents. *Death Studies,* 27(2), 143–165.

11. Fawcett, J. (1990). Targeting treatment in patients with mixed symptoms of anxiety and depression. *Journal of Clinical Psychiatry,* 51(11), 40–43.

12. Fontana, A., & Rosenheck, R. (1995). Attempted suicide among Vietnam veterans: A model of etiology in a community sample. *American Journal of Psychiatry,* 152(1), 102–109.

13. Gould, M., Jamieson, P., & Romer, D. (2003). Media contagion and suicide among the young. *American Behavioral Scientist,* 46(9), 1269–1284.

14. Gould, M. S. (2001). Suicide and the media. In H. Hendin & J. J. Mann (Eds.), The clinical science of suicide prevention. *Annals of the New York Academy of Sciences,* vol. 932 (pp. 200–224). New York, NY: New York Academy of Sciences.

15. Hendin, H., & Haas, A. P. (1991). Suicide and guilt as manifestations of PTSD in Vietnam combat veterans. *American Journal of Psychiatry,* 148(5), 586–591.

16. Kotler, M., Iancu, I., Efroni, R., & Amir, M. (2001). Anger, impulsivity, social support, and suicide risk in patients with

posttraumatic stress disorder. *Journal of Nervous & Mental Disease,* 189(3), 162–167.

17. Mann, J. J., Waternaux, C., Haas, G. L., & Malone, K. M. (1999). Toward a clinical model of suicidal behavior in psychiatric patients. *American Journal of Psychiatry,* 156(2), 181–189.

18. Melhem, N. M., Day, N., Shear, M. K., Day, R., Reynolds, C. F., & Brent, D. A. (2004). Traumatic grief among adolescents exposed to a peer's suicide. *American Journal of Psychiatry,* 161(8), 1411–1416.

19. Murphy, S. A., Johnson, L. C., Wu, L., Fan, J. J., & Lohan, J. (2003). Bereaved parents' outcomes 4 to 60 months after their children's deaths by accident, suicide, or homicide: A comparative study demonstrating differences. *Death Studies,* 27(1), 29–61.

20. Prigerson, H. G., Shear, M. K., Jacobs, S. C., Reynolds, C. F. I., Maciejewsk, P. K., Davidson, J. R., et al. (1999). Consensus criteria for traumatic grief: A preliminary empirical test. *British Journal of Psychiatry,* 174, 67–73.

21. Qin, P., Agerbo, E., & Mortensen, P. B. (2002). Suicide risk in relation to family history of completed suicide and psychiatric disorders: A nested case-control study based on longitudinal registers. *Lancet,* 360(9340), 1126–1130.

22. Robison, B. K. (2002). Suicide risk in Vietnam veterans with posttraumatic stress disorder. Unpublished Doctoral Dissertation, Pepperdine University.

23. Runeson, B., & Asberg, M. (2003). Family history of suicide among suicide victims. *American Journal of Psychiatry,* 160(8), 1525–1526.

24. Shaffer, D., Gould, M. S., Fisher, P., Trautman, P., Moreau, D., Kleinman, M., et al. (1996). Psychiatric diagnosis in child and adolescent suicide. *Archives of General Psychiatry,* 53(4), 339–348.

25. Soloff, P. H., Lynch, K. G., Kelly, T. M., Malone, K. M., & Mann, J. J. (2000). Characteristics of suicide attempts of patients with major depressive episode and borderline personality disorder:

A comparative study. *American Journal of Psychiatry,* 157(4), 601–608.

26. Stroebe, W., & Stroebe, M. (1987). Bereavement as a stressful life event: A paradigm for research on the stress-health relationship? In G. R. Semin (Ed.), *Issues in contemporary German social psychology: History, theories and application* (pp. 258–272). Thousand Oaks, CA: Sage Publications, Inc.

27. Thompson, M. E., Kaslow, N. J., Kingree, J. B., Puett, R., Thompson, N. J., & Meadows, L. (1999). Partner abuse and posttraumatic stress disorder as risk factors for suicide attempts in a sample of low-income, inner-city women. *Journal of Traumatic Stress,* 12(1), 59–72.

Chapter 45

Helping Friends in Trouble: Suicide Danger Signals

We all have bad days, or weeks, or even months. We all feel overwhelmed at times. Things usually get better. Sometimes that's hard to remember when you're down. But stress, depression, and even suicide happen in the lives of people young and old.

Problems get people down. We feel tense, fearful, or angry because things are changing—they seem out of control. It's hard to manage. More than 2,000 Minnesota junior and senior high school students were asked how they handle serious problems in their lives. Can you guess what they said? They either try to handle the problem themselves or talk to their friends. It's important to think about how to help yourself as well as a friend who comes to you.

How People React to Stress and Problems

Failure on a test, a fight with a friend, an argument with a parent, or a put-down by a teacher can be upsetting. Many things that cause problems are beyond our control: parents divorcing, a family moving away, the death of someone close to us, or family financial problems. We all know someone who has broken up with a boyfriend or girlfriend, feared pregnancy, gotten in trouble with the law, or felt utterly deserted and alone.

"Helping Friends in Trouble: Stress, Depression and Suicide," by Joyce Walker, © 2005 University of Minnesota Extension. Reprinted with permission.

There are three basic ways of reacting to the problem:

1. You can get angry—scream, shout, throw things, start a fight, or go on a rampage.

2. You can withdraw—take a drink, shut up in a room, take a pill, daydream, stop talking to everyone.

3. You can take charge—think out the problem, try to find a solution, ask for help, or work for change.

Unhealthy Ways to React to Problems

Aggression and anger get attention. Striking out at whomever seems responsible for the problem brings temporary relief. But aggressive actions, like drinking too much, driving recklessly, swearing at people, and breaking up things, can cause trouble in the long run. They don't usually solve the problem.

Withdrawal can also be destructive. It's normal to react, "Just leave me alone!" But if it goes on for a long time, we are without what we need most—sharing, understanding, and help. Alone with a problem, we feel like no one cares. The depression and anger become worse, and we begin to make bad choices instead of healthy ones.

Healthy Ways to React to Problems

When your stomach churns, your head aches, and fear creeps through your insides, your mind and body are reacting to stress. There are a number of things you can do, such as:

• talk to someone you trust;

• share what is bothering you;

• listen to music and relax;

• get some physical exercise;

• do something that normally gives you pleasure; or

• give yourself a chance to think.

These are first-aid actions. They don't solve the problem, but you can blow off some steam. Once that's done, it's a good idea to get in touch with someone you trust and respect. This could be a friend, a friend's parent, a coach, or someone you work with. Go have a good talk; lay out the problem and try to figure out some ways to solve it.

Warning Signs of Trouble

Be aware of real trouble signs. Any one of these alone, lasting only a short time, is normal. But if you know a friend with several of these problems lasting more than a couple of weeks, he or she may be nearing a crisis. The person needs help. The warning signs can include:

- avoiding friends, activities, school, or social events;
- totally unable to think of anything but the problem;
- unexpected outbursts of anger or crying;
- unable to sleep; always feeling exhausted, or irritated;
- unable to eat; or eating and vomiting;
- escaping by sleeping or daydreaming all the time;
- severe behavior change—quiet person becoming wild or active;
- person becoming withdrawn; or
- excessive use of drugs or alcohol.

There are four other signals that should be taken particularly seriously.

Suicide Danger Signals

- Threats or talk of killing himself or herself
- Preparing for death—giving away prized possessions, making a will, writing farewell letters, gathering pills, or saying goodbye
- Talking like there is no hope even in the future
- Acting or talking like not a single person cares; completely giving up on himself or herself and others

Support You Can Offer to Friends

- **Take the problem seriously:** Even if the problem doesn't seem real important to you, it may be important to him or her. Things may be piling up. Show the person you understand.
- **Don't put the person down:** It doesn't help to say, "Things will be better tomorrow" or "Keep your chin up!" The problem is real to him or her.

425

- **Encourage the person to talk to other people as well as to you:** Offer to go along with him or her to talk with some adult friend he or she can trust.

- **Offer to join the person in some activity he or she normally enjoys:** The person needs a chance to have some fun and get his or her mind cleared.

- **Let the person know you care:** He or she may try to put you off. Stay in touch. Reach out. Invite him or her to do things with you. Don't force the person to be cheerful. Stick with him or her.

Remember CLUES—Five Action Steps to Help a Troubled Person

- **C**—Connect. Make contact. Reach out, talk to him or her. Notice his or her pain.

- **L**—Listen. Take the time and really pay attention. You don't have to have all the answers. Just listen.

- **U**—Understand. Nod, pay attention, let him or her know you appreciate what he or she is going through.

- **E**—Express concern. Say that you care, you are worried, and you want to be helpful.

- **S**—Seek help. Tell the person you want to go with him or her to talk to a third person, preferably an adult with experience and the ability to help. Don't agree to be secretive. Enlarge the circle of support.

Dos and Don'ts If a Person Threatens Suicide

- Take the threat seriously. Insist on getting help. If the person doesn't agree to help himself or herself, then you need to go to someone who can help.

- Do not agree to keep suicide thoughts or threats a secret. Keeping the secret won't help the person. And you cannot bear the responsibility if the person does hurt or kill himself or herself.

- Don't try to call his or her bluff. It may not be one. Reinforce the fact that you care about the person and insist he or she get help.

- Let the person know you care he or she is alive.

Being a Helping Friend

It is important to remember that you cannot be responsible for another person's actions when he or she is stressed, depressed, or suicidal. Whether he or she is crying out for help or suffering silently in despair, only the person can help himself or herself. What you can do is be the most caring and responsible friend possible during the hard times. This means listening to concerns, supporting him or her, and helping the person get skilled help from a trusted and capable adult friend.

Part Five

Controlling and Reducing Stress

Chapter 46

Overview of Stress Management and Reduction Techniques

Stress management and stress reduction techniques help you to cope with stress resulting from events like divorce, losing your job, children getting into trouble, caring for a sick relative, preparing for an exam, or just your daily commute.

What is stress management?

Stress is a normal physical reaction that occurs when you feel threatened or overwhelmed. The perception of a threat is as stressful as a real threat. You perceive a situation as threatening or feel overwhelmed because you are dealing with an unusually large number of everyday responsibilities. With increasing demands of home and work life, many people are under enormous stress. Stress in one setting can affect stress levels in the other.

The stress response narrows your ability to think clearly and function effectively. It can disable you physically and emotionally. The goal of stress management is to bring your nervous system back into balance, giving you a sense of calmness and control in your life.

"Coping with Stress: Management, Prevention and Reduction," reprinted with permission from http://www.helpguide.org/mental/stress_management_relief _coping.htm. © 2007 Helpguide.org. All rights reserved. Helpguide provides a detailed list of related references for this article, including links to information from other websites. For a complete list of Helpguide's current resources related to stress signs and symptoms, causes of stress, burnout, and stress relief and relaxation techniques, visit www.helpguide.org.

Controlling your life means balancing various aspects of it—work, relationships, and leisure—as well as the physical, intellectual, and emotional parts. People who effectively manage stress consider life a challenge rather than a series of irritations, and they feel they have control over their lives, even in the face of setbacks.

There are no "one size fits all" solutions to managing stress. Every individual has a unique response to stress, so experiment with a variety of approaches to manage and reduce stress to learn what works best for you.

How can I change my lifestyle habits to manage stress better?

- **Get enough sleep:** Adequate sleep fuels your mind, as well as your body. Feeling tired will increase your stress because it may cause you to think irrationally.

- **Connect with others:** Develop a support system and share your feelings. Perhaps a friend, family member, teacher, clergy person, or counselor can help you see your problem in a different light. Talking with someone else can help clear your mind of confusion so that you can focus on problem solving.

- **Exercise regularly:** Find at least 30 minutes, three times per week, to do something physical. Nothing beats aerobic exercise to dissipate the excess energy. Physical activity plays a key role in reducing and preventing the effects of stress. During times of high stress, choose things you like to do. It also is beneficial to have a variety of exercise outlets. Be physically fit in ways appropriate for your age, rather than being sedentary.

- **Eat a balanced, nutritious diet:** Be mindful of what you put in your body. Healthy eating fuels your mind, as well as your body. Take time to eat breakfast in the morning; it will help keep you going throughout the day. Eating several balanced, nutritious meals throughout the day will give you the energy to think rationally and clearly. Well-nourished bodies are better prepared to cope with stress.

- **Reduce caffeine and sugar:** Avoid consuming too much caffeine and sugar. In excessive amounts, the temporary "highs" they provide often end in fatigue or a "crash" later. You'll feel more relaxed, less jittery or nervous, and you'll sleep better. In addition, you'll have more energy, less heartburn, and fewer muscle aches.

- **Don't self-medicate with alcohol or drugs:** While consuming alcohol or drugs may appear to alleviate stress, it is only temporary. When sober, the problems and stress will still be there. Don't mask the issue at hand; deal with it head on and with a clear mind.

- **Do something for yourself everyday:** Take time out from the hustle and bustle of life for leisure time. Too much work is actually inefficient and can lead to burnout. Recognize when you are most stressed and allow yourself some reasonable breaks. When things feel especially difficult, take a walk or change your scenery. Most importantly, have fun. Do things that make you happy.

How can I change my thinking and emotional responses to handle stress better?

- **Have realistic expectations:** Know your limits. Whether personally or professionally, be realistic about how much you can do. Set limits for yourself and learn to say "no" to more work and commitments.

- **Reframe problems:** See problems as opportunities. As a result of positive thinking, you will be able to handle whatever is causing your stress. Refute negative thoughts and try to see the glass as half full. It is easy to fall into the rut of seeing only the negative when you are stressed. Your thoughts can become like a pair of dark glasses, allowing little light or joy into your life.

- **Maintain your sense of humor:** This includes the ability to laugh at yourself. Watch a funny movie: the sillier the plot the better. The act of laughing helps your body fight stress in a number of ways.

- **Express your feelings instead of bottling them up:** In order to live a less stressful life, learn to calm your emotions. A good cry during periods of stress or sharing your concerns with someone you trust can be healthy ways to bring relief to your anxiety.

- **Don't try to control events or other people:** Many circumstances in life are beyond your control, particularly the behavior of others. Consider that we live in an imperfect world. Learn to accept what is, for now, until the time comes when perhaps you can change things.

- **Ask yourself "Is this my problem?"** If it isn't, leave it alone. If it is, can you resolve it now? Once the problem is settled, leave it alone. Don't agonize over the decision, and try to accept situations you cannot change.

How can I meet the challenges of stressful situations?

- **Manage time:** One of the greatest sources of stress is over-commitment or poor time management. Plan ahead. Make a reasonable schedule for yourself and include time for stress reduction as a regular part of your schedule. When you try to take care of everything at once it can seem overwhelming and as a result, you may not accomplish anything. Instead, make a list of what tasks you have to do, and then complete them one at a time, checking them off as they're completed.

- **Give priority to the most important tasks and do those first:** If a particularly unpleasant task faces you, tackle it early in the day and get it over with. You will experience less anxiety the rest of the day as a result. Most importantly, do not overwork yourself. Resist the temptation to schedule things back-to-back. All too often, we underestimate how long things will take.

- **Schedule time for both work and recreation:** Too much studying or working is actually inefficient and can lead to burn-out.

- **Delegate tasks and break up big projects:** Being efficient and effective means you must delegate tasks and prioritize, schedule, budget, and plan your precious time. Aim to work in short, intensive periods, which allow you to rest in between. Break big projects into smaller, more manageable tasks so you don't feel overwhelmed and nothing gets done as a result.

What are some more tips for coping with stress?

- **Take a mental vacation:** Take a moment to close your eyes and imagine a place where you feel relaxed and comfortable. Notice all the details of your chosen place, including pleasant sounds, smells, and the temperature. Or change your mental "channel" by reading a good book or playing relaxing music to create a sense of peace and tranquility.

- **Take a warm bath or shower:** Wash the stress away and give yourself some time by yourself to reflect and quiet the mind. Soaking in the bathtub can make you feel like you are a world away from your reality.

- **Use aromatherapy:** Originating in ancient China, aromatherapy is based on the healing properties of plants; from which concentrated aromatic oils are extracted. The vapors of these "essential oils" are then inhaled and carried via the bloodstream, which controls the release of hormones and emotions.

- **Care for a pet:** Petting an animal can help reduce stress and lower blood pressure.

- **Keep a journal:** One strategy that many people have found effective in coping with stress is keeping a journal, sometimes referred as a "stress diary." Writing thoughts down has a marvelous way of putting problems into perspective. Putting your worries into words may help you see that you don't really have that much to worry about, or it may help you get organized and

Table 46.1. Some Common Techniques for Stress Relief

Common Techniques for Stress Relief

Stress relief technique	Description
Diaphragmatic breathing (abdominal breathing)	Stress often causes our breathing to be shallow, which nearly always causes more stress because it puts less oxygen in the bloodstream and increases muscle tension. The next time you feel uptight, try taking a minute to slow down and breathe deeply. Breathe in through your nose and out through your mouth. Try to inhale enough so that your lower abdomen rises and falls. Count slowly as you exhale.
Progressive Muscle Relaxation (PMR)	Relaxation exercises help reduce anxiety and stress. First, you cause tension in certain muscle groups and then you totally relax them.
Meditation	Quiet the mind and engage in exercises that help you focus on your breathing, an object, or your body sensations. The goal is to relax the mind, body, and spirit.
Practice yoga for stress reduction	Yoga allows you to build up a natural response to stress and bring the relaxed state more into your daily life.
Practice tai chi for stress reduction	Tai chi focuses on the breath and the mind's attention in the present moment.
Use massage for stress relief	A massage provides deep relaxation and improves physiological processes. As the muscles relax, so does your entire body, as well as your over-stressed mind.

manage your stress, rather than letting it manage you. Regardless, keeping a journal should help you identify your concerns and establish a plan for moving forward. In your journal:

- List the situations that produce stress in your life (e.g., moving to a new location, work or school demands, balancing priorities, job promotion, etc.).

- Describe how you cope with each type of stressful experience.

- Evaluate your responses. Are they healthy or unhealthy, appropriate or unproductive?

When is professional help needed for stress management?

There's a fine line between feeling stressed out while still being able to function effectively, and the debilitating, even paralyzing phenomenon we think of as burnout or breakdown. The difference is between handling your stress on your own, and being unable to figure out what to do because the pressures of life have become so overwhelming. It's time to seek professional help if you:

- feel that stress is affecting your health;

- feel that it will never end;

- feel so desperate that you think about quitting your job, running away, taking a drug overdose, or injuring yourself;

- feel depressed, sad, tearful, or that life is not worth living;

- lose your appetite and find it difficult to sleep;

- are managing your stress level by eating, sleeping, drinking alcoholic beverages, smoking, or using recreational drugs;

- have worries, feelings, and thoughts that are difficult to talk about; or

- hear voices telling you what to do.

Chapter 47

Alternative Approaches to Maintaining Mental Health

What Are Alternative Approaches to Mental Health Care?

An alternative approach to mental health care is one that emphasizes the interrelationship between mind, body, and spirit. Although some alternative approaches have a long history, many remain controversial.

The National Center for Complementary and Alternative Medicine at the National Institutes of Health was created in 1992 to help evaluate alternative methods of treatment and to integrate those that are effective into mainstream health care practice. It is crucial, however, to consult with your health care providers about the approaches you are using to achieve mental wellness.

Self-Help

Many people with mental illnesses find that self-help groups are an invaluable resource for recovery and for empowerment. Self-help generally refers to groups or meetings that:

- involve people who have similar needs;
- are facilitated by a consumer, survivor, or other layperson;

Excerpted from "Alternative Approaches to Mental Health Care," by the Substance Abuse and Mental Health Services Administration (SAMHSA, www.samhsa .gov), part of the U.S. Department of Health and Human Services, April 2003.

- assist people to deal with a life-disrupting event, such as a death, abuse, serious accident, addiction, or diagnosis of a physical, emotional, or mental disability, for oneself or a relative;

- are operated on an informal, free-of-charge, and nonprofit basis;

- provide support and education; and

- are voluntary, anonymous, and confidential.

Diet and Nutrition

Adjusting both diet and nutrition may help some people with mental illnesses manage their symptoms and promote recovery. For example, research suggests that eliminating milk and wheat products can reduce the severity of symptoms for some people who have schizophrenia and some children with autism. Similarly, some holistic/natural physicians use herbal treatments, B-complex vitamins, riboflavin, magnesium, and thiamine to treat anxiety, autism, depression, drug-induced psychoses, and hyperactivity.

Pastoral Counseling

Some people prefer to seek help for mental health problems from their pastor, rabbi, or priest, rather than from therapists who are not affiliated with a religious community. Counselors working within traditional faith communities increasingly are recognizing the need to incorporate psychotherapy and/or medication, along with prayer and spirituality, to effectively help some people with mental disorders.

Animal-Assisted Therapies

Working with an animal (or animals) under the guidance of a health care professional may benefit some people with mental illness by facilitating positive changes, such as increased empathy and enhanced socialization skills. Animals can be used as part of group therapy programs to encourage communication and increase the ability to focus. Developing self-esteem and reducing loneliness and anxiety are just some potential benefits of individual-animal therapy.

Expressive Therapies

Art therapy: Drawing, painting, and sculpting help many people to reconcile inner conflicts, release deeply repressed emotions, and foster self-awareness, as well as personal growth. Some mental health providers use art therapy as both a diagnostic tool and as a way to help treat disorders such as depression, abuse-related trauma, and schizophrenia. You may be able to find a therapist in your area who has received special training and certification in art therapy.

Dance/movement therapy: Some people find that their spirits soar when they let their feet fly. Others—particularly those who prefer more structure or who feel they have "two left feet"—gain the same sense of release and inner peace from the Eastern martial arts, such as aikido and tai chi. Those who are recovering from physical, sexual, or emotional abuse may find these techniques especially helpful for gaining a sense of ease with their own bodies. The underlying premise to dance/movement therapy is that it can help a person integrate the emotional, physical, and cognitive facets of "self."

Music/sound therapy: It is no coincidence that many people turn on soothing music to relax or snazzy tunes to help feel upbeat. Research suggests that music stimulates the body's natural "feel good" chemicals (opiates and endorphins). This stimulation results in improved blood flow, blood pressure, pulse rate, breathing, and posture changes. Music or sound therapy has been used to treat disorders such as stress, grief, depression, schizophrenia, and autism in children, and to diagnose mental health needs.

Culturally Based Healing Arts

Traditional Oriental medicine (such as acupuncture, shiatsu, and Reiki), Indian systems of health care (such as Ayurveda and yoga), and Native American healing practices (such as the Sweat Lodge and Talking Circles) all incorporate the beliefs that:

- wellness is a state of balance between the spiritual, physical, and mental/emotional "selves";

- an imbalance of forces within the body is the cause of illness; and

- herbal/natural remedies, combined with sound nutrition, exercise, and meditation/prayer, will correct this imbalance.

Acupuncture: The Chinese practice of inserting needles into the body at specific points manipulates the body's flow of energy to balance the endocrine system. This manipulation regulates functions such as heart rate, body temperature, and respiration, as well as sleep patterns and emotional changes. Acupuncture has been used in clinics to assist people with substance abuse disorders through detoxification; to relieve stress and anxiety; to treat attention deficit and hyperactivity disorder in children; to reduce symptoms of depression; and to help people with physical ailments.

Ayurveda: Ayurvedic medicine is described as "knowledge of how to live." It incorporates an individualized regimen—such as diet, meditation, herbal preparations, or other techniques—to treat a variety of conditions, including depression, to facilitate lifestyle changes, and to teach people how to release stress and tension through yoga or transcendental meditation.

Yoga/meditation: Practitioners of this ancient Indian system of health care use breathing exercises, posture, stretches, and meditation to balance the body's energy centers. Yoga is used in combination with other treatment for depression, anxiety, and stress-related disorders.

Native American traditional practices: Ceremonial dances, chants, and cleansing rituals are part of Indian Health Service programs to heal depression, stress, trauma (including those related to physical and sexual abuse), and substance abuse.

Cuentos: Based on folktales, this form of therapy originated in Puerto Rico. The stories used contain healing themes and models of behavior such as self-transformation and endurance through adversity. Cuentos is used primarily to help Hispanic children recover from depression and other mental health problems related to leaving one's homeland and living in a foreign culture.

Relaxation and Stress Reduction Techniques

Biofeedback: Learning to control muscle tension and "involuntary" body functioning, such as heart rate and skin temperature, can be a path to mastering one's fears. It is used in combination with, or as an alternative to, medication to treat disorders such as anxiety, panic, and phobias. For example, a person can learn to "retrain" his or her breathing habits in stressful situations to induce relaxation and decrease hyperventilation. Some preliminary research indicates it may offer an additional tool for treating schizophrenia and depression.

Guided imagery or visualization: This process involves going into a state of deep relaxation and creating a mental image of recovery and wellness. Physicians, nurses, and mental health providers occasionally use this approach to treat alcohol and drug addictions, depression, panic disorders, phobias, and stress.

Massage therapy: The underlying principle of this approach is that rubbing, kneading, brushing, and tapping a person's muscles can help release tension and pent emotions. It has been used to treat trauma-related depression and stress. A highly unregulated industry, certification for massage therapy varies widely from state to state. Some states have strict guidelines, whereas others have none.

Technology-Based Applications

The boom in electronic tools at home and in the office makes access to mental health information just a telephone call or a mouse click away. Technology is also making treatment more widely available in once-isolated areas.

Telemedicine: Plugging into video and computer technology is a relatively new innovation in health care. It allows both consumers and providers in remote or rural areas to gain access to mental health or specialty expertise. Telemedicine can enable consulting providers to speak to and observe patients directly. It also can be used in education and training programs for generalist clinicians.

Telephone counseling: Active listening skills are a hallmark of telephone counselors. These also provide information and referral to interested callers. For many people telephone counseling often is a first step to receiving in-depth mental health care. Research shows that counseling from specially trained mental health providers reaches many people who otherwise might not get the help they need. Before calling, be sure to check the telephone number for service fees; a 900 area code means you will be billed for the call, an 800 or 888 area code means the call is toll-free.

Electronic communications: Technologies such as the internet, bulletin boards, and electronic mail lists provide access directly to consumers and the public on a wide range of information. On-line consumer groups can exchange information, experiences, and views on mental health, treatment systems, alternative medicine, and other related topics.

Radio psychiatry: Another relative newcomer to therapy, radio psychiatry was first introduced in the United States in 1976. Radio psychiatrists and psychologists provide advice, information, and referrals in response to a variety of mental health questions from callers. The American Psychiatric Association and the American Psychological Association have issued ethical guidelines for the role of psychiatrists and psychologists on radio shows.

Others: This information does not cover every alternative approach to mental health. A range of other alternative approaches—psychodrama, hypnotherapy, recreational, and Outward Bound-type nature programs—offer opportunities to explore mental wellness. Before jumping into any alternative therapy, learn as much as you can about it. In addition to talking with your health care practitioner, you may want to visit your local library, book store, health food store, or holistic health care clinic for more information. Also, before receiving services, check to be sure the provider is properly certified by an appropriate accrediting agency.

Chapter 48

Mind-Body Medicine and Its Effect on Stress Levels

Introduction

Mind-body medicine focuses on the interactions among the brain, mind, body, and behavior, and the powerful ways in which emotional, mental, social, spiritual, and behavioral factors can directly affect health. It regards as fundamental an approach that respects and enhances each person's capacity for self-knowledge and self-care, and it emphasizes techniques that are grounded in this approach.

Definition of Scope of Field

Mind-body medicine typically focuses on intervention strategies that are thought to promote health, such as relaxation, hypnosis, visual imagery, meditation, yoga, biofeedback, tai chi, qi gong, cognitive-behavioral therapies, group support, autogenic training, and spirituality. The field views illness as an opportunity for personal growth and transformation, and health care providers as catalysts and guides in this process.

Certain mind-body intervention strategies listed here, such as group support for cancer survivors, are well integrated into conventional care

From "Mind-Body Medicine: An Overview," by the National Center for Complementary and Alternative Medicine (NCCAM, nccam.nih.gov), part of the National Institutes of Health, August 2006.

and, while still considered mind-body interventions, are not considered to be complementary and alternative medicine.

Mind-body interventions constitute a major portion of the overall use of CAM by the public. In 2002, five relaxation techniques and imagery, biofeedback, and hypnosis, taken together, were used by more than 30 percent of the adult U.S. population. Prayer was used by more than 50 percent of the population.[1]

Background

The concept that the mind is important in the treatment of illness is integral to the healing approaches of traditional Chinese and Ayurvedic medicine, dating back more than 2,000 years. It was also noted by Hippocrates, who recognized the moral and spiritual aspects of healing, and believed that treatment could occur only with consideration of attitude, environmental influences, and natural remedies (ca. 400 B.C.). While this integrated approach was maintained in traditional healing systems in the East, developments in the Western world by the 16th and 17th centuries led to a separation of human spiritual or emotional dimensions from the physical body. This separation began with the redirection of science, during the Renaissance and Enlightenment eras, to the purpose of enhancing humankind's control over nature. Technological advances (e.g., microscopy, the stethoscope, the blood pressure cuff, and refined surgical techniques) demonstrated a cellular world that seemed far apart from the world of belief and emotion. The discovery of bacteria and, later, antibiotics further dispelled the notion of belief influencing health. Fixing or curing an illness became a matter of science (i.e., technology) and took precedence over, not a place beside, healing of the soul. As medicine separated the mind and the body, scientists of the mind (neurologists) formulated concepts, such as the unconscious, emotional impulses, and cognitive delusions, that solidified the perception that diseases of the mind were not "real," that is, not based in physiology and biochemistry.

In the 1920s, Walter Cannon's work revealed the direct relationship between stress and neuroendocrine responses in animals.[2] Coining the phrase "fight or flight," Cannon described the primitive reflexes of sympathetic and adrenal activation in response to perceived danger and other environmental pressures (e.g., cold, heat). Hans Selye further defined the deleterious effects of stress and distress on health.[3] At the same time, technological advances in medicine that could identify specific pathological changes, and new discoveries in pharmaceuticals, were occurring at a very rapid pace. The disease-based model, the search for a specific pathology, and the identification of external cures were paramount, even in psychiatry.

During World War II, the importance of belief reentered the web of health care. On the beaches of Anzio, morphine for the wounded soldiers was in short supply, and Henry Beecher, M.D., discovered that much of the pain could be controlled by saline injections. He coined the term "placebo effect," and his subsequent research showed that up to 35 percent of a therapeutic response to any medical treatment could be the result of belief.[4] Investigation into the placebo effect and debate about it are ongoing.

Since the 1960s, mind-body interactions have become an extensively researched field. The evidence for benefits for certain indications from biofeedback, cognitive-behavioral interventions, and hypnosis is quite good, while there is emerging evidence regarding their physiological effects. Less research supports the use of CAM approaches like meditation and yoga. The following is a summary of relevant studies.

Mind-Body Interventions and Disease Outcomes

Over the past 20 years, mind-body medicine has provided considerable evidence that psychological factors can play a substantive role in the development and progression of coronary artery disease. There is evidence that mind-body interventions can be effective in the treatment of coronary artery disease, enhancing the effect of standard cardiac rehabilitation in reducing all-cause mortality and cardiac event recurrences for up to 2 years.[5]

Mind-body interventions have also been applied to various types of pain. Clinical trials indicate that these interventions may be a particularly effective adjunct in the management of arthritis, with reductions in pain maintained for up to 4 years and reductions in the number of physician visits.[6] When applied to more general acute and chronic pain management, headache, and low-back pain, mind-body interventions show some evidence of effects, although results vary based on the patient population and type of intervention studied.[7]

Evidence from multiple studies with various types of cancer patients suggests that mind-body interventions can improve mood, quality of life, and coping, as well as ameliorate disease- and treatment-related symptoms, such as chemotherapy-induced nausea, vomiting, and pain.[8] Some studies have suggested that mind-body interventions can alter various immune parameters, but it is unclear whether these alterations are of sufficient magnitude to have an impact on disease progression or prognosis.[9,10]

Mind-Body Influences on Immunity

There is considerable evidence that emotional traits, both negative and positive, influence people's susceptibility to infection. Following systematic exposure to a respiratory virus in the laboratory, individuals who report higher levels of stress or negative moods have been shown to develop more severe illness than those who report less stress or more positive moods.[11] Recent studies suggest that the tendency to report positive, as opposed to negative, emotions may be associated with greater resistance to objectively verified colds. These laboratory studies are supported by longitudinal studies pointing to associations between psychological or emotional traits and the incidence of respiratory infections.[12]

Meditation and Imaging

Meditation, one of the most common mind-body interventions, is a conscious mental process that induces a set of integrated physiological changes termed the relaxation response. Functional magnetic resonance imaging (fMRI) has been used to identify and characterize the brain regions that are active during meditation. This research suggests that various parts of the brain known to be involved in attention and in the control of the autonomic nervous system are activated, providing a neurochemical and anatomical basis for the effects of meditation on various physiological activities.[13] Recent studies involving imaging are advancing the understanding of mind-body mechanisms. For example, meditation has been shown in one study to produce significant increases in left-sided anterior brain activity, which is associated with positive emotional states. Moreover, in this same study, meditation was associated with increases in antibody titers to influenza vaccine, suggesting potential linkages among meditation, positive emotional states, localized brain responses, and improved immune function.[14]

Physiology of Expectancy (Placebo Response)

Placebo effects are believed to be mediated by both cognitive and conditioning mechanisms. Until recently, little was known about the role of these mechanisms in different circumstances. Now, research has shown that placebo responses are mediated by conditioning when unconscious physiological functions such as hormonal secretion are involved, whereas they are mediated by expectation when conscious physiological processes such as pain and motor performance come into play, even though a conditioning procedure is carried out.

Positron emission tomography (PET) scanning of the brain is providing evidence of the release of the endogenous neurotransmitter dopamine in the brain of Parkinson disease patients in response to placebo.[15] Evidence indicates that the placebo effect in these patients is powerful and is mediated through activation of the nigrostriatal dopamine system, the system that is damaged in Parkinson disease. This result suggests that the placebo response involves the secretion of dopamine, which is known to be important in a number of other reinforcing and rewarding conditions, and that there may be mind-body strategies that could be used in patients with Parkinson disease in lieu of or in addition to treatment with dopamine-releasing drugs.

Stress and Wound Healing

Individual differences in wound healing have long been recognized. Clinical observation has suggested that negative mood or stress is associated with slow wound healing. Basic mind-body research is now confirming this observation. Matrix metalloproteinases (MMPs) and the tissue inhibitors of metalloproteinases (TIMPs), whose expression can be controlled by cytokines, play a role in wound healing.[16] Using a blister chamber wound model on human forearm skin exposed to ultraviolet light, researchers have demonstrated that stress or a change in mood is sufficient to modulate MMP and TIMP expression and, presumably, wound healing.[17] Activation of the hypothalamic-pituitary-adrenal (HPA) and sympathetic-adrenal medullary (SAM) systems can modulate levels of MMPs, providing a physiological link among mood, stress, hormones, and wound healing. This line of basic research suggests that activation of the HPA and SAM axes, even in individuals within the normal range of depressive symptoms, could alter MMP levels and change the course of wound healing in blister wounds.

Surgical Preparation

Mind-body interventions are being tested to determine whether they can help prepare patients for the stress associated with surgery. Initial randomized controlled trials—in which some patients received audiotapes with mind-body techniques (guided imagery, music, and instructions for improved outcomes) and some patients received control tapes—found that subjects receiving the mind-body intervention recovered more quickly and spent fewer days in the hospital.[18]

447

Behavioral interventions have been shown to be an efficient means of reducing discomfort and adverse effects during percutaneous vascular and renal procedures. Pain increased linearly with procedure time in a control group and in a group practicing structured attention, but remained flat in a group practicing a self-hypnosis technique. The self-administration of analgesic drugs was significantly higher in the control group than in the attention and hypnosis groups. Hypnosis also improved hemodynamic stability.[19]

Conclusion

Evidence from randomized controlled trials and, in many cases, systematic reviews of the literature, suggest that:

- Mechanisms may exist by which the brain and central nervous system influence immune, endocrine, and autonomic functioning, which is known to have an impact on health.

- Multicomponent mind-body interventions that include some combination of stress management, coping skills training, cognitive-behavioral interventions, and relaxation therapy may be appropriate adjunctive treatments for coronary artery disease and certain pain-related disorders, such as arthritis.

- Multimodal mind-body approaches, such as cognitive-behavioral therapy, particularly when combined with an educational/informational component, can be effective adjuncts in the management of a variety of chronic conditions.

- An array of mind-body therapies (e.g., imagery, hypnosis, relaxation), when employed presurgically, may improve recovery time and reduce pain following surgical procedures.

- Neurochemical and anatomical bases may exist for some of the effects of mind-body approaches.

Mind-body approaches have potential benefits and advantages. In particular, the physical and emotional risks of using these interventions are minimal. Moreover, once tested and standardized, most mind-body interventions can be taught easily. Finally, future research focusing on basic mind-body mechanisms and individual differences in responses is likely to yield new insights that may enhance the effectiveness and individual tailoring of mind-body interventions. In the meantime, there is considerable evidence that mind-body interventions, even as they are being studied today, have positive effects on psychological functioning and quality of life, and may be particularly helpful for patients coping with chronic illness and in need of palliative care.

References

1. Wolsko PM, Eisenberg DM, Davis RB, et al. Use of mind-body medical therapies. *Journal of General Internal Medicine.* 2004;19(1):43–50.

2. Cannon WB. *The Wisdom of the Body.* New York, NY: Norton; 1932.

3. Selye H. *The Stress of Life.* New York, NY: McGraw-Hill; 1956.

4. Beecher H. *Measurement of Subjective Responses.* New York, NY: Oxford University Press; 1959.

5. Rutledge JC, Hyson DA, Garduno D, et al. Lifestyle modification program in management of patients with coronary artery disease: the clinical experience in a tertiary care hospital. *Journal of Cardiopulmonary Rehabilitation.* 1999;19(4):226–234.

6. Luskin FM, Newell KA, Griffith M, et al. A review of mind/body therapies in the treatment of musculoskeletal disorders with implications for the elderly. *Alternative Therapies in Health and Medicine.* 2000;6(2):46–56.

7. Astin JA, Shapiro SL, Eisenberg DM, et al. Mind-body medicine: state of the science, implications for practice. *Journal of the American Board of Family Practice.* 2003;16(2):131–147.

8. Mundy EA, DuHamel KN, Montgomery GH. The efficacy of behavioral interventions for cancer treatment-related side effects. *Seminars in Clinical Neuropsychiatry.* 2003;8(4):253–275.

9. Irwin MR, Pike JL, Cole JC, et al. Effects of a behavioral intervention, Tai Chi Chih, on varicella-zoster virus specific immunity and health functioning in older adults. *Psychosomatic Medicine.* 2003;65(5):824–830.

10. Kiecolt-Glaser JK, Marucha PT, Atkinson C, et al. Hypnosis as a modulator of cellular immune dysregulation during acute stress. *Journal of Consulting and Clinical Psychology.* 2001;69(4):674–682.

11. Cohen S, Doyle WJ, Turner RB, et al. Emotional style and susceptibility to the common cold. *Psychosomatic Medicine.* 2003;65(4):652–657.

12. Smith A, Nicholson K. Psychosocial factors, respiratory viruses and exacerbation of asthma. *Psychoneuroendocrinology.* 2001;26(4):411–420.

13. Lazar SW, Bush G, Gollub RL, et al. Functional brain mapping of the relaxation response and meditation. *Neuroreport.* 2000;11(7):1581–1585.

14. Davidson RJ, Kabat-Zinn J, Schumacher J, et al. Alterations in brain and immune function produced by mindfulness meditation. *Psychosomatic Medicine.* 2003;65(4):564–570.

15. Fuente-Fernandez R, Phillips AG, Zamburlini M, et al. Dopamine release in human ventral striatum and expectation of reward. *Behavioural Brain Research.* 2002;136(2):359–363.

16. Stamenkovic I. Extracellular matrix remodelling: the role of matrix metalloproteinases. *Journal of Pathology.* 2003;200(4):448–464.

17. Yang EV, Bane CM, MacCallum RC, et al. Stress-related modulation of matrix metalloproteinase expression. *Journal of Neuroimmunology.* 2002;133(1-2):144–150.

18. Tusek DL, Church JM, Strong SA, et al. Guided imagery: a significant advance in the care of patients undergoing elective colorectal surgery. *Diseases of the Colon and Rectum.* 1997;40(2):172–178.

19. Lang EV, Benotsch EG, Fick LJ, et al. Adjunctive non-pharmacological analgesia for invasive medical procedures: a randomised trial. *Lancet.* 2000;355(9214):1486–1490.

Chapter 49

Massage Therapy

Massage therapy is a practice that dates back thousands of years. There are many types of massage therapy; all involve manipulating the muscles and other soft tissues of the body. In the United States, massage therapy is sometimes part of conventional medicine. In other instances, it is part of complementary and alternative medicine (CAM). This information provides a general overview of massage therapy used as CAM and suggests some resources you can use to learn more.

Conventional medicine is medicine as practiced by holders of M.D. (medical doctor) and D.O. (doctor of osteopathy) degrees and by their allied health professionals, such as physical therapists, psychologists, and registered nurses. An example of massage therapy as conventional medicine is using it to reduce a type of swelling called lymphedema.

CAM is a group of diverse medical and health care systems, practices, and products that are not presently considered to be part of conventional medicine. While some scientific evidence exists regarding some CAM therapies, for most there are key questions that are yet to be answered through well-designed scientific studies. An example of massage therapy as CAM is using it with the intent to enhance immune system functioning.

Excerpted from "Massage Therapy as CAM," a backgrounder from the National Center for Complementary and Alternative Medicine (NCCAM, nccam.nih .gov), part of the National Institutes of Health, NCCAM Publication No. D327, September 2006.

What Massage Therapy Is

The term massage therapy (also called massage, for short; massage also refers to an individual treatment session) covers a group of practices and techniques. There are over 80 types of massage therapy. In all of them, therapists press, rub, and otherwise manipulate the muscles and other soft tissues of the body, often varying pressure and movement. They most often use their hands and fingers, but may use their forearms, elbows, or feet. Typically, the intent is to relax the soft tissues, increase delivery of blood and oxygen to the massaged areas, warm them, and decrease pain.

A few popular examples of this therapy are as follows:

- In **Swedish massage**, the therapist uses long strokes, kneading, and friction on the muscles and moves the joints to aid flexibility.

- A therapist giving a **deep tissue massage** uses patterns of strokes and deep finger pressure on parts of the body where muscles are tight or knotted, focusing on layers of muscle deep under the skin.

- In **trigger point massage** (also called pressure point massage), the therapist uses a variety of strokes but applies deeper, more focused pressure on myofascial trigger points—"knots" that can form in the muscles, are painful when pressed, and cause symptoms elsewhere in the body as well.

- In **shiatsu massage**, the therapist applies varying, rhythmic pressure from the fingers on parts of the body that are believed to be important for the flow of a vital energy called qi.

Massage therapy (and, in general, the laying on of hands for health purposes) dates back thousands of years. References to massage have been found in ancient writings from many cultures, including those of Ancient Greece, Ancient Rome, Japan, China, Egypt, and the Indian subcontinent.

In the United States, massage therapy first became popular and was promoted for a variety of health purposes starting in the mid-1800s. In the 1930s and 1940s, however, massage fell out of favor, mostly because of scientific and technological advances in medical treatments. Interest in massage revived in the 1970s, especially among athletes.

More recently, a 2002 national survey on Americans' use of CAM (published in 2004) found that 5 percent of the 31,000 participants had used massage therapy in the preceding 12 months, and 9.3 percent had ever used it. According to recent reviews, people use massage for a wide variety of health-related intents: for example, to relieve pain (often from musculoskeletal conditions, but from other conditions as well); rehabilitate sports injuries; reduce stress; increase relaxation; address feelings of anxiety and depression; and aid general wellness.

Who Provides Massage Therapy?

A person who professionally provides massage therapy is most often called a massage therapist, although there are some other health care providers (such as chiropractors) who also have massage training. This text mainly uses the term massage therapist. Most massage therapists learn and practice more than one type of massage.

To learn massage, most therapists attend a school or training program, with a much smaller number training instead with an experienced practitioner. Many students are already licensed as another type of health care provider, such as a nurse.

There are about 1,300 massage therapy schools, college programs, and training programs in the United States. The course of study typically covers subjects such as anatomy and physiology (structure and function of the body); kinesiology (motion and body mechanics); therapeutic evaluation; massage techniques; first aid; business, ethical, and legal issues; and hands-on practice of techniques. These educational programs vary in many respects, such as length, quality, and whether they are accredited. Many require 500 hours of training, which is the same number of hours that many states require for certification. Some therapists also pursue specialty or advanced training.

At the end of 2004, 33 states and the District of Columbia had passed laws regulating massage therapy—for example, requiring that massage therapists graduate from an approved school or training program and pass the national certification exam in their field in order to practice. Cities and counties may have laws that apply as well. Professional organizations of massage therapists have not agreed upon the standards for recognizing that a massage therapist is properly and adequately trained.

What Massage Therapists Do in Treating Patients

Massage therapists work in a variety of settings, including private offices, hospitals, other clinical settings, nursing homes, studios, and sport and fitness facilities. Some also travel to patients' homes or workplaces to provide a massage.

Massage therapy treatments usually last for 30 to 60 minutes; less often, they are as short as 15 minutes or as long as 1.5 to 2 hours. For some conditions (especially chronic ones), therapists often advise a series of appointments. Therapists usually try to provide an environment that is as calm and soothing as possible (for example, by using dim lighting, soft music, and fragrances).

At the first appointment, a massage therapist will discuss your symptoms, medical history, the results you (and your health care provider, if applicable) desire, and possibly other factors such as your work and levels of stress. She will likely perform some evaluations through touch. If she finds nothing that would make a massage inadvisable, she will proceed with the massage. At any time, you can bring up questions or concerns.

During treatment, you will lie on a special padded table or sit on a stool or chair. You might be fully clothed (for example, for a "chair massage") or partially or fully undressed (in which case you will be covered by a sheet or towel; only the parts of your body that the therapist is currently massaging are exposed). Oil or powder helps reduce friction on the skin. The therapist may use other aids, such as ice, heat, fragrances, or machines. He may also provide recommendations for self-care, such as drinking fluids, learning better movement, and developing an awareness of your body.

Why People Use Massage Therapy

In the 2002 national survey on Americans' use of CAM, respondents who used a CAM therapy could choose from five reasons for using the therapy. The results for massage were as follows:

- They believed that massage combined with conventional medicine would help: 60 percent

- They thought massage would be interesting to try: 44 percent

- They believed that conventional medical treatments would not help: 34 percent

- Massage was suggested by a conventional medical professional: 33 percent

- They thought that conventional medicine was too expensive: 13 percent

Side Effects and Risks

Massage therapy appears to have few serious risks if appropriate cautions are followed. A very small number of serious injuries have been reported, and they appear to have occurred mostly because cautions were not followed or a massage was given by a person who was not properly trained.

Health care providers recommend that patients not have massage therapy if they have one or more of the following conditions:

- Deep vein thrombosis (a blood clot in a deep vein, usually in the legs)

- A bleeding disorder or taking blood-thinning drugs such as warfarin

- Damaged blood vessels

- Weakened bones from osteoporosis, a recent fracture, or cancer

- A fever

- Any of the following in an area that would be massaged:
  - An open or healing wound
  - A tumor
  - Damaged nerves
  - An infection or acute inflammation
  - Inflammation from radiation treatment

If you have one or more of the following conditions, be sure to consult your health care provider before having massage:

- Pregnancy
- Cancer
- Fragile skin, as from diabetes or a healing scar
- Heart problems
- Dermatomyositis, a disease of the connective tissue
- A history of physical abuse

Side effects of massage therapy may include:

- Temporary pain or discomfort

- Bruising
- Swelling
- A sensitivity or allergy to massage oils

Some Other Points to Consider about Massage Therapy as CAM

Massage therapy should not be used to replace your regular medical care or to delay seeing a doctor about a medical problem.

Before you decide about having massage therapy, ask the therapist about:

- Her training, experience, and any licenses or credentials
- Any medical conditions you have and whether she has had any specialized training or experience with them
- The number of treatments that might be needed
- Cost
- Insurance coverage, if any

If a massage therapist suggests using other CAM practices (herbs or other supplements, a special diet, etc.), discuss it first with your regular health care provider.

How Massage Therapy Might Work

Scientists are studying massage to understand what effects massage therapy has on patients, how it has those effects, and why. Some aspects of this are better understood than others. For example, it is known that:

- When certain forces are applied to the muscles, changes occur in the muscles (although those changes are not clearly understood or agreed upon).
- Massage therapy typically enhances relaxation and reduces stress. Stress makes some diseases and conditions worse.

There are many more aspects that are not yet known or well understood scientifically, however. Some of the proposed theories are that massage:

- Might provide stimulation that may help block pain signals sent to the brain (the "gate control theory" of pain reduction).

- Might shift the patient's nervous system away from the sympathetic and toward the parasympathetic. The sympathetic nervous system helps mobilize the body for action. When a person is under stress, it produces the fight-or-flight response (the heart rate and breathing rate go up, for example; the blood vessels narrow; and muscles tighten). The parasympathetic nervous system creates what some call the "rest and digest" response (the heart rate and breathing rate slow down, for example; the blood vessels dilate; and activity increases in many parts of the digestive tract).

- Might stimulate the release of certain chemicals in the body, such as serotonin or endorphins.

- Might cause beneficial mechanical changes in the body—for example, by preventing fibrosis (the formation of scar-like tissue) or increasing the flow of lymph (a fluid that travels through the body's lymphatic system and carries cells that help fight disease).

- Might improve sleep, which has a role in pain and healing.

- Might provide some health benefit from the interaction between therapist and patient.

- More well-designed studies are needed to understand and confirm these theories and other scientific aspects of massage.

NCCAM-Sponsored Research on Massage

Some recent examples of NCCAM-sponsored research on massage include:

- How massage affects healthy people, and whether these effects are different depending on how many massages are given and how often.

- The effects of massage on chronic neck pain, and comparing the benefits of conventional therapeutic massage with usual medical treatment.

- Massage for cancer patients at the end of life, to see if massage helps relieve depression, improves emotional well-being and quality of life, and eases the process of dying.

- Whether massage given at home by a trained family member helps reduce pain from sickle cell anemia.

Chapter 50

Meditation and Other Relaxation Techniques

Chapter Contents

Section 50.1

Meditation for Health Purposes

From "Meditation for Health Purposes," a publication by the National Center for Complementary and Alternative Medicine (NCCAM, www .nccam.nih.gov), part of the National Institutes of Health, February 2006.

Introduction

Meditation for health purposes is a mind-body practice in complementary and alternative medicine (CAM). There are many types of meditation, most of which originated in ancient religious and spiritual traditions. Generally, a person who is meditating uses certain techniques, such as focusing attention (for example, on a word, an object, or the breath); a specific posture; and an open attitude toward distracting thoughts and emotions. Meditation can be practiced for various reasons—for example, with an intent to increase physical relaxation, mental calmness, and psychological balance; to cope with one or more diseases and conditions; and for overall wellness. This text provides a general introduction to meditation.

Complementary and alternative medicine is medicine used outside of conventional medicine as practiced in the United States—that is, by holders of Doctor of Medicine (M.D.) and Doctor of Osteopathy (D.O.) degrees and their allied health professionals. Complementary medicine is used along with conventional medicine, and alternative medicine is used instead of conventional medicine. Some conventional medicine practitioners are also practitioners of CAM.

What Meditation Is

The term meditation refers to a group of techniques, most of which started in Eastern religious or spiritual traditions. These techniques have been used by many different cultures throughout the world for thousands of years. Today, many people use meditation outside of its traditional religious or cultural settings, for health and wellness purposes.

In meditation, a person learns to focus his attention and suspend the stream of thoughts that normally occupy the mind. This practice is believed to result in a state of greater physical relaxation, mental calmness, and psychological balance. Practicing meditation can change how a person relates to the flow of emotions and thoughts in the mind.

Most types of meditation have four elements in common:

- **A quiet location:** Many meditators prefer a quiet place with as few distractions as possible. This can be particularly helpful for beginners. People who have been practicing meditation for a longer period of time sometimes develop the ability to meditate in public places, like waiting rooms or buses.

- **A specific, comfortable posture:** Depending on the type being practiced, meditation can be done while sitting, lying down, standing, walking, or in other positions.

- **A focus of attention:** Focusing one's attention is usually a part of meditation. For example, the meditator may focus on a mantra (a specially chosen word or set of words), an object, or the breath.

- **An open attitude:** Having an open attitude during meditation means letting distractions come and go naturally without stopping to think about them. When distracting or wandering thoughts occur, they are not suppressed; instead, the meditator gently brings attention back to the focus. In some types of meditation, the meditator learns to observe the rising and falling of thoughts and emotions as they spontaneously occur.

Meditation is practiced both on its own and as a component of some other therapies, such as yoga, tai chi, and qi gong. This text focuses on meditation practiced on its own.

Meditation for Health Purposes

Meditation used as CAM is a type of mind-body medicine (one of the four domains, or areas of knowledge, in CAM). Generally, mind-body medicine focuses on:

- the interactions among the brain, the rest of the body, the mind, and behavior and

- the ways in which emotional, mental, social, spiritual, and behavioral factors can directly affect health.

461

People use meditation for various health problems, such as:

- anxiety;
- pain;
- depression;
- mood and self-esteem problems;
- stress;
- insomnia; and
- physical or emotional symptoms that may be associated with chronic illnesses and their treatment, such as:
  - cardiovascular (heart) disease;
  - HIV/AIDS; and
  - cancer.

Meditation is also used for overall wellness.

A large national survey on Americans' use of CAM, released in 2004, found that nearly 8 percent of the participants had used meditation specifically for health reasons during the year before the survey.

Examples of Meditation

Mindfulness meditation and the Transcendental Meditation technique (also known as TM) are two common approaches to meditation. They are also two types of meditation being studied in NCCAM-sponsored research projects.

Mindfulness meditation originated in Buddhism. It is based on the concept of being mindful, or having an increased awareness and total acceptance of the present. While meditating, the meditator is taught to bring all her attention to the sensation of the flow of the breath in and out of the body. The intent might be described as focusing attention on what is being experienced, without reacting to or judging that experience. This is seen as helping the meditator learn to experience thoughts and emotions in normal daily life with greater balance and acceptance.

TM originated in the Vedic tradition in India. It is a type of meditation that uses a mantra (a word, sound, or phrase repeated silently) to prevent distracting thoughts from entering the mind. The intent of TM might be described as allowing the mind to settle into a quieter state and the body into a state of deep rest. This is seen as ultimately leading to a state of relaxed alertness.

Looking at How Meditation May Work

Practicing meditation has been shown to induce some changes in the body, such as changes in the body's "fight or flight" response. The system responsible for this response is the autonomic nervous system (sometimes called the involuntary nervous system). It regulates many organs and muscles, including functions such as the heartbeat, sweating, breathing, and digestion, and does so automatically.

The autonomic nervous system is divided into two parts:

- The sympathetic nervous system helps mobilize the body for action. When a person is under stress, it produces the fight-or-flight response: the heart rate and breathing rate go up, for example, the blood vessels narrow (restricting the flow of blood), and muscles tighten.

- The parasympathetic nervous system creates what some call the "rest and digest" response. This system's responses oppose those of the sympathetic nervous system. For example, it causes the heart rate and breathing rate to slow down, the blood vessels to dilate (improving blood flow), and activity to increase in many parts of the digestive tract.

While scientists are studying whether meditation may afford meaningful health benefits, they are also looking at how it may do so. One way some types of meditation might work is by reducing activity in the sympathetic nervous system and increasing activity in the parasympathetic nervous system.

Scientific research is using sophisticated tools to learn more about what goes on in the brain and the rest of the body during meditation and diseases or conditions for which meditation might be useful. There is still much to learn in these areas. One avenue of research is looking at whether meditation is associated with significant changes in brain function. A number of researchers believe that these changes account for many of meditation's effects.

Side Effects and Risks

Meditation is generally safe. There have been a small number of reports that intensive meditation could cause or worsen symptoms in people who have certain psychiatric problems, but this question has not been fully researched. Individuals who are aware of an underlying psychiatric disorder and want to start meditation should speak with a mental health professional before doing so.

Any person who is interested in using meditation as CAM should consider the following:

- Meditation should never delay the time it takes you to see your health care provider about having a medical problem diagnosed or treated, and it should not be used as the only treatment without first consulting your provider.

- It is important to discuss any CAM therapies you are considering or using (including meditation) with your provider for a complete treatment plan and your safety.

- If you are interested in learning meditation, ask about the training and experience of the instructor.

- Find out whether there have been any research studies published on meditation for the health condition you are interested in.

NCCAM-Supported Research

Some recent studies supported by NCCAM have been investigating:

- the potential effectiveness of the transcendental meditation technique to prevent and treat heart disease;

- mindfulness-based stress reduction to relieve symptoms of rheumatoid arthritis and, in a different study, chronic lower back pain;

- what happens to the brain's activity and structures during Buddhist insight meditation (which includes mindfulness) in a study that uses a brain scan called fMRI (functional magnetic resonance imaging); and

- the long-term impact of meditation on basic emotional and cognitive functions and on mechanisms in the brain that are involved in these functions.

Section 50.2

Autogenic Training: Improving Body Awareness and Relaxation

"AT Questions and Answers," © 2006 British Autogenic Society.
Reprinted with permission.

What is AT?

AT stands for autogenic therapy. Autogenic means 'generated from within.' AT offers a non-drug approach to preventing and treating a wide range of both organic and psychosomatic illnesses and psychological issues. It is a self-help technique that brings about profound relaxation and relief from the negative effects of stress. Quite simply, it retrains the mind to calm itself. AT was developed 85 years ago by the psychiatrist and neurologist Dr. Johannes Schultz, and has been available in the UK [United Kingdom] for over 25 years. It is one of the most scientifically proven complementary therapies, but remains one of the least known.

Who is AT for?

AT is suitable for people engaged in all areas of life, including those in the world of sport and creative arts. It is particularly useful for busy managers and business executives, and just about anybody who may find himself or herself in a stressful life situation, including parents of young children. AT has even been proven useful in facilitating less stressful pregnancies, childbirth, and accelerating post-delivery healing.

How is AT learned?

A typical AT course run by a trained and qualified Autogenic Therapist comprises 8–10 weekly, one-hour sessions. Each individual is always monitored in case any variations from the standard form are necessary. Following an initial assessment, individuals are taught a series of simple, easily learned mental exercises that allow the mind to calm itself by switching off the body's stress responses. Once learned it is a skill for life and simple to do almost anywhere: on planes, at work, or while at the dentist's.

How effective is AT?

A huge number of scientific papers document the effectiveness of AT. It is known to have numerous psychological applications including anxiety states, insomnia, depression, posttraumatic stress disorder (PTSD), as well as medical applications such as skin conditions, asthma, hypertension, colitis, arthritis, migraine, and irritable bowel syndrome (IBS), among others. People who have learned AT commonly report better health and emotional balance, greater coping ability, increased well-being, improved quality of sleep, and reduction of anxiety levels.

Chapter 51

Reducing Stress with Nutrition and Exercise

Chapter Contents

Section 51.1

Handling Stress with Good Nutrition

"Handling Stress . . . Nutrition Tips," © 2000 Wisconsin Department of Health and Family Services, Division of Public Health (http://dhfs .wisconsin.gov). Reprinted with permission. Reviewed by David A. Cooke, M.D., April 2007.

Good nutrition can increase your ability to manage stress.

Poor nutrition could lead to fatigue, weakness, and a reduced ability to concentrate. Healthy eating helps you fight off colds and infection.

Here are some tips that will help to keep you at your best when dealing with stress. Check those that you want to work on and put this list on your refrigerator today as a reminder.

- **Eat right:** Eat regular meals—3 times a day. Use the food guide pyramid to help you choose.

- **Control portion sizes:** Avoid eating too much or too little. For some, stress makes them want to snack all day, while others don't want to eat at all.

- **Eat breakfast:** Start your day off with a healthy breakfast each morning to give you the energy you need to face the day's challenges.

- **Think ahead** so that healthy foods are available to prepare for meals and snacks. Make a shopping list and stick to it.

- **Limit calorie-loaded "comfort" foods:** Although some foods may bring back happy memories, over-consumption may cause you to feel guilty.

Other Things to Remember

- **Eat 5 a day for better health:** Try to eat at least 5 servings of vegetables and fruits every day.

- **Go easy on the caffeine:** Too much caffeine can contribute to feelings of anxiety. Try gradually reducing caffeine by drinking decaffeinated coffee or tea and caffeine-free soft drinks. Choose fruit and vegetable juices, fat-free or low-fat milk, and water as beverages.

- **Avoid high doses of vitamins:** Vitamin pills can't relieve stress. One "regular" vitamin/mineral supplement that contains 100% of the daily value (DV) may improve your overall health. Megadoses of vitamins (10 times the DV) could be dangerous.

- **Be careful with herbal products:** Talk to your health care provider or pharmacist before using products that claim to relieve stress.

Before Stress Gets the Best of You

- Share your feelings with someone you trust. This person might be a friend, relative, or clergy.

- Talk to your health care provider, a social worker, or a mental health professional.

- You can also find help by calling the National Institute of Mental Health Information Line at 866-615-6464 or visiting their website at www.nimh.nih.gov.

- In your local community, contact "First Call for Help" hotline (check white pages for local number) or call the local mental health center.

Section 51.2

Exercise for Stress Relief

This information is by Major Leo Mahony, MPT, from Targeting Health: Stress Management, September 2000, from the U.S. Army Center for Health Promotion and Preventive Medicine. Reviewed by David A. Cooke, M.D., April 2007.

Exercise and physical activity are powerful and readily available tools for preventing and treating symptoms of stress. The old adages "run for your life" and "burn off some steam" merit serious consideration. It is truly possible to walk, bike, run, lift, and stretch your way to a happier less stressful lifestyle. The first step is up to you: make a realistic activation plan for being more active.

The Exercise-Stress Connection

Studies are beginning to show that physical activity enhances psychological well-being and relieves symptoms of depression and anxiety. Here are some of the factors involved:

- Regular exercise helps one to feel in control. This sense of control over the body may translate to an improved sense of control over other aspects of life, a key defense against stress.

- Exercise promotes well-being and relaxation. Regular exercisers demonstrate higher levels of self-esteem and confidence and maintain a sense of self-discipline. The individual acts upon the belief, "I am in charge of myself and can improve my health and fitness."

- Moderate physical activity is a natural, physiological outlet for a body in the "fight or flight" state of arousal frequently associated with stress. It cleanses the body of adrenaline, can lower the blood pressure, and relaxes tight muscles. Exercise produces neurotransmitters called endorphins in the brain. These are the body's own natural tranquilizers. Endorphins can make one feel calm and relaxed during and for up to three hours after moderate physical activity. This elevation in mood has been referred to as the runners' high but is also experienced by those involved in other forms of exercise.

- Exercise can cause many people who are physically active to give up unhealthy and stressful habits that interfere with exercise. Smokers may cut down or quit because smoking hinders aerobic performance. Others may eat more nutritiously to improve performance. The chronically busy individual may "work in" a workout to increase energy, alertness, and productivity—clearly a sound business investment with ample rewards.

- Exercise can be a group or solo activity. Some individuals seek and develop alliances with other exercisers, which may provide social support—another stress reliever. Others may prefer some private time to exercise alone to "clear the head." Still others prefer some of both, depending on mood and circumstances. People of all ages can realize these benefits.

Before Starting an Exercise Program

Precautions: Physical activity is an excellent stress management tool when used correctly and safely. However, an inconsistent (sporadic) or hasty ("too much too soon") program invites injury—from trauma to overuse—which can add to stress rather than alleviating it.

Considerations: Most adults do not need to be examined by a health care provider before starting a moderate-level physical activity program. Exceptions include: men over the age of 40; women over the age of 50; those with one or more cardiac risk factors; and those with signs or symptoms of cardiac, pulmonary, or metabolic disease. Programs for children should be age-appropriate so as not to exceed strength or coordination abilities, jeopardize normal growth, or pose a serious threat of injury or disability.

Helpful Hints

- **Start slowly:** Begin exercising at your current level and gradually increase the pace or the length of your workouts over time. A helpful rule of thumb for a safe progression is no greater than 10 percent increase in total weekly repetitions, resistance, distance, or time. Unfortunately, many exercisers must stop a program because of an overuse injury; they attempted too much, too soon. While some morning soreness after a workout is normal, anything beyond this or occurring longer than 24 hours is probably indicative of a hasty progression. Starting slow can be encouraging rather than discouraging.

- **Set realistic goals:** Stop exercising your excuses and start exercising your body! Small steps taken today will help you achieve long-range goals, but it won't happen overnight and it won't happen if you don't start. Daily walks, slow stretching, and a light toning routine can ease you into a realistic plan.

- **Do it now:** Many extremely busy people do live healthy lifestyles and exercise regularly. The key is in making fitness a priority. The commitment is the key. Waiting until things are less stressful won't work. Find an activity and/or routine that you like and get started. Make and keep an appointment with exercise. The most popular exercise time for the chronically busy is first thing in the morning, before the rest of the world tries to derail you.

- **Write it down:** Many people obtain personal reward and additional motivation by documenting their health and fitness accomplishments. Fitness notes can be as simple as an exercise diary or as innovative as computer software programs that provide personalized feedback with flashy displays and printouts. The best method is whatever motivates you to be consistent.

- **Stay on track:** Don't get discouraged if you miss an occasional workout. We all have days where in spite of best intentions, we did not accomplish all our objectives. Injury, travel, and obligations may force a missed workout. In the context of a lifetime, several days or weeks off is no big deal but don't take a month or two to resume your program. Reaffirm the priority of health and regular exercise and get back on track again as soon as you can.

- **Enjoy yourself:** Working out is something you should enjoy and look forward to. Select a variety of activities that energize you enough to continue performing on a regular basis. Many people make exercise a family activity. This can be a great way to spend quality time with family or friends while establishing healthy habits that last a lifetime.

Chapter 52

Yoga and Tai Chi for Stress Relief

Exercise is good for the mind, not just the body. Exercise can help with stress relief because it provides a way for the body to release tension and pent-up frustration. The Eastern practices of Yoga and tai chi are effective stress-reducing forms of exercise.

Whenever we encounter a stressful event, our bodies undergo a series of hormonal and biochemical changes that put us in 'alarm mode.' Our heart rate increases, adrenaline rushes through our bloodstream, and our digestive and immune systems temporarily shut down. If the stressors continue and we stay on high alert for a prolonged period of time, we experience exhaustion and burnout. None of us can avoid stress, but we can return to a state of balance and regulation through a variety of means, including deep breathing, meditation, yoga, and exercise. These activities provide calming and relaxing sensory input for stress relief and can be selected according to lifestyle and preference.

How do breathing exercises relieve stress?

When you're facing a stressful situation, you can reduce your stress

"Stress Relief: Yoga, Meditation, and Other Relaxation Techniques," reprinted with permission from http://www.helpguide.org/mental/stress_relief_meditation _yoga_relaxation.htm. © 2007 Helpguide.org. All rights reserved. Helpguide provides a detailed list of related references for this article, including links to information from other websites. For a complete list of Helpguide's current resources related to stress signs and symptoms, causes of stress, burnout, and stress relief and relaxation techniques, visit www.helpguide.org.

simply by deep breathing. Deep breathing involves not only the lungs but also the abdomen. To experience abdominal breathing, sit comfortably with your back straight. Put one hand on your chest and the other on your stomach. Inhale through your nose and the hand on your stomach should begin to rise. Your other hand should move very little. Exhale as much air as you can while contracting your abdominal muscles. Once again, the hand on your stomach should move in as you exhale, but your other hand should move very little.

If you have a hard time breathing from your abdomen sitting up, lie on the floor, put a small book on your stomach, and try to breathe so that the book rises as you inhale and falls as you exhale. Breathing techniques can be practiced almost anywhere and can be combined with other relaxation exercises, such as aromatherapy and music. All you really need is 10 minutes a day and a place to stretch out.

How does progressive muscle relaxation work?

You can combine deep breathing with the controlled contracting and relaxing of muscles to achieve an additional level of relief from stress:

- Loosen your clothing and get comfortable.

- Tighten the muscles in your toes. Hold for a count of 10. Relax and enjoy the release of tension.

- Flex the muscles in your feet. Hold for a count of 10. Relax.

- Move slowly up through your body—legs, abdomen, back, neck, face—contracting and relaxing muscles as you go.

- Breathe deeply and slowly.

What can meditation do to relieve stress?

When you meditate you bring together all of the mind's energies and focus them on a word, a sound, a symbol, a comforting image, or your own breathing. The optimal setting for meditation is a quiet, clean place. People typically meditate sitting on the floor or in a chair with their eyes closed.

Meditation involves both effort and passive participation. It takes effort to bring your attention back to your chosen focus but you also become simply a witness to everything that happens: random thoughts, sensory input, body sensations, such as itches and cramps and external stimuli. As a result, you incorporate them into the meditation experience. All meditation practices involve the development of mindfulness—being fully engaged in whatever is happening in the present moment, without analyzing or otherwise "over-thinking" the experience.

A variation of traditional meditation involves guided imagery or visualization. If you use this method, you'll imagine a scene in which you feel at peace, able to let go of all concerns and tensions. In guided imagery, audio instructions help you visualize the scene, focus your thoughts, and relax.

You don't have to be seated or still to meditate. In walking meditation, mindfulness involves being focused on the physicality of each step—the sensation of your feet touching the ground, the rhythm of your breath while moving, feeling the wind against your face.

What is yoga and how can it help with stress relief?

Yoga is a broad term for a series of personal practices, which bring together your physical, mental, and spiritual resources with the goal of attaining a state of wholeness and completeness. The term yoga is a Sanskrit word meaning "to unite."

There are many forms of yoga, and all have a spiritual component. Most Westerners practice Hatha yoga, which focuses on the physical aspects. Yoga teaches you a series of stationary and moving poses called asanas and a form of breath control known as pranayama, as well as concentration techniques.

Yoga postures are designed to balance the different systems of the body, including the central nervous, the endocrine (glandular), and the digestive systems. By slowing down your mental activity, taking your mind off the causes of stress, and having you gently stretch your body in ways that massage your internal organs, yoga helps you create dynamic peacefulness within yourself.

Health Benefits of Yoga

- Improves flexibility and joint mobility
- Strengthens and tones muscles
- Increases stamina
- Improves digestion
- Lowers cholesterol and blood sugar levels
- Improves circulation
- Boosts immune response

Mental Benefits of Yoga

- Increases positive body awareness
- Relieves chronic stress patterns in the body
- Relaxes the mind and body
- Centers attention
- Sharpens concentration
- Frees the spirit

It's healthy to challenge yourself in assuming yoga positions, but don't extend yourself beyond what feels comfortable, and always back off on a pose at the first sign of pain.

While instructional CDs and DVDs are available, you'll get the best results by attending classes at a yoga studio or hiring a private teacher. The Yoga Alliance provides an international, searchable list of Registered Teachers who hold Registered Yoga Teacher credentials.

What is tai chi and how can it offer stress relief?

Tai chi is a self-paced, non-competitive series of slow, gentle, flowing body movements that emphasize concentration, relaxation, and the conscious circulation of vital energy throughout the body. Though tai chi was first developed as a martial art during the 13th century, it is primarily practiced today as a way of calming the mind, conditioning the body, and reducing stress. As in meditation, tai chi practitioners focus on their breathing and keeping their attention in the present moment.

As the Mayo Clinic points out, tai chi is considered less strenuous and challenging than yoga and is generally safe for people of all ages and levels of fitness. Because the movements are low impact, it's often appealing to older adults, people with joint pain, and those recovering from injuries. It can also improve balance and reduce the risk of falls. Once you have learned the moves, you can practice it anywhere, at any time, by yourself or with others; and without special clothing or gear.

Health Benefits of Tai Chi

- Reduced stress
- Greater body awareness
- Increased strength and stamina

- Easier breathing and better sleep
- Slower bone loss in postmenopausal women
- Improved balance and coordination
- Better cardiovascular fitness
- Chronic pain relief

The International Taoist Tai Chi Society provides a world directory of tai chi practitioners as a resource to find qualified instruction near where you live, or check your local listings for an instructor.

How does massage therapy ease stress?

A professional massage can provide soothing, deep relaxation and can improve physiological processes such as circulation. As the tense muscles relax, so does your entire body, as well as your over-stressed mind. According to the American Massage Therapy Association (AMTA), the most common type of massage is Swedish massage, which is specifically meant to relax and energize you through stroking and kneading the muscles.

Another common type of massage is shiatsu, also known as acupressure. Therapists use their fingers to manipulate the body's pressure points to open channels that can release fresh energy and carry away spent energy and toxins. You may consider visiting the consumer section of AMTA's website to learn more about what massage can do for you, what to expect from a massage, and how to find a qualified massage therapist.

If regular massage therapy is out of your price range, try giving yourself a massage. Table 52.1 has examples from Northwestern University Health Services:

How can cardiovascular exercise relieve stress?

If you're trying to manage or relieve stress, you owe it to yourself to work up a sweat on a regular basis because vigorous exercise helps the mind as much as it benefits the body.

Exercise relieves stress in several ways:

- It allows the body to release tension and pent-up frustration.
- It raises the output of endorphins, "feel-good" brain chemicals that ward off depression.
- It decreases the output of stress hormones.

477

- It helps you get better sleep.

- It relaxes muscles and lowers your resting pulse rate.

- It makes you feel better about yourself.

You can start with as little as 15 minutes, twice a week. However, 20 to 60 minutes, five or more times a week is recommended for optimal stress management.

Table 52.1. Self-Massage Techniques

Scalp Soother	Place your thumbs behind your ears while spreading your fingers on top of your head. Move your scalp back and forth slightly by making circles with your fingertips for 15 to 20 seconds.
Easy on the Eyes	Close your eyes and place your ring fingers directly under your eyebrows, near the bridge of your nose. Slowly increase the pressure for 5 to 10 seconds, then gently release. Repeat 2 to 3 times.
Sinus Pressure Relief	Place your fingertips at the bridge of your nose. Slowly slide your fingers down your nose and across the top of your cheekbones to the outside of your eyes.
Shoulder Tension Relief	Reach one arm across the front of your body to your opposite shoulder. Using a circular motion, press firmly on the muscle above your shoulder blade. Repeat on the other side.

Table 52.2. Common Exercise Problems and Solutions

Excuse	Solution
I don't have time to exercise.	Incorporate exercise into something you're already doing, such as running errands or watching TV.
I'm too tired to exercise.	Start small and slow: a 10-minute stroll will become a brisk half hour trot.
I have trouble with weight-bearing exercise.	To spare your knees, try cycling or an elliptical machine. If any weight-bearing activity is a problem, try swimming.
Working out is boring.	Work out with a friend or use a workout machine that allows you to read, listen to music, or watch TV while exercising.
I can't afford equipment or gym membership.	Walking and jogging cost nothing. Also, cleaning your house counts as exercise.

Getting motivated to exercise can be difficult. Table 52.2 shows some common problems and solutions to them.

Ask your health care provider to recommend an exercise program that fits your needs, especially if you're over 35. If you have heart problems, high blood pressure, or problems with your bones or joints, you should also seek advice from a doctor.

How can your sensory organs help you relieve stress?

You can use sensory stimuli to help you reduce stress. Methods include:

- Listening to soothing music.
- Taking a long, hot bath or shower.
- Looking at a beautiful scene or picture.
- Using aromatherapy, or various scents, to evoke physical responses.

By enlisting your body as an ally, you may be better able to reduce and relieve your levels of stress.

Chapter 53

Herbs Used to Reduce Stress and Anxiety Symptoms

Chapter Contents

Section 53.1

Kava

"Kava—*Piper methysticum*" is a fact sheet published by the National Center for Complementary and Alternative Medicine (NCCAM, nccam.nih .gov), part of the National Institutes of Health, June 1, 2006.

Introduction

This text provides basic information about the herb kava—common names, uses, potential side effects, and resources for more information. Kava is native to the islands of the South Pacific and is a member of the pepper family.

Common Names

Kava kava, awa, kava pepper; Latin Names—*Piper methysticum*

What It Is Used For

• Kava has been used as a ceremonial beverage in the South Pacific for centuries.

• Kava has also been used to help people fall asleep and fight fatigue, as well as to treat asthma and urinary tract infections.

• Topically (on the skin), kava has been used as a numbing agent.

• Today, kava is used primarily for anxiety, insomnia, and menopausal symptoms.

How It Is Used

The root and rhizome (underground stem) of kava are used to prepare beverages, extracts, capsules, tablets, and topical solutions.

What the Science Says

• Although scientific studies provide some evidence that kava may be beneficial for the management of anxiety, the U.S. Food and Drug Administration (FDA) has issued a warning that using kava supplements has been linked to a risk of severe liver damage.

- Kava is not a proven therapy for other uses.

- NCCAM-funded studies on kava were suspended after the FDA issued its warning.

Side Effects and Cautions

- Kava has been reported to cause liver damage, including hepatitis and liver failure (which can cause death).

- Kava has been associated with several cases of dystonia (abnormal muscle spasm or involuntary muscle movements).

- Kava may interact with several drugs, including drugs used for Parkinson's disease.

- Long-term and/or heavy use of kava may result in scaly, yellowed skin.

- Avoid driving and operating heavy machinery while taking kava because the herb has been reported to cause drowsiness.

- Tell your health care providers about any herb or dietary supplement you are using, including kava. This helps to ensure safe and coordinated care.

Sources

National Center for Complementary and Alternative Medicine. *Kava Linked to Liver Damage.* National Center for Complementary and Alternative Medicine Website. Accessed at http://nccam.nih.gov/health/alerts/kava on March 30, 2006.

Kava. Natural Medicines Comprehensive Database Website. Accessed March 30, 2006.

Kava *(Piper methysticum G. Forst).* Natural Standard Database Website. Accessed March 30, 2006.

Kava kava rhizome (root). In: Blumenthal M, Goldberg A, Brinckman J, eds. *Herbal Medicine: Expanded Commission E Monographs.* Newton, MA: Lippincott Williams & Wilkins; 2000:221–225.

Kava (*Piper methysticum*). In: Coates P, Blackman M, Cragg G, et al., eds. *Encyclopedia of Dietary Supplements*. New York, NY: Marcel Dekker; 2005:373–380.

Food and Drug Administration. *Kava-Containing Dietary Supplements May Be Associated With Severe Liver Injury*. Food and Drug Administration Website. Accessed at http://www.cfsan.fda.gov/~dms/addskava .html on March 30, 2006.

Pittler MH, Ernst E. Kava extract versus placebo for treating anxiety. *Cochrane Database of Systematic Reviews*. 2003;(1):CD003383. Accessed at http://www.cochrane.org on April 25, 2006.

Section 53.2

Valerian

"Valerian—*Valeriana officinalis*" is a fact sheet published by the National Center for Complementary and Alternative Medicine (NCCAM, nccam.nih .gov), part of the National Institutes of Health, May 30, 2006.

Introduction

This text provides basic information about the herb valerian—common names, uses, potential side effects, and resources for more information. Valerian is a plant native to Europe and Asia; it is also found in North America.

Common Names

Valerian, all-heal, garden heliotrope; Latin Names—*Valeriana officinalis*

What It Is Used For

- Valerian has long been used for sleep disorders and anxiety.
- Valerian has also been used for other conditions, such as headaches, depression, irregular heartbeat, and trembling.

How It Is Used

The roots and rhizomes (underground stems) of valerian are typically used to make supplements, including capsules, tablets, and liquid extracts, as well as teas.

What the Science Says

- Research suggests that valerian may be helpful for insomnia, but there is not enough evidence from well-designed studies to confirm this.

- There is not enough scientific evidence to determine whether valerian works for anxiety or for other conditions, such as depression and headaches.

- NCCAM is funding a study to look at the effects of valerian on sleep in healthy older adults and in people with Parkinson disease.

Side Effects and Cautions

- Studies suggest that valerian is generally safe to use for short periods of time (for example, 4 to 6 weeks).

- No information is available about the long-term safety of valerian.

- Valerian can cause mild side effects, such as headaches, dizziness, upset stomach, and tiredness the morning after its use.

- Tell your health care providers about any herb or dietary supplement you are using, including valerian. This helps to ensure safe and coordinated care.

Sources

Office of Dietary Supplements and National Center for Complementary and Alternative Medicine. *Questions and Answers About Valerian for Insomnia and Other Sleep Disorders.* Office of Dietary Supplements Website. Accessed May 3, 2006.

Valerian. Natural Medicines Comprehensive Database Website. Accessed May 3, 2006.

Valerian *(Valeriana officinalis L.).* Natural Standard Database Website. Accessed May 3, 2006.

Valerian root *(Valeriana officinalis)*. In: Blumenthal M, Goldberg A, Brinckman J, eds. *Herbal Medicine: Expanded Commission E Monographs*. Newton, MA: Lippincott Williams & Wilkins; 2000:394–400.

Awang DVC, Leung AY. Valerian. In: Coates P, Blackman M, Cragg G, et al., eds. *Encyclopedia of Dietary Supplements*. New York, NY: Marcel Dekker; 2005:687–700.

Chapter 54

Controlling Anger before It Controls You

We all know what anger is, and we've all felt it: whether as a fleeting annoyance or as full-fledged rage.

Anger is a completely normal, usually healthy, human emotion. But when it gets out of control and turns destructive, it can lead to problems—problems at work, in your personal relationships, and in the overall quality of your life. And it can make you feel as though you're at the mercy of an unpredictable and powerful emotion. This information is meant to help you understand and control anger.

What Is Anger?

The Nature of Anger

Anger is "an emotional state that varies in intensity from mild irritation to intense fury and rage," according to Charles Spielberger, Ph.D., a psychologist who specializes in the study of anger. Like other emotions, it is accompanied by physiological and biological changes; when you get angry, your heart rate and blood pressure go up, as do the levels of your energy hormones, adrenaline, and noradrenaline.

Anger can be caused by both external and internal events. You could be angry at a specific person (Such as a coworker or supervisor) or event (a traffic jam, a canceled flight), or your anger could be caused

Copyright © 1992 by the American Psychological Association. Reprinted with permission. Reviewed by David A. Cooke, M.D., April 2007.

by worrying or brooding about your personal problems. Memories of traumatic or enraging events can also trigger angry feelings.

Expressing Anger

The instinctive, natural way to express anger is to respond aggressively. Anger is a natural, adaptive response to threats; it inspires powerful, often aggressive, feelings and behaviors, which allow us to fight and to defend ourselves when we are attacked. A certain amount of anger, therefore, is necessary to our survival.

On the other hand, we can't physically lash out at every person or object that irritates or annoys us; laws, social norms, and common sense place limits on how far our anger can take us.

People use a variety of both conscious and unconscious processes to deal with their angry feelings. The three main approaches are expressing, suppressing, and calming. Expressing your angry feelings in an assertive—not aggressive—manner is the healthiest way to express anger. To do this, you have to learn how to make clear what your needs are, and how to get them met, without hurting others. Being assertive doesn't mean being pushy or demanding; it means being respectful of yourself and others.

Anger can be suppressed, and then converted or redirected. This happens when you hold in your anger, stop thinking about it, and focus on something positive. The aim is to inhibit or suppress your anger and convert it into more constructive behavior. The danger in this type of response is that if it isn't allowed outward expression, your anger can turn inward—on yourself. Anger turned inward may cause hypertension, high blood pressure, or depression.

Unexpressed anger can create other problems. It can lead to pathological expressions of anger, such as passive-aggressive behavior (getting back at people indirectly, without telling them why, rather than confronting them head on) or a personality that seems perpetually cynical and hostile. People who are constantly putting others down, criticizing everything, and making cynical comments haven't learned how to constructively express their anger. Not surprisingly, they aren't likely to have many successful relationships.

Finally, you can calm down inside. This means not just controlling your outward behavior, but also controlling your internal responses, taking steps to lower your heart rate, calm yourself down, and let the feelings subside.

As Dr. Spielberger notes, "when none of these three techniques work, that's when someone—or something—is going to get hurt."

Anger Management

The goal of anger management is to reduce both your emotional feelings and the physiological arousal that anger causes. You can't get rid of, or avoid, the things or the people that enrage you, nor can you change them, but you can learn to control your reactions.

Are You Too Angry?

There are psychological tests that measure the intensity of angry feelings, how prone to anger you are, and how well you handle it. But chances are good that if you do have a problem with anger, you already know it. If you find yourself acting in ways that seem out of control and frightening, you might need help finding better ways to deal with this emotion.

Why Are Some People More Angry than Others?

According to Jerry Deffenbacher, Ph.D., a psychologist who specializes in anger management, some people really are more "hotheaded" than others are; they get angry more easily and more intensely than the average person does. There are also those who don't show their anger in loud spectacular ways but are chronically irritable and grumpy. Easily angered people don't always curse and throw things; sometimes they withdraw socially, sulk, or get physically ill.

People who are easily angered generally have what some psychologists call a low tolerance for frustration, meaning simply that they feel that they should not have to be subjected to frustration, inconvenience, or annoyance. They can't take things in stride, and they're particularly infuriated if the situation seems somehow unjust: for example, being corrected for a minor mistake.

What makes these people this way? A number of things. One cause may be genetic or physiological: There is evidence that some children are born irritable, touchy, and easily angered, and that these signs are present from a very early age. Another may be sociocultural. Anger is often regarded as negative; we're taught that it's all right to express anxiety, depression, or other emotions but not to express anger. As a result, we don't learn how to handle it or channel it constructively.

Research has also found that family background plays a role. Typically, people who are easily angered come from families that are disruptive, chaotic, and not skilled at emotional communications.

Is It Good to Let It All Hang Out?

Psychologists now say that this is a dangerous myth. Some people use this theory as a license to hurt others. Research has found that "letting it rip" with anger actually escalates anger and aggression and does nothing to help you (or the person you're angry with) resolve the situation.

It's best to find out what it is that triggers your anger, and then to develop strategies to keep those triggers from tipping you over the edge.

Strategies to Keep Anger at Bay

Relaxation

Simple relaxation tools, such as deep breathing and relaxing imagery, can help calm down angry feelings. There are books and courses that can teach you relaxation techniques, and once you learn the techniques, you can call upon them in any situation. If you are involved in a relationship where both partners are hot-tempered, it might be a good idea for both of you to learn these techniques.

Some simple steps you can try:

- Breathe deeply, from your diaphragm; breathing from your chest won't relax you. Picture your breath coming up from your gut.

- Slowly repeat a calm word or phrase such as "relax" or "take it easy." Repeat it to yourself while breathing deeply.

- Use imagery; visualize a relaxing experience, from either your memory or your imagination.

- Nonstrenuous, slow yoga-like exercises can relax your muscles and make you feel much calmer.

- Practice these techniques daily. Learn to use them automatically when you're in a tense situation.

Cognitive Restructuring

Simply put, this means changing the way you think. Angry people tend to curse, swear, or speak in highly colorful terms that reflect their inner thoughts. When you're angry, your thinking can get very exaggerated and overly dramatic. Try replacing these thoughts with more rational ones. For instance, instead of telling yourself, "Oh, it's awful, it's terrible, everything's ruined," tell yourself, "It's frustrating, and it's understandable that I'm upset about it, but it's not the end of the world and getting angry is not going to fix it anyhow."

Be careful of words like "never" or "always" when talking about yourself or someone else. "This !&*%@ machine never works," or "You're always forgetting things" are not just inaccurate, they also serve to make you feel that your anger is justified and that there's no way to solve the problem. They also alienate and humiliate people who might otherwise be willing to work with you on a solution.

Remind yourself that getting angry is not going to fix anything and that it won't make you feel better (and may actually make you feel worse).

Logic defeats anger, because anger, even when it's justified, can quickly become irrational. So use cold hard logic on yourself. Remind yourself that the world is "not out to get you," you're just experiencing some of the rough spots of daily life. Do this each time you feel anger getting the best of you, and it'll help you get a more balanced perspective. Angry people tend to demand things: fairness, appreciation, agreement, willingness to do things their way. Everyone wants these things, and we are all hurt and disappointed when we don't get them, but angry people demand them, and when their demands aren't met, their disappointment becomes anger. As part of their cognitive restructuring, angry people need to become aware of their demanding nature and translate their expectations into desires. In other words, saying, "I would like" something is healthier than saying, "I demand" or "I must have" something. When you're unable to get what you want, you will experience the normal reactions—frustration, disappointment, hurt—but not anger. Some angry people use this anger as a way to avoid feeling hurt, but that doesn't mean the hurt goes away.

Problem Solving

Sometimes, our anger and frustration are caused by very real and inescapable problems in our lives. Not all anger is misplaced, and often it's a healthy, natural response to these difficulties. There is also a cultural belief that every problem has a solution, and it adds to our frustration to find out that this isn't always the case. The best attitude to bring to such a situation, then, is not to focus on finding the solution, but rather on how you handle and face the problem.

Make a plan, and check your progress along the way. Resolve to give it your best, but also not to punish yourself if an answer doesn't come right away. If you can approach it with your best intentions and efforts and make a serious attempt to face it head on, you will be less likely to lose patience and fall into all-or-nothing thinking, even if the problem does not get solved right away.

Better Communication

Angry people tend to jump to—and act on—conclusions, and some of those conclusions can be very inaccurate. The first thing to do if you're in a heated discussion is slow down and think through your responses. Don't say the first thing that comes into your head, but slow down and think carefully about what you want to say. At the same time, listen carefully to what the other person is saying and take your time before answering.

Listen, too, to what is underlying the anger. For instance, you like a certain amount of freedom and personal space, and your significant other wants more connection and closeness. If he or she starts complaining about your activities, don't retaliate by painting your partner as a jailer, a warden, or an albatross around your neck.

It's natural to get defensive when you're criticized, but don't fight back. Instead, listen to what's underlying the words: the message that this person might feel neglected and unloved. It may take a lot of patient questioning on your part, and it may require some breathing space, but don't let your anger—or a partner's—let a discussion spin out of control. Keeping your cool can keep the situation from becoming a disastrous one.

Using Humor

"Silly humor" can help defuse rage in a number of ways. For one thing, it can help you get a more balanced perspective. When you get angry and call someone a name or refer to them in some imaginative phrase, stop and picture what that word would literally look like. If you're at work and you think of a coworker as a "dirtbag" or a "single-cell life form," for example, picture a large bag full of dirt (or an amoeba) sitting at your colleague's desk, talking on the phone, going to meetings. Do this whenever a name comes into your head about another person. If you can, draw a picture of what the actual thing might look like. This will take a lot of the edge off your fury; and humor can always be relied on to help unknot a tense situation.

The underlying message of highly angry people, Dr. Deffenbacher says, is "things oughta go my way!" Angry people tend to feel that they are morally right, that any blocking or changing of their plans is an unbearable indignity and that they should NOT have to suffer this way. Maybe other people do, but not them!

When you feel that urge, he suggests, picture yourself as a god or goddess, a supreme ruler, who owns the streets and stores and office space, striding alone and having your way in all situations while others defer to you. The more detail you can get into your imaginary scenes, the more chances you have to realize that maybe you are being unreasonable; you'll also realize how unimportant the things you're angry about really are. There are two cautions in using humor. First, don't try to just "laugh off" your problems; rather, use humor to help yourself face them more constructively. Second, don't give in to harsh, sarcastic humor; that's just another form of unhealthy anger expression.

What these techniques have in common is a refusal to take yourself too seriously. Anger is a serious emotion, but it's often accompanied by ideas that, if examined, can make you laugh.

Changing Your Environment

Sometimes it's our immediate surroundings that give us cause for irritation and fury. Problems and responsibilities can weigh on you and make you feel angry at the "trap" you seem to have fallen into and all the people and things that form that trap.

Give yourself a break. Make sure you have some "personal time" scheduled for times of the day that you know are particularly stressful. One example is the working mother who has a standing rule that when she comes home from work, for the first 15 minutes "nobody talks to Mom unless the house is on fire." After this brief quiet time, she feels better prepared to handle demands from her kids without blowing up at them.

Some Other Tips for Easing up on Yourself

Timing: If you and your spouse tend to fight when you discuss things at night—perhaps you're tired, or distracted, or maybe it's just habit—try changing the times when you talk about important matters so these talks don't turn into arguments.

Avoidance: If your child's chaotic room makes you furious every time you walk by it, shut the door. Don't make yourself look at what infuriates you. Don't say, "well, my child should clean up the room so

493

I won't have to be angry!" That's not the point. The point is to keep yourself calm.

Finding alternatives: If your daily commute through traffic leaves you in a state of rage and frustration, give yourself a project—learn or map out a different route, one that's less congested or more scenic. Or find another alternative, such as a bus or commuter train.

Do You Need Counseling?

If you feel that your anger is really out of control, if it is having an impact on your relationships and on important parts of your life, you might consider counseling to learn how to handle it better. A psychologist or other licensed mental health professional can work with you in developing a range of techniques for changing your thinking and your behavior.

When you talk to a prospective therapist, tell her or him that you have problems with anger that you want to work on, and ask about his or her approach to anger management. Make sure this isn't only a course of action designed to "put you in touch with your feelings and express them"—that may be precisely what your problem is. With counseling, psychologists say, a highly angry person can move closer to a middle range of anger in about 8 to 10 weeks, depending on the circumstances and the techniques used.

What about Assertiveness Training?

It's true that angry people need to learn to become assertive (rather than aggressive), but most books and courses on developing assertiveness are aimed at people who don't feel enough anger. These people are more passive and acquiescent than the average person; they tend to let others walk all over them. That isn't something that most angry people do. Still, these books can contain some useful tactics to use in frustrating situations.

Remember, you can't eliminate anger—and it wouldn't be a good idea if you could. In spite of all your efforts, things will happen that will cause you anger; and sometimes it will be justifiable anger. Life will be filled with frustration, pain, loss, and the unpredictable actions of others. You can't change that; but you can change the way you let such events affect you. Controlling your angry responses can keep them from making you even more unhappy in the long run.

Chapter 55

Stress on the Road

Chapter Contents

Section 55.1

What Is Aggressive Driving and Road Rage?

"What Is Aggressive Driving?" is from the tip sheet "Aggressive Driving: Fact-Tip Sheet With Talking Points," published by the National Highway Traffic Safety Administration (NHTSA), October 2000. Reviewed by David A. Cooke, M.D., April 2007.

Aggressive driving is defined as a progression of unlawful driving actions such as:

- speeding: exceeding the posted limit or driving too fast for conditions;

- improper or excessive lane changing, failing to signal intent, failing to see that movement can be made safely; or

- improper passing: failing to signal intent, using an emergency lane to pass, or passing on the shoulder.

The "aggressive driver" fails to consider the human element involved. The anonymity of being behind the wheel gives aggressive drivers a false sense of control and power; therefore, they seldom take into account the consequences of their actions.

Aggressive driving vs. road rage: There is a difference. Aggressive driving is a traffic offense; road rage is a criminal offense.

Road rage is defined as "an assault with a motor vehicle or other dangerous weapon by the operator or passenger(s) of another motor vehicle or an assault precipitated by an incident that occurred on a roadway."

Road rage requires willful and wanton disregard for the safety of others.

A national survey sponsored by NHTSA of 6,000 drivers over the age of 16 showed that the public supports increased enforcement including photo enforcement, increasing sanctions, increasing intervention by vehicle occupants and increasing public awareness of risks, as ways of reducing these types of unsafe driving practices.

The posted speed limit is a law that applies to all traffic lanes. Technically speaking, there is no fast lane or slow lane. In at least 21 states, slower traffic is expected to keep right, except for emergency vehicles, which are permitted to exceed the posted speed limit, but only when their lights and sirens are on. In some states, laws specify "keep right except to pass."

According to NHTSA's Traffic Safety Facts 1998, approximately 6,335,000 crashes occur in the United States each year. It is unknown exactly how many of those crashes are caused by aggressive driving. Estimates indicate the number to be substantial, based on the violations committed by the drivers of the vehicles involved in the crashes and reported by law enforcement agencies as the contributing factor of the crash.

Section 55.2

Tips for Reducing Aggressive Driving

"Are You an Aggressive Driver?" is a brochure by the National Highway Traffic Safety Administration (NHTSA), October 2000. Reviewed by David A. Cooke, M.D., April 2007.

Are You an Aggressive Driver?

Do you:

- **express frustration?** Taking out your frustrations on your fellow motorists can lead to violence or a crash.

- **fail to pay attention when driving?** Reading, eating, drinking, or talking on the phone can be a major cause of roadway crashes.

- **tailgate?** This is a major cause of crashes that can result in serious deaths or injuries.

- **make frequent lane changes?** If you whip in and out of lanes to advance ahead, you can be a danger to other motorists.

- **run red lights?** Do not enter an intersection on a yellow light. Remember flashing red lights should be treated as a stop sign.

- **speed?** Going faster than the posted speed limit, being a "road racer," and going too fast for conditions are some examples of speeding.

Plan Ahead and Allow Yourself Extra Time

- **Concentrate:** Don't allow yourself to become distracted by talking on your cellular phone, eating, drinking, or putting on makeup.

- **Relax:** Tune the radio to your favorite relaxing music. Music can calm your nerves and help you to enjoy your time in the car.

- **Drive the posted speed limit:** Fewer crashes occur when vehicles are traveling at or about the same speed.

- **Identify alternate routes:** Try mapping out an alternate route. Even if it looks longer on paper, you may find it is less congested.

- **Use public transportation:** Public transportation can give you some much-needed relief from life behind the wheel.

- **Just be late:** If all else fails, just be late.

When Confronted with Aggressive Drivers

- **Get out of the way:** First and foremost make every attempt to get out of their way.

- **Put your pride aside:** Do not challenge them by speeding up or attempting to hold your own in your travel lane.

- **Avoid eye contact:** Eye contact can sometimes enrage an aggressive driver.

- **Gestures:** Ignore gestures and refuse to return them.

- **Report serious aggressive driving:** You or a passenger may call the police. But, if you use a cell phone, pull over to a safe location.

Chapter 56

Reducing Stress in the Workplace

Chapter Contents

Section 56.1

What Employers and Managers Can Do to Reduce Stress at Work

"Job Stress Management: Stress Causes & Effects; Tips for Workplace Stress Reduction," by Ellen Jaffe-Gill, M.A., Robert Segal, M.A., Jaelline Jaffe, Ph.D., reprinted with permission from http://www.helpguide.org/ mental/work_stress_management.htm. © 2007 Helpguide.org. All rights reserved. Helpguide provides a detailed list of related references for this article, including links to information from other websites. For a complete list of Helpguide's current resources related to stress signs and symptoms, causes of stress, burnout, and stress relief and relaxation techniques, visit www.helpguide.org.

Workplace stress has a negative impact on the business as well as on the individual employee. The increase in job stress creates emotional, financial, and safety concerns for employers and managers. The bottom line: workplace stress management and stress reduction make sense.

Stress in the workplace is not a new phenomenon, but it is a greater threat to employee health and well-being than ever before. While technology has made aspects of many jobs easier, it has also added to the anxieties of office life through information overload, heightened pressure for productivity, and a threatening sense of impermanence in the workplace. In 1996, the World Health Organization labeled stress a "worldwide epidemic." Today, workplace stress is estimated to cost American companies more than $300 billion a year in poor performance, absenteeism, and health costs.

What is workplace stress?

Stress—the responses our bodies and minds have to the demands placed on them—is a normal part of life and a normal part of any job. Without stress, we wouldn't meet deadlines, strive to hit sales or production targets, or line up new clients. Meeting the demands and challenges of a job is part of what makes work interesting and satisfying, and it's often what allows people to develop new skills and advance in their careers. In the workplace, we regularly experience stress-causing situations, react to them with heightened tension, then return to a more relaxed state when the crisis, big or small, is resolved. However, problems occur when stress is so overwhelming or constant that the tension never abates and we never get to relax.

What we think of as "job stress" is what happens when:

- The challenges and demands of work become excessive.

- The pressures of the workplace surpass workers' abilities to handle them.

- Satisfaction becomes frustration and exhaustion.

When stress crosses the line from normal to excessive, it can trigger physical and emotional responses that are harmful to employees and businesses alike. And unfortunately, for many people "stress" has become synonymous with "work."

What causes stress in the workplace?

Some jobs are stressful by definition because they're physically dangerous (such as firefighting or criminal justice), involve matters of life and death (emergency functions), or are psychologically demanding (social work, teaching). But people who stamp metal or crunch numbers can also be subject to stress on the job.

Workplace stress is usually the result of high demands on the job, real or perceived lack of control concerning those demands, poor day-to-day organization and communication, and an unsupportive work environment.

Table 56.1 lays out many of the factors that lead to job stress:

What are the health effects of job stress?

There is a clear connection between workplace stress and physical and emotional problems. According to the National Institute for Occupational Safety and Health, early warning signs of job stress include:

- headache;
- sleep disturbance;
- upset stomach;
- difficulty concentrating;
- irritability;

- low morale; or
- poor relations with family and friends.

While these early signs are relatively easy to recognize, it may be harder to see how job stress affects chronic health problems, since chronic conditions develop over time and may be influenced by factors other than stress. Still, evidence suggests that workplace stress

Table 56.1. Factors That Lead to Job Stress

Types of Job Stressors	Examples
Specific work factors	• Excessive workload. • Tedious or meaningless tasks. • Long hours and low pay. • Infrequent rest breaks. • Unreasonable performance demands.
Physical environment	• Noise and overcrowding. • Poor air quality. • Ergonomic problems. • Health and safety risks (heavy equipment, toxic chemicals).
Organizational practices	• Unclear responsibilities or expectations. • Conflicting job demands. • Multiple supervisors. • Lack of autonomy or participation in decision-making. • Inefficient communication patterns. • Lack of family-friendly policies.
Workplace change	• Fear of layoff. • Frequent personnel turnover. • Lack of preparation for technological changes. • Poor chances for advancement or promotion. • Tensions brought about by greater workplace diversity.
Interpersonal relationships	• Distant, uncommunicative supervisors. • Poor performance from subordinates. • Office politics, competition, and other conflicts among staff. • Bullying or harassment. • Problems caused by excessive time away from family.

plays an important role in several types of ongoing health problems, especially:

- cardiovascular disease;
- musculoskeletal conditions; and
- psychological disorders.

What can managers or employers do to reduce stress at work?

Stress on the job creates high costs for businesses and institutions, reducing morale, productivity, and earnings. Clearly, it is in every employer's best interests—fiscal and otherwise—to reduce workplace stress as much as possible. Businesses can lower and prevent job stress through two methods:

- stress management programs and training for employees and
- organizational changes that improve working conditions.

Stress management: Nearly half of large American corporations provide their employees with stress management training and Employee Assistance Programs (EAPs). EAPs are designed to help workers with personal problems that may be adversely affecting their on-the-job performance. The confidential services include counseling, mental health assessment and referrals, workshops on topics such as time management and relaxation, and legal and financial assistance.

Read *The EAP Buyer's Guide* for advice on selecting the right EAP for your business, and browse the *EAP Directory* of national and international credentialed EAP providers.

Organizational change: While EAPs can be very beneficial to workers, the relief they provide may be superficial and short-lived if important root causes of stress in the work environment are not addressed. Lasting stress reduction is brought about by institutional change. "Managers are the key holders of corporate culture," Michael Peterson, a professor at University of Delaware, told *FDU magazine.* "They perpetuate it." While stress management techniques like yoga are great, he said, "if your boss is draconian, exercise is not going to help."

No meaningful job or workplace is, or should be expected to be, stress-free. However, less stress occurs when a business or institution encourages employee participation from the bottom up, implements policies that take employee needs into account, and empowers employees to do their best.

Look at Table 56.2 for a list of ways in which an organization can foster low levels of job stress and high levels of productivity:

What can employees do to reduce job stress?

While organizational change comes from management, there are still many things employees—individually or collectively—can do to reduce workplace stress.

Stand up for Yourself

- *Get a job description:* If your employer hasn't provided a specific, written description of your job, ask for one, or, better, ask to negotiate one. According to the American Psychological Association,

Table 56.2. Changing the Organization to Reduce Job Stress

Improve communication

- Share information with employees to reduce uncertainty about their jobs and futures.
- Clearly define employees' roles and responsibilities.
- Make communication friendly and efficient, not mean-spirited or petty.

Consult your employees

- Give workers opportunities to participate in decisions that affect their jobs.
- Consult employees about scheduling and work rules.
- Be sure the workload is suitable to employees' abilities and resources; avoid unrealistic deadlines.
- Show that individual workers are valued.

Offer rewards and incentives

- Praise good work performance verbally and institutionally.
- Provide opportunities for career development.
- Promote an "entrepreneurial" work climate that gives employees more control over their work.

Cultivate a friendly social climate

- Provide opportunities for social interaction among employees.
- Establish a zero-tolerance policy for harassment.
- Make management actions consistent with organizational values.

the act of negotiating a job description "does more to dispel a sense of powerlessness than anything else we know. You can object to what and insist on what you do want. If there is a compromise, it's because you agreed to it. With a clear job description, your expectations are spelled out, as are your boss's."

- *Change your job:* If you like where you're working but your job is too stressful, ask if the company can tailor the job to your skills or move you to a less pressured slot.

- *Get support:* Use the local, state, and federal agencies created to support workers' interests—and your union, if you belong to one—to back you up in situations that expose you to unnecessary danger, unsafe or unhealthful conditions, or undue harassment. While some locations and agencies are more sympathetic to employees' rights than others, sometimes simply mentioning that you know where to turn for help is enough to start an employer thinking about improvement.

- *Get a new job:* If the level of stress at your job is harming your health and your relationships, and you don't see any prospect of real change, it may be time to move on.

Eliminate Self-Defeating Behaviors

Many of us make job stress worse with patterns of thought or behavior that keep us from relieving pressure on ourselves. If you can turn around these self-defeating habits, you'll find employer-imposed stress easier to handle.

- *Resist perfectionism:* No project, situation, or decision is ever perfect, and you put undue stress on yourself by trying to do everything perfectly. When you set unrealistic goals for yourself or try to do too much, you're setting yourself up to fall short. Do your best, and you'll do fine.

- *Clean up your act:* If you're always running late, set your clocks and watches fast and give yourself extra time. If your desk is a mess, file and throw away the clutter; just knowing where everything is saves time and cuts stress. Make to-do lists and cross off items as you accomplish them. Plan your day and stick to the schedule—you'll feel less overwhelmed.

- *Flip your negative thinking:* If you see the downside of every situation and interaction, you'll find yourself drained of energy and motivation. Try to think positively about your work, avoid negative-thinking co-workers, and pat yourself on the back about small accomplishments, even if no one else does.

Find Ways to Dispel Stress

Quintessential Careers offers these tips for reducing stress:

- *Get time away:* If you feel stress building, take a break. Walk away from the situation. Take a stroll around the block, sit on a park bench, or spend a few minutes meditating. Exercise does wonders for the psyche. But even just finding a quiet place and listening to your iPod can reduce stress.

- *Talk it out:* Sometimes the best stress-reducer is simply sharing your stress with someone close to you. The act of talking it out—and getting support and empathy from someone else—is often an excellent way of blowing off steam and reducing stress.

- *Cultivate allies at work:* Just knowing you have one or more co-workers who are willing to assist you in times of stress will reduce your stress level. Just remember to reciprocate and help them when they are in need.

- *Find humor in the situation:* When you—or the people around you—start taking things too seriously, find a way to break through with laughter. Share a joke or funny story.

Section 56.2

Coping with Techno-Stress: Tips on Managing Cellular Phones, E-mail, and Other Gadgets in Your Life

"Managing Techno-Stress," © 2006 American Institute of Architects (www.aia.org). Reprinted with permission.

The very gadgets designed to make life easier can actually cause an added dimension of stress. It's frustrating when the faxes, e-mails, and voice mails pile up; annoying when phones don't stop ringing; and infuriating when equipment breaks down.

When your cell phone rings, do you tense up, wondering who wants what from you now or why you are receiving this call at dinner? Do you receive a staggering number of e-mails, voice messages, and faxes every day? And while you're on the phone returning calls, they continue to pile up.

Cell phones are indispensable in case of a highway emergency, to catch up on calls when waiting in traffic or at the airport, and to keep in close touch with family, friends, and business associates. They ring in the office, at school, restaurants, movies, and even at church! People walk down the street talking on the phone. As great as they are, cell phones (especially other people's) can be very annoying.

Tips on Managing Cell Phone Use

- Turn off your phone at concerts, theaters, movies, restaurants, church, and weddings and funerals. Turn it off whenever you need peace and quiet for a while.

- If the phone must be on, set it to vibrate and inform your companions that you have an important call coming in.

- When the call comes in, answer it with your most quiet "inside voice" and go to a private area (vestibule, parking lot) to complete your call.

- If other people talk loudly on their phone in a restaurant, ask the waiter or manager to invite the person to take their call in a private area.

Tips on Keeping Your E-mail under Control

E-mail is a great way to stay in touch with friends and family members who live in different time zones or even just around the corner. In the business world, e-mail has eliminated tons of paper.

- Limit e-mail time. Retrieve and read e-mail only twice a day.

- Respond, forward, and delete immediately. Print lengthy items to be read later. Save only those e-mails that are critical.

- Automate tasks. Create an automated signature, automated responses, and lists for forwarding.

- Preview e-mail messages. Just a glance at the subject line may tell you whether you can delete it. Delete messages from anyone you don't know to prevent receiving an e-mail virus.

- Keep your e-mail address confidential to avoid spamming.

Tips on Managing Stress at Home

There are ways to decrease stress levels at home as well. It's important to avoid being constantly on call by the office or by others making demands on your time.

- Turn off all the phones at family mealtimes and children's bath and story time.

- Keep your phone number unlisted to reduce unsolicited calls or use caller ID.

- Develop a hobby, such as gardening, reading, or caring for a pet.

- Turn off the television.

- Try stress busters such as relaxation tapes, yoga, meditation, and exercise.

By taking charge of technology, you won't become a slave to equipment or information or be on call 24 hours a day. Minimize stress by curtailing intrusions for at least one hour a day and do something you enjoy instead.

Chapter 57

Social Support Provides Stress Relief

Chapter Contents

Section 57.1

Finding Support through Self-Help Groups

From the National Women's Health Information Center's Pick Your Path to Health Campaign, 1995–2001. Reviewed by David A. Cooke, M.D., March 2007.

"My years as a medical practitioner, as well as my own first-hand experience, have taught me how important self-help groups are in assisting their members in dealing with problems, stress, hardship, and pain. Today, the benefits of mutual aid are experienced by millions of people who turn to others with a similar problem to attempt to deal with their isolation, powerlessness, alienation, and the awful feeling that nobody understands."—*Former Surgeon General C. Everett Koop*

The popularity of self-help groups has grown enormously over the last decade—and for good reason. Researchers and participants alike point to the benefits of self-help groups, and physicians, appreciating the value that self-help groups offer patients, are referring individuals to these venues for added "medicine." Today, millions of Americans turn to their peers for support, guidance, and empathy as they battle a host of conditions ranging from weight loss and codependency to alcoholism and bereavement.

A self-help group, also known as a mutual help group or a support group, generally has four characteristics:

- Mutual help is the primary goal of the environment.

- Members own and run the group themselves; while there may be a professional involved, he or she fills a supportive role and is not the leader of the group.

- Members share the same problem or experience.

- There is no or minimal cost for participating in the group.

The benefits of self-help groups are undeniable. Many studies point to the benefits of mutual support in helping members deal with the

510

realities of having a serious illness, understanding an emotional trauma, resisting addiction, or pursuing healthier relationships.

Consider these research findings:

- One half as many former psychiatric inpatients required rehospitalization after participating in a support group for 10 months than did former psychiatric patients who did not take part in a support group.

- One year after being admitted into a substance abuse treatment agency, African-American participants in a self-help program (Alcoholic Anonymous or Narcotics Anonymous) reported significantly more improvements in their medical, alcohol, and drug problems than did African-American patients who did not participate in self-help groups after treatment.

- Individuals who participated in a peer-led weight-loss group lost an equal amount of weight as individuals who participated in a similar group led by a professional (but they spent only half the money!).

- In a study of 57 African Americans who had been members of self-help groups for sickle-cell anemia, researchers found that the members who had been involved the longest reported fewest psychological problems associated with the disease, particularly in work and relationship areas.

Whatever the problem—whether it be physical, mental, emotional, or spiritual—there is likely to be a self-help group in your area where individuals are coming together in a shared pursuit for greater health and peace. Check out the American Self-Help Clearinghouse's Self-Help Sourcebook Online at http://mentalhelp.net/selfhelp for more information and details about how to find (or set up) a support group in your community. Take this step to lead you down the path to a healthier lifestyle.

Section 57.2

Religious Beliefs Can Protect Psychological Well-Being during Stressful Experiences

"Research shows how religious beliefs can protect psychological well-being during stressful experience," Copyright © 2006 by the American Psychological Association. Reprinted with permission.

According to a recent study, faith-based positive religious resources can protect psychological well-being through enhanced hope and perceived social support during stressful experiences, like undergoing cardiac surgery. Furthermore, having negative religious thoughts and struggles may hinder recovery. These results were presented at the 114th annual convention of the American Psychological Association (APA).

Although the connection between religiosity and health-related well-being has been studied for years, recent research found that the connection between religion and well-being is more complex than past studies suggested. Lead author Amy L. Ai, Ph.D., of the University of Washington and coauthor Crystal Park, Ph.D., of the University of Connecticut, sought to better understand the mechanisms through which religious coping styles operate by studying the postoperative adjustment of 309 cardiac patients at the University of Michigan Medical Center.

The researchers found that perceived social support and hope contributed to less depression and anxiety for postoperative patients who used positive religious coping styles in their everyday lives. "The contribution of social support to hope suggests that those who perceive more support at this critical moment may feel more hopeful about their recovery," said Dr. Ai. Acts of positive religious coping include religious forgiveness, seeking spiritual support, collaborative religious coping (fellowship with others who share the same beliefs), spiritual connection, religious purification, and thoughts of religious benevolence.

Negative coping styles are associated with the inability of patients to protect their psychological well-being against the distress of depression and anxiety that tend to predict poor postoperative recovery in the literature. This relationship is related to poor mental health at both preoperative and postoperative times, indicating ongoing faith-based struggles. Negative coping patterns consist of spiritual discontent, thoughts of punishing God, insecurity, demonic thoughts, interpersonal religious discontent, religious doubt, and discontented spiritual relations.

"These pathways appear to be key in understanding how religious coping styles may be helpful or harmful to a person's ability to handle stressful situations. These findings imply that health and mental health professionals should be more attentive to faith factors as inspirational or motivational springboards in some contexts," said Dr. Ai.

Chapter 58

Strategies for Managing Family Stress

Chapter Contents

Section 58.1

Make Time for Yourself So You Can Care for Others

Excerpted from "Make Time for Yourself," from the National Women's Health Information Center's (NWHIC, www.womenshealth.gov) Pick Your Path to Health Campaign, 1995–2001. Reviewed by David A. Cooke, M.D., March 2007.

Think for a moment. When was the last time you did something just for you? The holidays have come and gone along with many New Year's resolutions. But was making time for yourself among them?

For better health, set aside at least a couple of hours every week just for you. Ending each day stressed and overly fatigued is not healthy. Stress plays a role in high blood pressure. Doctors also link stress to migraine headaches, colds, heart disease, and many other illnesses. Taking a little bit of time to take care of yourself may be the single most important thing you can do to reduce stress and prevent serious illness.

Whatever their income level, many women find that leisure time doesn't come easily, particularly for single mothers who bear most of the responsibilities of family life. Caught up in maintaining a job, caring for children and older parents, pursuing a degree, or keeping a home in order, women often consider leisure time a luxury.

Take Care of Your Body and Mind

Taking time for yourself goes beyond the things that you would normally do such as eating a nutritious diet and sleeping well. "We don't want the message to be that this is one more thing that women have to do," says Amy Allina, Program and Policy Director for the National Women's Health Network. This is an opportunity to make small adjustments in your life so you don't feel overwhelmed.

If you are already taking time for yourself, keep doing it until it becomes an integral part of your routine. If you are looking for ways to get started, here are some suggestions:

- Start small. You won't be able to take huge blocks of time for yourself on a regular basis, but even 15 minutes, every other day will be a good habit-forming start.

- Seek connections that soothe your soul. Participate in a women-only retreat once a year—secular or religious—to renew your commitment to your well-being.

- Be realistic about what you can accomplish in a day. Plan room for unexpected demands on your time and events you can't control.

- Trade a few hours of child care with a neighbor every month. If you are married or have a significant other, trade child-care duties with a friend specifically so you can have a leisurely date.

- Ask someone to relieve you at least once a week if you take care of an ill family member.

- Send your children to bed early. They will begin the next day refreshed, and you can use the time to do something other than chores.

- Redistribute responsibilities with your partner if you are the only person caring for the children and tending to household needs.

- If your after-work social life seems too hectic, learn to say no; stay home and enjoy a hot bath instead.

And if leading a fast-paced life and taking care of others is what you truly love, just make sure your own needs are still being met. When you choose to do things you enjoy, you'll lead yourself down a path to better health year-round.

Section 58.2

Tips on Reducing Stress for Family Caregivers

"Tips on Reducing Stress for Family Caregivers," © 2006 North Dakota State University Extension Service (http://www.ext.nodak.edu). Reprinted with permission.

Caregiving provided to aging family members is often associated with stress and burnout. Although providing direct care to an adult family member can result in significant stress, it should also be remembered that this experience can have positive benefits as well. Both the rewards and the challenges of the caregiving experience should be honestly considered.

Suggested Benefits of Caregiving

It can be helpful to discuss how the caregiving experience has provided positive benefits to both the caregiver and the care recipient. This focus on the positive aspects of the experience can help give perspective and needed hope when stress increases. According to research, there are specific positive things associated with caregiving by many who pass through this experience.

Positive Benefits to the Caregiver

- Developing closer relationships with the person they care for and having sufficient time to be together

- Increased understanding of a parent or family member and the ability to forgive or heal past difficulties

- Greater patience with individuals and life challenges

- Personal growth as an individual due to being challenged and stretched in emotional and other ways

Positive Benefits to the Care Recipient

- Opportunity to receive assistance in a setting that is caring and personal

- Greater individualized care and attention than in other work settings

- Sharing of life experiences and close relationships with people who are close to them and who they appreciate

Areas of Stress Impact Related to Family Caregiving

The caregiving experience does impose demands on family members, and at times they may need to deal with significant levels of stress. Identifying specific areas of stress in caregiving allows for intervention to reduce or alleviate stress as it continues.

- Physical Demands—direct care, lifting, bathing, feeding, etc.

- Financial Demands—medical costs, equipment, hired help, lost income

- Emotional Burdens—feeling isolated, alone, without time for oneself

- Relationship Challenges—sibling conflict, conflict with dependent adult, etc.

Caregiving involves providing direct physical and emotional support to a family member or other adult who has become dependent and needs some care and assistance. The level of caregiving can vary from occasional monitoring of how a person is doing to full-time, round-the-clock care for a bed-bound individual. Caregiving can be a healthy and fulfilling experience. However, at times it can also bring burdens that lead to stress, exhaustion, anger, and even abuse. Awareness of the stresses that may accompany caregiving and tips for dealing with such stresses can be helpful to caregivers and family members.

Physical Demands and Direct Care as a Source of Stress

Caregiving often involves basic, practical aspects of care such as helping someone bathe or dress, moving from a bed to a wheelchair, or other physical demands. When these tasks are performed for a dependent adult, the resulting demands and labor can be challenging and stressful to a caregiver. Stress sources of physical demands and suggested coping tips include:

Stress Sources of Physical Demands

- Creating a safe physical environment, preventing falls

- Providing first aid and medical assistance as possible
- Bathing a care recipient
- Assisting with oral hygiene
- Dressing a care recipient
- Assisting with toileting needs
- Feeding or assistance with eating, nutrition needs
- Meal planning and preparation
- Lifting, turning, or transferring a care recipient
- Routine housework
- Management of behavior with care recipients who have cognitive impairment
- Other physical challenges

Suggested Coping Tips

- Learn how to properly care for your family member. Get training so you know how to perform needed skills, which will make your work easier and safer.
- Practice healthy habits, including a balanced diet, regular exercise, sufficient sleep, and visits to the doctor.
- When needed, get help with physical tasks from other care providers, neighbors, or sources of help.
- Work to keep your care recipient as independent as possible to reduce your stress and maintain dignity.
- Utilize adaptive or assistive equipment with specific needs.

Tips on Caring for Yourself

Plan ahead for those times when you will be stressed as a caregiver. It happens to everyone. If you have a plan of action, you will be better prepared to deal with stress so it does not interfere in your life or the care you are providing. No one will be helped if you become sick from too much stress.

A few tips include:

- Take a walk or ride a bike
- Take a bubble bath

- Engage in a favorite activity
- Allow for some quiet personal time
- Read a favorite book
- Talk with a friend
- Listen to soothing music
- Watch the sunset
- Share favorite memories with a friend
- Watch a favorite movie

Financial Demands and Management as a Source of Stress

Caregiving often takes a financial toll on caregivers and families. Financial demands that caregivers experience may include costs of medical care or payment for hired help. Also, at times caregivers can become directly involved in management of a person's financial affairs with banking, saving, or other issues. Stress sources of financial demands and suggested coping tips include:

Stress Sources of Financial Demands

- Costs of medical care and treatment
- Costs of adaptive or assistive equipment that is needed
- Costs of hired help
- Lost income
- Reduced work hours
- Loss of employee benefits
- Management of financial concerns for care recipients
- Planning for long-term care financial needs

Suggested Coping Tips

- Evaluate and utilize programs that assist with medical and treatment costs related to family caregiving.
- Identify programs that provide assistive technology at reduced fees or on loan.
- Discuss financial needs and impacts with other family members.

- Plan ahead for projected medical costs or treatment needs.
- Work with financial planning specialists as needed.

Emotional Burdens as a Source of Stress

Caregiving can be a tiresome experience that feels emotionally challenging, especially if it continues over an extended period. Emotional demands are the hidden cost of caregiving and may be the most severe in their stress impact. Stress sources of emotional demands and suggested coping tips include:

Stress Sources of Emotional Demands

- Feeling alone, unaided, or unappreciated
- A sense of isolation and frustration
- Insufficient time for oneself and personal activities
- Fatigue and emotional irritability
- Anger or frustration at perceived unfairness of a situation
- Discouragement or personal depression
- Loss of opportunities
- Feeling overburdened with demands from care recipient or others
- Lack of control over circumstances

Suggested Coping Tips

- Find someone you trust and talk about your feelings or frustrations.
- Be realistic about the demands of caregiving and turn to others for help.
- Set aside time for self-care and personal renewal.
- Take advantage of respite care services and get a break for a few hours or a couple of days.
- Join a caregiver support group so you can share feelings, learn about resources, and reduce stress.
- Get assistance from others.

Relationship Challenges as a Source of Stress

Caregiving changes the normal patterns of family life and can sometimes result in relationship challenges that make life more stressful. For example, adult siblings may disagree about a care plan or an adult child and dependent parent might have conflict about the level of care or monitoring required. Stress sources of relationship challenges and suggested coping tips include:

Stress Sources of Relationship Challenges

- Feeling overburdened by care responsibilities so you become resentful of the care recipient
- Conflict with care recipient about care demands or plans
- Disagreement with family members about care responsibilities or plans
- Insufficient time and energy for other family relationships
- Difficulties with spouse due to care demands
- Criticism or lack of help from other family members related to caregiving
- Limited communication about needs

Suggested Coping Tips

- Focus on positive experiences with the care recipient such as sharing memories or doing a life story.
- Involve the care recipient as much as possible in discussion of guidelines for care.
- Express needs and issues clearly to other family members related to caregiving responsibilities.
- Take time for other family relationships.
- Participate in a support network for caregivers and get respite care.
- Have each family member participate in caregiving and express appreciation for each other.

Section 58.3

Program for Parents of Preemies Reduces Stress

This information was provided by KidsHealth, one of the largest resources online for medically reviewed health information written for parents, kids, and teens. For more articles like this one, visit www.KidsHealth.org, or www.TeensHealth.org. © 2006 The Nemours Foundation. This text was reviewed by Steven Dowshen, M.D., August 2006.

Between the worries about their child's health and development, daily or almost-daily trips to the hospital, and the concerns about sky-high medical bills, parents of preterm babies have a lot on their minds. These stresses may increase a parent's risk for depression and anxiety and affect parenting once a baby comes home from the hospital. Could a special class help moms and dads cope with the demands of preemie parenting?

Researchers from the University of Oslo in Norway compared two groups of parents of newborn babies. The parents of 71 premature infants, known as the intervention group, were assigned to attend eight sessions of a parenting class before the baby's discharge from the hospital. During the class, the parents could openly discuss their feelings, experiences, and grief over not having a full-term pregnancy and delivery. The researchers and neonatal nurses also encouraged parents to learn about their infant's hunger and distress cues.

At home, nurses visited the families four times to teach parents about preemie development and improve interaction between the parents and the infants.

Parents in the intervention group were compared with parents of 69 premature babies who didn't receive the special parenting classes, as well as with parents of 74 babies born full-term. Parents in all groups answered questions about their stress levels when their babies were 6 months and 12 months of age (the parents of preterm babies completed the surveys 6 months after the babies would have been considered full-term).

Compared with the parents of preterm babies who didn't attend parenting classes, parents who took the classes reported that they had less stress when the children were 12 months' corrected age. Both moms and dads of preemies in the intervention group said their children had fewer problems with hyperactivity and attachment compared with parents who didn't attend the parenting classes. Overall, moms and dads of premature infants who attended the parenting classes had stress levels similar to parents of full-term infants.

What This Means to You

According to the results of this study, parents of premature infants who learn about their infant's cues and have a place to vent their feelings may experience stress levels on par with parents of full-term infants. If your child was born prematurely and you feel you need help with your parenting skills or you feel depressed or anxious, the nurses or doctors in the neonatal unit or your doctor can help you find someone to talk to. For more information about your child's physical growth or emotional development, talk to your doctor.

Source: Per Ivar Kaaresen, M.D.; John A. Ronning, Ph.D.; Stein Erik Ulvund, Ph.D.; Lauritz B. Dahl, M.D., Ph.D.; *Pediatrics,* July 2006.

Section 58.4

Controlling and Minimizing Holiday Stress

"Managing Family Stress during the Holidays" is from the National Women's Health Information Center's (NWHIC, www.womenshealth.gov) Pick Your Path to Health Campaign, 1995–2001. Reviewed by David A. Cooke, M.D., April 2007.

This holiday season make a special list. And check it twice! No! Not the kind of list that asks for presents, but one that helps you and your family navigate the stress the holiday season brings. Regardless of how few activities you have planned, stress can creep into your family life because many factors intensify during the holidays.

And women, who usually have multiple demands in their lives, often don't find the time to think about how stressed they are.

As a mother, wife, daughter, sister, friend, employee, employer, and volunteer, you have myriad responsibilities. Your list may be quite long and overwhelming, but slowing down, thinking about how you will handle all the tasks, making a plan, and asking for assistance will help you survive the holidays.

Reverend Alice Davis, Executive Minister of Shiloh Baptist Church in Washington, D.C., says that one of the major sources of stress for women is gift giving. "We tend to give expensive gifts that sometimes we can't afford. Gift giving doesn't have to be expensive. We tend to overspend, and we should not do it because overspending will give us stress the rest of the year."

Stress is unavoidable, but it can be controlled and minimized. Set the tone early, and your family will follow your lead:

- Set a budget for gift giving to avoid overspending.

- Make presents at home such as bookmarks, cookies, tree ornaments, or holiday cards.

- Find free activities to share with your family.

- Avoid the pressure to buy a gift for every child and adult in your family.

- Institute a family gift exchange to ease money tensions.

Stress does not come only from holiday-related activities. An ill family member, loneliness during the holidays, unresolved grudges with family members, weight-related issues, drinking problems, and work may all contribute to stress.

It is key, however, to identify the issues that cause you stress. If seeing that cousin who has not spoken to you in years is stressful, then try to put the situation in perspective:

- You can't mend a relationship in one day, but the holiday season may lend itself to a renewed spirit of forgiveness.

- Limit the length of your visit or conversation with a person who upsets you.

- Try to enjoy the company of family members you miss.

- Children's happiness is contagious; enjoy their company.

- Focus on the blessings your family has received during the year.

Stress not only reduces your quality of life but it can develop into depression, which is common, especially among women, during the holidays. Consider some of these recommendations to help you get started with your plan to reduce and manage stress:

- Share the list of tasks you need to accomplish. Enlist the help of your significant other, your children, other family members, and friends.

- Attend celebrations that bring you peace and joy.

- Share the holidays with a neighbor, volunteer at a shelter, or adopt a family in need.

- Do something just for yourself.

- Have family get-togethers and focus on the positive.

- Have a potluck holiday celebration so no one feels overwhelmed with all the preparations.

- Shop early to avoid the crowds.

- If you don't celebrate the holidays, prepare mentally for the activities that surround you. Find something to do that you really like, holiday-related or not, and have fun.

- Don't worry about a perfectly clean house; enjoy the clutter of the holidays!

Use these tips to reduce stress and to lead you down a path to better health on your way to a brand new year!

Chapter 59

Helping Children and Teens Manage Stress

Chapter Contents

Section 59.1

Adults Can Help Kids Cope with Stress

"Ideas for Helping Kids Deal with Stress," © 2001 North Dakota State University Extension Service (http://www.ext.nodak.edu). Reprinted with permission. Reviewed by David A. Cooke, M.D., April 2007.

Adults Can Help Kids Dealing with Stress

Parents and other adults play significant roles in helping children who are dealing with stress. They provide an example for children, act as a resource in helping children cope, and give guidance and support in managing emotions. Trying to return to a "normal" routine after problems occur can be difficult since some of these problems may last for weeks or months. However, parents and other adults need to be attentive to children's needs in helping them overcome fears or reestablish a sense of security. Parents tend to set the atmosphere that will help children cope or remain overly stressed.

Ideas for Helping Children

There are a variety of strategies that parents or other adults can use in helping children deal with stress. These may include:

- **Hold the child and provide physical comfort:** Children may naturally seek the comfort and security that comes from being held. Give children extra hugs, smiles, and hand-holding. Set aside time just to sit next to children, put your arm around them, or hold them on your lap and talk with them about their feelings.

- **Give your child verbal reassurance:** It is important for children to hear messages of support. Remember to tell them often that you love them, that everything will work out, and that they are taken care of.

- **Be honest with the child about your feelings:** It helps children to know that parents may share some of their feelings. Answer your child's questions in a simple, straightforward way. Share your own thoughts and feelings as appropriate.

- **Ask your child to share his or her own thoughts and feelings:** Listen. Parents can help children by encouraging their expression of feelings and listening carefully to them. Ask them to tell you if they feel scared, angry, or frustrated. Help them realize such feelings are normal and that they can be worked out. Ask them for their ideas on how they might help with family needs or service.

- **Read books together that involve dealing with challenges:** A very effective technique is to buy, check out, or borrow books that show children or families dealing with challenges and overcoming them. Ask children what they think about the characters and how they respond. Compare your own situation. Read books several times or leave them out for children to look at.

- **Use humor to lighten circumstances:** Laugh. Laugh some more! Humor, smiles, and laughter relieve tension, especially for children.

- **Have children write or tell a story or draw a picture about the family experience:** Children often express emotion and deal with stressful situations through play or expressive behavior. Ask children to tell you a story about the problems or help them write a story about it. Record this and read it back to them. You may also have children draw pictures about the experience. Ask them about the picture and what it means.

- **Provide materials for dramatic play related to the experience:** Often children will gain a sense of control over difficult situations through dramatic play. Make available props or materials they can use to play the roles of firefighters, doctors or nurses, construction workers, safety personnel, or other helpers. Help facilitate such play as appropriate, and give children feedback about what they express.

- **Establish and maintain consistent routines that provide security and familiarity to children:** As much as possible, adults should create and maintain some routines that children can rely on for security. This might include a particular routine at lunch, nap time, dinner, or bed time. It might involve reading stories each night, rough-and-tumble playing, or playing family games. Use these times to build security and reassure children.

- **Help children express and cope with grief or feelings of loss:** Some children may have lost valued items or toys due to damage. It is natural for them to feel a sense of loss. Allow children to express their loss or frustration, and acknowledge the reality of their feelings. Plan to replace a lost object if appropriate.

- **Develop a plan with children for action to take in case of future problems or stress:** Children feel empowered if they know beforehand what might be done to respond to a concern. This may include a home evacuation drill, knowledge of contact information for safety experts, or simply greater understanding of potential weather-related concerns such as thunderstorms. Discuss such issues with children and involve them in making plans that will aid in responding to future challenges. Practice emergency procedures so children are familiar with them.

- **Involve children in clean-up or repair activities as appropriate:** It can be helpful to give children something to do in responding to stress. Children benefit from feeling that they are making a contribution. As possible, find an appropriate activity that children or youth can do to help clean up, repair, or otherwise assist with responding to a stressful situation. Perhaps they can perform a service activity for others in need.

- **Show an example of self-control and positive response to stress:** Children learn how to respond to stress by watching adults. Adults ought to set an example of self-control, maturity, and positive resolution in dealing with challenges. This will comfort children and create a secure atmosphere for them.

Taking Action to Reduce Stress

Set aside time to specifically think about the conditions in your own family and what things you can do to help your children deal with stress. Make a plan and follow up on the activities. Share what you have done with others who may be facing challenges.

Section 59.2

De-Stressing Strategies for Kids

"Feelin' Frazzled?" is a publication for kids by the Centers for Disease Control and Prevention (CDC), www.bam.gov, 2001. Reviewed by David A. Cooke, M.D., April 2007.

Finding yourself in a hectic situation, whether it's forgetting your homework or missing your ride home, can really stress you out. Are you looking for a safety net for those days that seem to get worse by the second? Could you really use some advice on how to destress both your body and your mind? Knowing how to deal can be half the battle. Check out these 10 tips to keep you cool, calm, and collected.

Put Your Body in Motion

Moving from the chair to the couch while watching TV is not being physically active. Physical activity is one of the most important ways to keep stress away by clearing your head and lifting your spirits. Physical activity also increases endorphin levels—the natural "feel-good" chemicals in the body which leave you with a naturally happy feeling.

Whether you like full-fledged games of football, tennis, or roller hockey, or you prefer walks with family and friends, it's important to get up, get out, and get moving.

Fuel Up

Start your day off with a full tank—eating breakfast will give you the energy you need to tackle the day. Eating regular meals (this means no skipping dinner) and taking time to enjoy them (nope, eating in the car on the way to practice doesn't count) will make you feel better, too.

Make sure to fuel up with fruits, vegetables, proteins (peanut butter, a chicken sandwich, or a tuna salad), and grains (wheat bread, pasta, or some crackers)—these will give you the power you need to make it through those hectic days.

Don't be fooled by the jolt of energy you get from sodas and sugary snacks—this only lasts a short time, and once it wears off, you may feel sluggish and more tired than usual. For that extra boost of energy to sail through history notes, math class, and after-school activities, grab a banana, some string cheese, or a granola bar for some power-packed energy.

LOL

Some say that laughter is the best medicine—well, in many cases, it is! Did you know that it takes 15 facial muscles to laugh? Lots of laughing can make you feel good—and, that good feeling can stay with you even after the laughter stops. So, head off stress with regular doses of laughter by watching a funny movie or cartoons, reading a joke book (you may even learn some new jokes), or even make up your own riddles. Laughter can make you feel like a new person.

Everyone has those days when they do something really silly or stupid—instead of getting upset with yourself, laugh out loud! No one's perfect. Life should be about having fun. So, lighten up.

Have Fun with Friends

Being with people you like is always a good way to ditch your stress. Get a group together to go to the movies, shoot some hoops, or play a board game—or just hang out and talk. Friends can help you work through your problems and let you see the brighter side of things.

Spill to Someone You Trust

Instead of keeping your feelings bottled up inside, talk to someone you trust or respect about what's bothering you. It could be a friend, a parent, someone in your family, or a teacher. Talking out your problems and seeing them from a different view might help you figure out ways to deal with them. Just remember, you don't have to go it alone.

Take Time to Chill

Pick a comfy spot to sit and read, daydream, or even take a snooze. Listen to your favorite music. Work on a relaxing project like putting together a puzzle or making jewelry.

Stress can sometimes make you feel like a tight rubber band—stretched to the limit. If this happens, take a few deep breaths to help yourself unwind. If you're in the middle of an impossible homework problem, take a break. Finding time to relax after (and sometimes during) a hectic day or week can make all the difference.

Catch Some Zzzs

Fatigue is a best friend to stress. When you don't get enough sleep, it's hard to deal—you may feel tired, cranky, or you may have trouble thinking clearly. When you're overtired, a problem may seem much bigger than it actually is. You may have a hard time doing a school assignment that usually seems easy, you don't do your best in sports or any physical activity, or you may have an argument with your friends over something really stupid.

Sleep is a big deal. Getting the right amount of sleep is especially important for kids your age. Because your body (and mind) is changing and developing, it requires more sleep to recharge for the next day. So don't resist, hit the hay!

Keep a Journal

If you're having one of those crazy days when nothing goes right, it's a good idea to write things down in a journal to get it off of your chest—like how you feel, what's going on in your life, and things you'd like to accomplish. You could even write down what you do when you're faced with a stressful situation, and then look back and think about how you handled it later. So, find a quiet spot, grab a notebook and pen, and start writing.

Get It Together

Too much to do but not enough time? Forgot your homework? Feeling overwhelmed or discombobulated? Being unprepared for school, practice, or other activities can make for a very stressful day.

Getting everything done can be a challenge, but all you have to do is plan a little and get organized.

Lend a Hand

Get involved in an activity that helps others. It's almost impossible to feel stressed out when you're helping someone else. It's also a great way to find out about yourself and the special qualities you never knew you had. Signing up for a service project is a good idea, but helping others is as easy as saying hello, holding a door, or volunteering to keep a neighbor's pet. If you want to get involved in a more organized volunteer program, try working at a local recreation center, or helping with an after school program. The feeling you will get from helping others is greater than you can imagine.

Most importantly, don't sweat the small stuff. Try to pick a few really important things and let the rest slide—getting worked up over every little thing will only increase your stress. So, toughen up and don't let stressful situations get to you! Remember, you're not alone—everyone has stresses in their lives. It's up to you to choose how to deal with them.

Section 59.3

Is Your Child Too Busy?

This information was provided by KidsHealth, one of the largest resources online for medically reviewed health information written for parents, kids, and teens. For more articles like this one, visit www.KidsHealth.org, or www.TeensHealth.org. © 2005 The Nemours Foundation. This information was reviewed by Mary L. Gavin, M.D., January 2005.

- "She's not really good at soccer and she doesn't really like it, but all her friends are doing it," reports the mother of a 9-year-old.

- "If I miss a practice, even for a doctor's appointment, I get benched," a 13-year-old says.

- "If my son didn't have an after-school activity every day of the week, he'd sit around eating junk and playing video games," the father of a 10-year-old says worriedly.

- "I don't really like lacrosse, but I have to do it because it'll look good on my college transcript," a 16-year-old explains.

- "She wants to take gymnastics, art, dance, and cooking, and she goes to afternoon religious school twice a week. I'm not pushing her. She has to eliminate something!" exclaims the mother of a 7-year-old.

- "I don't have anything scheduled on Sunday afternoons. That's when I have my life," a 14-year-old reasons.

Clearly, some kids have too much to do and not enough time to do it. And it's hard to tell if it's the parents pushing or the kids trying to keep up with their peers. Whatever the culprit, one thing's for sure—something's got to give for some kids. Is your child too busy?

Why Are Kids So Busy?

For some families, kids may be driving the schedule because they don't want to feel left out. Teens may feel pressure to boost their roster of activities to get into the college of their choice.

Some parents may feel that they have to keep their kids constantly occupied, rather than give them a chance to play, explore, and learn on their own. Parents may also feel the need to sign their kids up for one more class or team for fear that their children may be missing something the other kids are getting.

Parents usually just want whatever seems best for their kids. Even when intentions are good, though, a child can easily become over-scheduled. The pressure to participate in a handful of activities all the time and to "keep up with the Joneses" can be physically and emotionally exhausting, for parents and kids alike.

Of course, organized activities and sports are beneficial for kids for a number of reasons. They foster social skills and provide opportunities for play and exercise. They promote cultural enrichment and teach sportsmanship, self-discipline, and conflict resolution. Most of all, they're fun! The key is keeping them that way, and making sure that kids—and their parents—aren't becoming overwhelmed.

How Can I Tell If My Child Is Too Busy?

Sooner or later, too-busy children will begin to show signs of being over-scheduled. Every child is different, but over-scheduled kids may:

- feel tired, anxious, or depressed;

- complain of headaches and stomachaches, which may be due to stress, missed meals, or lack of sleep; or

- fall behind on their schoolwork, causing their grades to drop.

Over-scheduling can also take a toll on kids' friendships and social lives. Family life also can suffer when too many people are running in too many directions. When one parent is driving to basketball practice and the other is carpooling to dance class, meals are missed. As a result, some families rarely eat dinner together and parents and kids may not be taking the time to stay connected. Plus, the weekly grind of chauffeuring kids all over the place and getting to one class, game, or practice after another can be downright tiresome and stressful for parents.

Tips for Busy Families

Even those parents who try to help their children cut back on some activities can run up against coaches who won't tolerate absences and kids who want to keep up with their friends. However, it's important for parents to step back and make sure that their children aren't experiencing activity overload.

The key is to schedule things in moderation and choose activities with your child's age, temperament, interests, and abilities in mind. If something's too advanced, the experience may be frustrating. If it isn't engaging, your child will probably be bored. And if your child doesn't want to do it in the first place, he or she may do it only to please you, which defeats the whole purpose.

Depending on the age and interests of your child, you can set reasonable limits on extracurricular activities and help make them more enjoyable for both you and your child. Here are some simple suggestions:

- **Agree on some ground rules before you sign up for too much:** For instance, plan to play one sport per season, or limit activities to two afternoons or evenings during the school week.

- **Before you say yes, make sure your child knows how much time is required for an activity:** For example, will there be time to practice between lessons? Does your child realize that soccer practice is twice a week, right after school until dinnertime? Then there's the weekly game, too. Will his or her homework suffer?

- **Keep a calendar to stay organized:** Display it on the refrigerator or other prominent spot in the home so that the whole family can stay up-to-date. And if you find an empty space on the calendar, leave it alone!

- **Even if your child's signed up for the season, let him or her miss one or two sessions:** Sometimes taking the opportunity to hang out on a beautiful day is more important than going to one more activity, even if you've already paid for it.

- **Try to carpool with other parents to make life easier:**
Try to balance activities for all of your children—and yourself.
It hardly seems fair to expend time and energy carting one kid
to activities, leaving little time for the other. And don't forget to
take time for yourself, to do the things you enjoy, and to spend
time together as a family.

- **Create family time:** If it seems like you're eating pizza on the
run every night, make a plan so that everyone can be home for
dinner at the same time—even if it means eating a little later.
Make sure to schedule family fun time too, whether it's playing
a board game together or going on bike ride or hike.

- **Set priorities:** School should come first. If your child is having
a hard time keeping up academically, your child may need to
drop an activity.

- **Know when to draw the line and say no:** If your child is already doing a lot and really wants to participate in another activity, talk about what other activity or activities need to be dropped
to make the desired one happen.

- **Don't underestimate the importance of downtime:** Everyone needs a chance to relax, reflect on the day, or just do nothing.

Slowing It Down

Take a moment and think about your child's life. If you think your
child is over-scheduled, sit down together and decide where you can
cut back. If it's very structured, with school, after-school activities, and
homework being the weekday norm, consider helping your child create time to blow off some steam.

Riding a bike, taking a walk, playing a game, listening to music, or
just doing nothing for a while will give your child some much-needed
rest. And never forget how important it is for kids to simply get together to play. Kids just need time to be kids.

Section 59.4

Dealing with Media Stress:
How to Talk to Your Child about the News

"How to Talk to Your Child about the News" was provided by KidsHealth, one of the largest resources online for medically reviewed health information written for parents, kids, and teens. For more articles like this one, visit www.KidsHealth.org, or www.TeensHealth.org. © 2005 The Nemours Foundation. This information was reviewed by Mary L. Gavin, M.D., September 2005.

Although news gleaned from television, radio, or the internet can be a positive educational experience for kids, problems can arise when the images presented are violent or news stories touch on disturbing topics. Recent news about Hurricane Katrina and the earthquake in South Asia could potentially make a child worry that a natural disaster is going to hit home, or be fearful of a part of daily life—like rain and thunderstorms—that he or she never even thought about before.

Reports on subjects such as natural disasters, child abductions, homicides, terrorist attacks, school violence, or a politician's sex life can teach kids to view the world as a confusing, threatening, or unfriendly place.

How can you deal with these disturbing stories and images? Talking to your child about what he or she watches or hears will help your child put frightening information into a more balanced and reasonable context.

How Kids Perceive the News

Unlike movies or entertainment programs, news is real. But depending on your child's age or maturity level, he or she may not yet understand the distinctions between fact and fantasy. By the time a child reaches 7 or 8, however, what he or she watches on TV can seem all too real. For some youngsters, the vividness of a sensational news story can be internalized and transformed into something that might happen to them. A child watching a news story about a bombing on a bus or a subway might worry, "Could I be next? Could that happen to me?"

Natural disasters or stories of other types of devastation can be personalized in the same manner. A child in Massachusetts who sees a house being swallowed by floods from a hurricane in Louisiana may spend a sleepless night worrying about whether his home will be OK in a rainstorm. A child in Chicago, seeing news about an attack on subways in London, may get scared about using public transportation around town. TV has the effect of shrinking the world and bringing it into your own living room.

By concentrating on violent stories, television news can also promote a "mean-world" syndrome, which can give children a misrepresentation of what the world and society are actually like.

Talking about the News

To calm children's fears about the news, parents should be prepared to deliver what psychologists call "calm, unequivocal, but limited information." This means delivering the truth, but only as much truth as the child needs to know. The key is to be as truthful, yet as inexplicit as you can be. There's no need to go into more details than your child is interested in.

Although it's true that some things—like a natural disaster—can't be controlled, parents should still give children space to share their fears. Encourage your child to talk openly about what scares him or her.

Older children are less likely to accept an explanation at face value. Their budding skepticism about the news and how it's produced and sold might mask anxieties they have about the stories it covers. If an older child is bothered about a story, help him or her cope with these fears. An adult's willingness to listen will send a powerful message.

Teens also can be encouraged to consider why a frightening or disturbing story was on the air: Was it to increase the program's ratings because of its sensational value or because it was truly newsworthy? In this way, a scary story can be turned into a worthwhile discussion about the role and mission of the news.

Tips for Parents

Keeping an eye on your child's TV news habits can go a long way toward monitoring the content of what he or she hears and sees. Here are some additional tips:

541

- Recognize that news doesn't have to be driven by disturbing pictures. Public television programs, newspapers, or newsmagazines specifically designed for children can be less sensational—and less upsetting—ways of getting information to children.

- Discuss current events with your child on a regular basis. It's important to help kids think through stories they hear about. Ask questions: What do you think about these events? How do you think these things happen? These questions can encourage conversation about non-news topics as well.

- Put news stories in proper context. Showing that certain events are isolated or explaining how one event relates to another helps a child make better sense of what he or she hears. Broaden the discussion from a disturbing news item to a larger conversation: Use the story of a natural disaster as an opportunity to talk about philanthropy, cooperation, and the ability of people to cope with overwhelming hardship.

- Watch the news with your child to filter stories as he or she watches them.

- Anticipate when guidance will be necessary and avoid shows that aren't appropriate for your child's age or level of development.

- If you're uncomfortable with the content of the news or if it's inappropriate for your child's age, turn off the TV or radio.

- Talk about what you can do to help. In the case of a news event like a natural disaster, your child may gain a sense of control and feel more secure if you find out about donations you can make or other ways that you can help those who you have heard about are in need.

Section 59.5

What Parents Can Do about School-Related Stress

"School-Related Stress," © 2007 Child Abuse Prevention Fund—Children's Hospital and Health System (www.capfund.org). All rights reserved. Reprinted with permission.

School can be a stressful experience for children. Experiencing a certain amount of stress is a normal part of child development, and all children and adolescents will experience school-related stress at some point or another. Many children worry and get stressed about being accepted, grades, transitions to new schools and classes, bullies, not knowing the answer, and the overall pressure to succeed.

Children react to stress in different ways based on their age, developmental stage, and reason for the stress. Some children react by changing behaviors, perhaps becoming withdrawn or acting out aggressively. Others may regress to behaviors they have grown out of, such as thumb sucking. Stress also can cause headaches, stomachaches, and sleep problems.

You can't remove all the stresses in your child's life, but you can help your child learn to cope with stress by looking for warning signs and providing him or her with tools to reduce and control stress.

What Parents Can Do

- Establish rituals and routines. A set schedule provides children with a sense of comfort and security.

- Make sure that your child gets plenty of rest, and provide nutritious meals to help your child's brain to function at its best.

- Spend time talking to your child about his or her problems and concerns. What may seem like a small problem to you may be very important to your child. Help your child find solutions and make good decisions by giving examples of ways to solve the problem.

- Don't overcommit your child with too many extracurricular activities, but provide opportunities for non-school related activities that allow him or her to be in a social setting, such as scouts and church groups.

- Have fun with your child and spend time doing activities that he or she likes. This will help your child refocus some of his or her energy on more positive things.

- Plan downtime for your child. Allow time in your child's schedule when he or she does not have to do anything or be anywhere.

- Pay attention to your child's verbal and nonverbal cues that things are getting overwhelming.

- Communicate with your child's teachers or caregivers and discuss possible sources of stress and solutions to help your child deal with it.

- Set a good example by handling your own stress in a positive way. Children learn by example and may deal with stress in the same ways they see adults handle it.

Section 59.6

Tips for Teens about Test-Related Anxiety

"Test Anxiety" was provided by TeensHealth, one of the largest resources online for medically reviewed health information written for parents, kids, and teens. For more articles like this one, visit www.TeensHealth.org, or www.KidsHealth.org. © 2004 The Nemours Foundation. This information was reviewed by D'Arcy Lyness, Ph.D., February 2007.

You've participated in class, done all of your homework, studied hard, and you think you have a grip on the material. But then the day of the test comes. Suddenly, you blank out, freeze up, zone out, or feel so nervous that you can't get it together to respond to those questions you knew the answers to just last night.

If this sounds like you, you may have a case of test anxiety—that nervous feeling that people sometimes get when they're about to take a test.

It's pretty normal to feel a little nervous and stressed before a test. Just about everyone does. And a touch of nervous anticipation can actually help you get revved and keep you at peak performance while you're taking the test. But for some people, this normal anxiety is more intense. The nervousness they feel before a test can be so strong that it interferes with their concentration or performance.

What is test anxiety?

Test anxiety is actually a type of performance anxiety—a feeling someone might have in a situation where performance really counts or when the pressure's on to do well. For example, a person might experience performance anxiety when he or she is about to try out for the school play, sing a solo on stage, get into position at the pitcher's mound, step onto the platform in a diving meet, or go into an important interview.

Like other situations in which a person might feel performance anxiety, test anxiety can bring on "butterflies," a stomachache, or a tension headache. Some people might feel shaky, sweaty, or feel their heart beating quickly as they wait for the test to be given out. A student with really strong test anxiety may even feel like he or she might pass out or throw up.

Test anxiety is not the same as doing poorly on a certain test because your mind is on something else. Most people know that having other things on their minds—such as a breakup or the death of someone close—can also interfere with their concentration and prevent them from doing their best on a test.

What causes it?

All anxiety is a reaction to anticipating something stressful. Like other anxiety reactions, test anxiety affects the body and the mind. When you're under stress, your body releases the hormone adrenaline, which prepares it for danger (you may hear this referred to as the "fight or flight" reaction). That's what causes the physical symptoms, such as sweating, a pounding heart, and rapid breathing. These sensations might be mild or intense.

Focusing on the bad things that could happen also fuels test anxiety. For example, someone worrying about doing poorly might think thoughts like, "What if I forget everything I know?" or "What if the test is too hard?" Too many thoughts like these leave no mental space for thinking about the test questions. People with test anxiety can also feel stressed out by their physical reaction and think things like "What if I throw up?" or "Oh no, my hands are shaking."

Just like other types of anxiety, test anxiety can create a vicious circle: The more a person focuses on the bad things that could happen, the stronger the feeling of anxiety becomes. This makes the person feel worse and, because his or her head is full of distracting thoughts and fears, it can increase the possibility that the person will do worse on the test.

Who's likely to have test anxiety?

People who worry a lot or who are perfectionists are more likely to have trouble with test anxiety. People with these traits sometimes find it hard to accept mistakes they might make or to get anything less than a perfect score. In this way, even without meaning to, they might really pressure themselves. Test anxiety is bound to thrive in a situation like this.

Students who aren't prepared for tests but who care about doing well are also likely to experience test anxiety. If you know you're not prepared, it's a no-brainer to realize that you'll be worried about doing poorly. People can feel unprepared for tests for several reasons: They may not have studied enough, they may find the material difficult, or perhaps they feel tired because they didn't get enough sleep the night before.

What can you do?

Test anxiety can be a real problem when someone is so stressed out over a test that he or she can't get past the nervousness to focus on the test questions and do his or her best work. Feeling ready to meet the challenge, though, can keep test anxiety at a manageable level.

Use a little stress to your advantage: Stress is your body's warning mechanism—it's a signal that helps you prepare for something important that's about to happen. So use it to your advantage. Instead of reacting to the stress by dreading, complaining, or fretting about the test with friends, take an active approach. Let stress remind you to study well in advance of a test. Chances are, you'll keep your stress from spinning out of control. After all, nobody ever feels stressed out by thoughts that they might do well on a test.

Ask for help: Although a little test anxiety can be a good thing, an overdose of it is another story entirely. If sitting for a test gets you so stressed out that your mind goes blank and causes you to miss answers that you know, then your level of test anxiety probably needs some attention. Your teacher, your school guidance counselor, or a tutor can be useful resources to talk to if you always get extreme test anxiety.

Be prepared: Some students think that going to class is all it should take to learn and do well on tests. But there's much more to learning than just hoping to soak everything up in class. That's why good study habits and skills are so important—and why no amount of cramming or studying the night before a test can take the place of the deeper level of learning that happens over time with regular study.

Many students find that their test anxiety is reduced when they start to study better or more regularly. It makes sense—the more you know the material, the more confident you'll feel. Having confidence going into a test means you expect to do well. When you expect to do well, you'll be able to relax into a test after the normal first-moment jitters pass.

Watch what you're thinking: If expecting to do well on a test can help you relax, what about when people expect they won't do well? Watch out for any negative messages you might be sending yourself about the test. They can contribute to your anxiety.

If you find yourself thinking negative thoughts ("I'm never any good at taking tests," or "It's going to be terrible if I do badly on this test"), replace them with positive messages. Not unrealistic positive messages, of course, but ones that are practical and true, such as "I've studied hard and I know the material, so I'm ready to do the best I can." (Of course, if you haven't studied, this message won't help!)

Accept mistakes: Another thing you can do is to learn to keep mistakes in perspective—especially if you're a perfectionist or you tend to be hard on yourself. Everyone makes mistakes, and you may have even heard teachers or coaches refer to mistakes as "learning opportunities." Learning to tolerate small failures and mistakes—like that one problem you got wrong in the math pop quiz—is a valuable skill.

Take care of yourself: It can help to learn ways to calm yourself down and get centered when you're tense or anxious. For some people, this might mean learning a simple breathing exercise. Practicing breathing exercises regularly (when you're not stressed out) helps your body see these exercises as a signal to relax.

And, of course, taking care of your health—such as getting enough sleep, exercise, and healthy eats before a test—can help keep your mind working at its best.

Everything takes time and practice, and learning to beat test anxiety is no different. Although it won't go away overnight, facing and dealing with test anxiety will help you learn stress management, which can prove to be a valuable skill in many situations besides taking tests.

Chapter 60

Stress Management for People with Physical Disabilities

By Jennifer Gray-Stanley

Though we all encounter many types of stress in our daily life, we must remember that ultimately, we have control over how it affects us. Through awareness and education, negative stressors can be managed, and positive stressors can be utilized as an impetus for change and added creativity in your life. As managing stress in your life requires proactive and consistent behavioral change, this text addresses how to adopt such changes on a gradual basis.

Defining Stress

A "stressor" consists of anything that causes stress, including physical, emotional, and environmental problems and barriers. These include, but are not limited to factors such as disability, illness, fear, worry, pollution, and noise (Powell & George-Warren, 1994; Seaward, 2006). Hans Seyle, stress researcher, defined stress as "the nonspecific response of the body to any demand made on it"(1973). This refers to how I react to any demand that affects my system from a

"Defining Stress," April 2006. This article is reproduced from the National Center on Physical Activity and Disability at www.ncpad.org. It may be freely distributed in its entirety as long as it includes this notice but cannot be edited, modified, otherwise altered without the express written permission of NCPAD. Contact NCPAD at 1-800-900-8086 for additional details. Copyright 2006 The Board of Trustees of the University of Illinois.

physical, mental, and/or emotional perspective. Stress can be defined in both positive (good stress—eustress) and negative (bad stress—distress) forms. Eustress or positive stress is the optimal amount of stress which can provide us with the energy to perform a task well, such as public speaking, engaging in competition, or completing a job interview. Exercise and physical activity can also be considered a positive stressor, although over-training can lead to injury. Additional variations of defining stress include hyperstress, an excess of stress, or hypostress, insufficient stress. Balance should be sought among all types of stress (Manning et al., 1999). Thus, particularly for managing negative stressors, successful stress management helps us to develop an awareness of stress in our lives, and how we respond to and manage these stressors.

Richard Lazarus further developed these definitions by stating that stress is a condition or feeling experienced when a person perceives that "demands exceed the personal and social resources that the individual is able to mobilize" (Lazarus & Folkman, 1984). Certainly, what is stressful one day may not be stressful the next. And each person perceives stress differently than does the next.

Stress Management Assessment

The first step to developing a stress management plan includes a thorough assessment of the stress you are currently experiencing. The following resources include checklists and exercises to help you familiarize yourself with your current stress levels. Choose the exercises that are most applicable to your current circumstances, whether that be work stress or specific symptoms experienced.

Quick Stress Management Checklists

Quick Stress Assessment

Check all statements which apply to you:

- Do you schedule more activities than you can handle into a day's work?

- Do you worry chronically?

- Are you addicted to excitement, stimulation?

- Do you tend to be overly concerned about what people think?

- Are you a multitasker?

- Are you an overachiever or perfectionist?

- Do you neglect to practice self-nurturing activities?

Affirmative responses to any of the above statements indicate a need for improved awareness and management of your current stress levels.

Holmes-Rahe Social Readjustment Rating Scale

The following scale allows you to estimate your general life stress values. A checklist is listed for both adult and youth stress. Circle the scores of the events that relate to you, and add them up for a total score.

Listing Problematic Stressors

Using Table 60.1 and Table 60.2 as guides, write down key stressors in your life that are of concern to you. Make these lists as detailed as possible, as they can serve as a basis for forming a coherent stress management program. This should fall into multiple areas, including:

- work;

- personal relationships or family life; and

- habits, i.e., eating, exercising.

Recognizing Signs of Stress

Stress unchecked can have an insidious effect physically, mentally, and spiritually. Consider how you feel from physical, emotional, and behavioral standpoints, and write it down. Use the following table from MayoClinic.com as a guide: https://www.mayoclinic.com/health/stress-symptoms/SR00008_D. Recognition of such symptoms is critical to managing your stress levels. Consider symptoms from physical, emotional, and behavioral sources.

- Physical symptoms: headache, fatigue, high blood pressure, shortness of breath

- Emotional symptoms: anxiety, worrying, depression, mood swings, depression

- Behaviors: increased smoking or alcohol use, overeating

The Influence of Personality

Personality must also be factored into the stress equation. The way one interprets and processes stress in one's life has a tremendous impact on the health outcomes realized. While some persons assume a more serious and competitive approach to life, others are more easy-going.

Type A & B personality types: Cardiologists Meyer Friedman and Ray Rosenman created the Western Collaborative Group Study epidemiological project in the 1950s and 1960s, where they developed

Table 60.1. Adult Stress Scale (continued on next page)

Death of spouse	100
Foreclosure of mortgage or loan	100
Divorce	60
Sleep less than 8 hours per night	60
Menopause	60
Separation from living partner	60
Jail term or probation	60
Death of close family member other than spouse	60
Serious personal injury or illness	45
Marriage or establishing life partnership	45
Fired at work	45
Marital or relationship reconciliation	40
Retirement	40
Change in health of immediate family member	40
Work more than 40 hours per week	35
Pregnancy or causing pregnancy	35
Sex difficulties	35
Gain of new family member	35
Business or work role change	35
Change in financial state	35
Death of a close friend (not a family member)	30
Change in number of arguments with spouse or life partner	30
Mortgage or loan for a major purpose	25

the typology of type A and B personalities. While type A personality qualities include physical and mental acuity, a quick pace, competitiveness, impatience, and difficulty relaxing and waiting, type B personalities exhibit a more relaxed approach to life and its challenges. Not surprisingly, individuals with type B personalities experience less stress and are less likely to develop heart disease than are those with type A personalities (Manning et al., 1999).

Hardiness/resilience. Being hardy or resistant to stress typifies a person who can remain healthy and balanced despite an ample work load. Essentially, this person lives in alignment with inner values. Susan

Table 60.1. Adult Stress Scale (continued)

Change in responsibilities at work	25
Trouble with in-laws, or with children	25
Outstanding personal achievement	25
Spouse begins or stops work	20
Begin or end school	20
Change in living conditions (visitors in the home, change in roommates, remodeling house)	20
Change in personal habits (diet, exercise, smoking, etc.)	20
Chronic allergies	20
Change in work hours or conditions	15
Moving to new residence	15
Presently in premenstrual period	15
Change in schools	15
Change in religious activities	15
Change in social activities (more or less than before)	15
Minor financial loan	10
Change in frequency of family get-togethers	10
Vacation	10
Presently in winter holiday season	10
Minor violation of the law	5

Total Score

Scoring: 0–149: low stress level; 150–199: mild life changes; 200–299: moderate stress level; 300 +: high stress level.

Kobasa typified the concept of the hardy personality in 1979, involving the traits of commitment, control, and challenge. Essentially, hardy people live according to their values and commitments to self, family,

Table 60.2. Youth Stress Scale (continued on next page)

Death of parent, spouse, boyfriend/girlfriend	100
Divorce (of yourself or your parents)	65
Puberty	65
Pregnancy (or causing pregnancy)	65
Marital separation or breakup with boyfriend/girlfriend	60
Jail term or probation	60
Death of other family member (other than spouse, parent or boyfriend/girlfriend)	60
Broken engagement	55
Engagement	50
Serious personal injury or illness	45
Marriage	45
Entering college or beginning next level of school (starting junior high or high school)	45
Change in independence or responsibility	45
Any drug and/or alcoholic use	45
Fired at work or expelled from school	45
Change in alcohol or drug use	45
Reconciliation with mate, family, or boyfriend/girlfriend (getting back together)	40
Trouble at school	40
Serious health problem of a family member	40
Working while attending school	35
Working more than 40 hours per week	35
Changing course of study	35
Change in frequency of dating	35
Sexual adjustment problems (confusion of sexual identify)	35
Gain of new family member (new baby born or parent remarries)	35
Change in work responsibilities	35

work, the community, and other goals. They assume responsibility for both personal successes and failures, and believe that they have the power to influence the course of one's destiny. Moreover, obstacles or

Table 60.2. Youth Stress Scale (continued)

Change in financial state	30
Death of a close friend (not a family member)	30
Change to a different kind of work	30
Change in number or arguments with mate, family or friends	30
Sleep less than 8 hours per night	25
Trouble with in-laws or boyfriend's or girlfriend's family	25
Outstanding personal achievement (awards, grades, etc.)	25
Mate or parents start or stop working	20
Begin or end school	20
Change in living conditions (visitors in the home, remodeling house, change in roommates)	20
Change in personal habits (start or stop a habit like smoking or dieting)	20
Chronic allergies	20
Trouble with the boss	20
Change in work hours	15
Change in residence	15
Change to a new school (other than graduation)	10
Presently in premenstrual period	15
Change in religious activity	15
Going in debt (you or your family)	10
Change in frequency of family gatherings	10
Vacation	10
Presently in winter holiday season	10
Minor violation of the law	5
Total Score	

Scoring: 0–149: low stress level; 150–199: mild life changes; 200–299: moderate stress level; 300 +: high stress level.

problems are viewed as challenges and an opportunity for further growth, rather than threats.

Take a personality hardiness test at the following website: http://www.retirementlifestyle.com/lifeplanning/personalitytest.htm

Modalities to Decrease Stress

A plethora of modalities exist to help you manage your stress levels, assuming that you incorporate these new behaviors into your lifestyle on a regular basis. They include, but are not limited to relaxation, positive thinking, goal setting and time management, as well as regular exercise and proper nutrition. This section includes some techniques for adoption into daily routines from Powell & George-Warren (1994) and the resources section below. Note that information on physical activity and nutrition will not be covered here. For this information, refer to the National Center on Physical Activity and Disability (NPCAD) website (www.ncpad.org) or call their free hotline at 800-900-8086 for this and other health promotion resources.

Relaxation: Getting Started

Relaxation can be practiced in many different forms and environments. To begin, consider a few guidelines:

- Locate a quiet environment where you feel comfortable. Use a blanket if necessary to stay warm.

- Situate yourself in a comfortable position. A seated position is preferred over lying down, so that one does not have the tendency to fall asleep.

- Reserve a regular time each day for practicing relaxation.

- Focus on a word, phrase, sound, or the rhythm of your breath that is repeated regularly throughout the session. It is natural for your mind to wander: simply focus again.

- Use a timer if necessary, so that you can focus on your relaxation practice rather than the time you are allocating to it.

- To learn proper techniques, practice with relaxation tapes from your local library, or take a class in your community, such as meditation, qi gong, and various forms of yoga. For example, see NPCAD's fact sheet on Yoga for Persons with Disabilities at http://www.ncpad.org/exercise/fact_sheet.php?sheet=345.

Positions for Practicing Relaxation Exercises

Sitting

- Sit in a comfortable chair where your back is supported, your feet are on the ground, and your knees are bent.

- Your head should feel as if it is a helium balloon, and your spine should lengthen, as if it is floating up freely.

Lying Down

- Lie flat with your arms comfortably resting at your side.

- Your legs should rest slightly apart.

- A blanket can be used to keep warm.

- Use a small pillow under your neck and/or under your knees, if you experience any strain in this position.

Breathing Guidelines

- Watch how a baby breathes, with her/his abdomen rising and falling. Place your hand on your belly/abdomen area, and practice breathing from this area, as you watch your hand rise and fall.

- Use your nose to inhale and then exhale through your nose or mouth.

- Breathe initially while lying down, and then practice from a sitting or standing position.

- Consult the following websites: http://swamij.com/breath.htm or http://www.ianprattis.com/meditations/sohummed.htm for tips on proper breathing guidelines and additional exercises.

Quick Exercises

Each of these simple exercises can be practiced throughout the day when you have
limited time but desire the benefits of relaxation.

In-out breathing: Breathe slowly and steadily. As you inhale, silently say "in" and as you exhale, silently say "out". Repeat for 5 to 10 minutes. Preferred mantras, terms, or images can be substituted for "in-out," if desired.

Self-massage: Use your fingers, hands, and fists to massage your facial muscles, neck, shoulders, arms, and/or hands. Focus on areas experiencing tension. During massage, practice deep breathing.

Relaxation response: This exercise can be practiced with the eyes open or closed. Breathe deeply from your abdomen. Hold for two to three seconds. Exhale slowly. While exhaling, let your jaw and shoulders drop. Experience the relaxation response in your arms and hands, as well as throughout your body.

Walking/wheeling meditation: Being conscious of your breathing while walking or wheeling can be an ideal exercise to focus your attention on the present, in order to relax your body and clear your mind. Begin walking or wheeling until you establish a comfortable pace. Become aware of the number of steps or pushes you take between breaths. For example: breathe in 1-2-3-4, exhale out 1-2-3-4.

Progressive relaxation: To learn a complete progressive relaxation series, go to http://www.guidetopsychology.com/pmr.htm, http://www.healthy.net/scr/article.asp?Id=1773, http://www.healthy.net/scr/article.asp?Id=1983, or follow the exercises indicated in Manning et al. (1999). To practice a tension-relaxation procedure, try the following: Focus on the muscle group you would like to target, such as your right arm. Inhale and squeeze this muscle group as hard as possible for about 8 seconds. Then, exhale as you release the tension. Experience the sensation as the tightness flows out of your arm, and through your hand and fingertips. Relax for at least 15 seconds, and then repeat the tension-relaxation procedure again for another muscle group.

Positive Thinking and Speaking

Similar to a computer, we save our ideas and beliefs within our consciousness, which have an effect on how we conduct and experience our life. Everyone has positive and negative thoughts, yet listening to positive thoughts can help you realize a positive disposition. It just takes practice. It is important to realize that the quality of the input from our consciousness can only be as beneficial as the input. If our mind operates like a "Yes" machine, accepting all that we input into it, we must fill our mind with positive, life-enhancing messages. The following exercises can be practiced to reaffirm the positive messages that you input in your mind.

Affirmations

Affirmations can be practiced throughout each day to reprogram positive messaging to your consciousness. Use words, prayers, poems, or sentences of your own that convey a positive message for you. Use the following guidelines to develop your own affirmation practice:

- State affirmations in the present tense, as if it has already has happened, and you are witnessing this occurring in your life.

- Use the pronoun "I," or your own name.

- Repeat positive, life enhancing messages within a positive context. Do not, for example, utilize negative terms within the affirmation, "My neck is not in pain."

- Be specific about the messages you want to realize in your life.

- Say affirmations aloud and speak while looking into a mirror to make a stronger connection with the message. Tape record the affirmations to establish a stronger sensory connection with the message. Make use of prerecorded affirmation tapes/CDs. Note: Do not listen to such tapes/CDs while driving or using heavy machinery.

- Write down your affirmations and display note cards in places where they are easily visible for you, such as on your computer monitor, vanity, and car dashboard.

Visualization

Visualization is a technique that can be practiced to envision what you would like to materialize in your life, whether it be better health, a clearer career focus, greater internal peace, or other qualities or outcomes.

- Relax. Find a quiet environment free of distractions. Wear comfortable clothing.

- Think about your goal.

- Imagine details: How will you feel? What will you be wearing? Who will accompany you?

- If necessary, record your impressions in a small notebook.

- Return to these images as much as possible throughout the day. Use affirmations to enhance and reaffirm your visualization exercises.

- To become more proficient, attend workshops, listen to visualization audiotapes, and consult books from your local library.

Goal Planning and Time Management

Goal planning and time management allows you to prioritize goals for your life, and how you are currently managing your time in order to achieve those goals. Note that determining your goals can be exercised in conjunction with visualization exercises.

Determining Your Goals

- Envision your goal and write it down. Don't worry about correct spelling and grammar.

- Is there anything you need to achieve these goals in terms of knowledge and skills?

- Is there anything that could prevent you from accomplishing this goal?

- Who can help you in attaining this goal? Friends? Family? Co-workers?

- Detail steps to achieving your goal, with a realistic time frame.

- Visualize yourself in the future as already having achieved this goal.

- Once you have achieved any goal, it is important to acknowledge this by rewarding yourself in a tangible way, i.e., going for a walk with your friend, reading a good book, etc.

Set Time Management Priorities

Most of us perceive that our demands exceed our resources, necessitating our need to set priorities that will guide our actions. Each day on your to-do list, determine which tasks are A, B, and C priority according to the following definitions. Note that these priorities can fluctuate on a day-to-day basis.

- *Priority A:* "Must Do": High importance. These tasks have immediate deadlines attached to them and/or are critical for advancement.

- *Priority B:* "Should Do": Medium importance. These tasks contribute to project development but do not have immediate deadlines.

- *Priority C:* "Could Do": Less important. Can be rescheduled to do at another time.

It may also be helpful to schedule certain tasks for when you are experiencing the most or least optimal energy level during the day. For example, focus on activities necessitating higher intellectual acuity at your peak times, whereas routine office work can be done later, or delegated to others, if possible.

Time Allocations

- Sketch a large circle onto a blank piece of paper. In a pie chart format, color code slices to what percentage of time you are allocating to various activities throughout the day. Break down categories in ways that seem most useful, i.e., work, housework, leisure, exercise/health promotion, sleep, etc. This can give you a proportional representation for how you are spending your time.

- In a notebook, write down all your activities over the course of the day, including phone calls, e-mails, meetings, family responsibilities, transportation, socializing, etc. Review them and color code the time you are prioritizing your projects instead of others' emergencies.

Simple Yet Effective Time Management Tips

- Determine your core values to determine your immediate and long-term goals and a to-do list of daily tasks.

- Use a simple, written to-do list: Prioritize your essential tasks and work on them sequentially. Make sure it is written down and portable.

- Eliminate time wasters: consolidate errands, eliminate unnecessary meetings, etc.

- Do your most undesirable tasks first while you are full of energy, which should give you energy to do other tasks.

- Say "no" to some tasks, and delegate those you need not do yourself.

- Strive for excellence, but know when perfectionism is unnecessary and impeding your progress.

- Consolidate time for returning telephone calls, e-mails, and handling mail and paperwork: By designating specific times for these tasks, they are less likely to interfere with deadlines and important projects.

- Stick to a schedule: Schedule ample time for sleeping, eating, running errands, and managing household tasks so that you will not feel rushed.

- Plan for emergencies: Get up 10 to 15 minutes earlier to account for the unexpected. Have extra sets of car and house keys for emergencies.

Stress Management Plan

Considering the stress management assessment that you have completed above, create mini action plans on addressing these stressors in a proactive way. Remember that making lasting behavioral change takes time to adopt on a permanent basis. Thus, propose doable goals that you can adopt in the time available.

Examples of a few mini action plans could include the following:

- Institute an exercise program by going for a 20 to 30 minute walk or roll in your wheelchair at lunchtime. See the NCPAD website (www.ncpad.org) or call NCPAD at 800-900-8086 for a myriad of examples of accessible exercises that can be practiced in limited time periods.

- Take regular breaks and move regularly. Practice flexibility exercises at your desk with your arms, neck, and shoulders. A 5-minute break to the water cooler can also assist you with relaxation.

- Make a to-do list, and rotate your tasks on a daily and weekly basis.

- Start a daily practice of gratitude and mindfulness by recording one or two things you are grateful for in a small notebook. This practice can help you orient to a more positive outlook.

- Begin a relaxation program by practicing relaxation exercises in short 5-minute intervals throughout the day, such as in the morning, at lunchtime, late afternoon, and at bedtime. If possible, use a watch with an alarm feature so that you can completely release in the 5 minutes designated for your relaxation. Even closing your eyes and focusing on your breathing for a few minutes while sitting at your desk can help to affect a relaxation response.

- If you have a tendency to snack on food which is high in sugar and fat, prepare healthy snacks, such as cut-up vegetables with hummus, low-fat yogurt, whole-wheat toast with peanut butter, a slice of cheese with whole-wheat crackers, fruit. See NPCAD's nutrition corner (http://www.ncpad.org/nutrition/) for additional ideas on healthy snacks.

Conclusion

A good stress management practice is developed through finding stress management modalities that suit you well and practicing them on a regular basis. Remember that just a limited amount of practice can have immeasurable effects on your well-being.

Part Six

Additional Help and Information

Chapter 61

Glossary of Stress-Related Terms

acute: Symptoms or signs that begin and worsen quickly; not chronic.

adrenal gland: A small gland that makes steroid hormones, adrenaline, and noradrenaline. These hormones help control heart rate, blood pressure, and other important body functions. There are two adrenal glands, one on top of each kidney. Also called suprarenal gland.

alternative medicine: Practices used instead of standard treatments. They generally are not recognized by the medical community as standard or conventional medical approaches. Alternative medicine includes dietary supplements, megadose vitamins, herbal preparations, special teas, acupuncture, massage therapy, magnet therapy, spiritual healing, and meditation.

anxiety: Feelings of fear, dread, and uneasiness that may occur as a reaction to stress. A person with anxiety may sweat, feel restless and tense, and have a rapid heartbeat. Extreme anxiety that happens often over time may be a sign of an anxiety disorder.

anxiety disorder: A disorder that causes a person to be filled with fearfulness and uncertainty. Anxiety disorders last at least 6 months

This glossary contains terms excerpted from glossaries and documents produced by the following government agencies: National Cancer Institute (NCI); National Center for Complementary and Alternative Medicine (NCCAM); National Center for Posttraumatic Stress Disorder (NCPTSD); National Institute of Mental Health (NIMH); National Institutes of Health (NIH); and the U.S. Department of Health and Human Services (HHS).

and can get worse if they are not treated. Anxiety disorders commonly occur along with other mental or physical illnesses, including alcohol or substance abuse, which may mask anxiety symptoms or make them worse.

arousal symptoms: A constant feeling of alertness after a traumatic event that occurs in people with posttraumatic stress disorder. Arousal symptoms can cause difficulty sleeping, outbursts of anger or irritability, and difficulty concentrating.

autogenic training: Autogenic training consists of imagining a peaceful environment and comforting bodily sensations. Six basic focusing techniques are used: heaviness in the limbs, warmth in the limbs, cardiac regulation, centering on breathing, warmth in the upper abdomen, and coolness in the forehead.

avoidance symptoms: Efforts people make to avoid a traumatic event. Individuals with posttraumatic stress disorder may try to avoid situations that trigger memories of the traumatic event.

biofeedback: A method of learning to voluntarily control certain body functions such as heartbeat, blood pressure, and muscle tension with the help of a special machine. This method can help control pain and stress.

burnout: The reaction of the body and mind to persistent stress. It can lead to aversion toward activities and people that are part of life in and out of work. Signs and symptoms of burnout may include exhaustion, cynicism, and ineffectiveness.

chronic: A disease or condition that persists or progresses over a long period of time.

cognitive-behavioral therapy (CBT): A type of therapy used in treating anxiety disorders. The cognitive part helps people change the thinking patterns that support their fears, and the behavioral part helps people change the way they react to anxiety-provoking situations.

complementary medicine: Practices often used to enhance or complement standard treatments. They generally are not recognized by the medical community as standard or conventional medical approaches. Complementary medicine may include dietary supplements, megadose vitamins, herbal preparations, special teas, acupuncture, massage therapy, magnet therapy, spiritual healing, and meditation.

cortisol: Hormone produced by the adrenal gland. Cortisol raises the blood sugar level and helps a stressed person's body respond to the increased demands of stress.

cytokines: A substance that is produced by cells of the immune system and can affect the immune response.

distress: Extreme mental or physical pain or suffering.

epinephrine: A hormone and neurotransmitter. Also called adrenaline.

generalized anxiety disorder: An anxiety disorder that is characterized by chronic anxiety, exaggerated worry and tension, even when there is little or nothing to provoke it.

hormone: A chemical made by glands in the body. Hormones circulate in the bloodstream and control the actions of certain cells or organs. Some hormones can also be made in a laboratory.

hypothalamic-pituitary-adrenal (HPA) system: The hypothalamus is the area of the brain where stress signals get routed. When a person is under stress, the HPA axis is activated, and after a number of steps, the hypothalamus releases a substance called corticotropin releasing factor (CRF). CRF then releases adrenocorticotropin hormone (ACTH) from the pituitary gland. Finally, ACTH releases cortisol from the adrenal gland, along with a number of other neurosteroids.

irritable bowel syndrome: A disorder characterized most commonly by cramping, abdominal pain, bloating, constipation, and diarrhea. IBS causes a great deal of discomfort and distress, but it does not permanently harm the intestines and does not lead to a serious disease.

kava: An herb native to the islands of the South Pacific and a member of the pepper family. Today kava is used primarily for anxiety, insomnia, and menopausal symptoms.

meditation: Meditation for health purposes is a mind-body practice in complementary and alternative medicine (CAM). There are many types of meditation, most of which originated in ancient religious and spiritual traditions. Generally, a person who is meditating uses certain techniques, such as focusing attention (for example, on a word, an object, or the breath); a specific posture; and an open attitude toward distracting thoughts and emotions. Meditation can be practiced for various reasons—for example, with an intent to increase physical relaxation, mental calmness, and psychological balance; to cope with one or more diseases and conditions; and for overall wellness.

mindfulness meditation: A type of meditation that originated in Buddhism. It is based on the concept of being mindful, or having an increased awareness and total acceptance of the present. While meditating, the meditator is taught to bring all his or her attention to the sensation of the flow of the breath in and out of the body. The intent might be described as focusing attention on what is being experienced, without reacting to or judging that experience. This is seen as helping the meditator learn to experience thoughts and emotions in normal daily life with greater balance and acceptance.

neurotransmitters: A chemical that is made by nerve cells and used to communicate with other cells, including other nerve cells and muscle cells.

numbing symptoms: Individuals with posttraumatic stress disorder may find it difficult to be in touch with their feelings or express emotions toward other people. For example, they may feel emotionally "numb" and may isolate from others.

obsessive-compulsive disorder: An anxiety disorder that is characterized by recurrent, unwanted thoughts (obsessions) and/or repetitive behaviors (compulsions). Repetitive behaviors such as hand-washing, counting, checking, or cleaning are often performed with the hope of preventing obsessive thoughts or making them go away. Performing these so-called rituals, however, provides only temporary relief, and not performing them markedly increases anxiety.

panic disorder: An anxiety disorder that is characterized by unexpected and repeated episodes of intense fear accompanied by physical symptoms that may include chest pain, heart palpitations, shortness of breath, dizziness, or abdominal distress.

parasympathetic nervous system: The part of the body that creates what some call the "rest and digest" response. This system's responses oppose those of the sympathetic nervous system. For example, it causes the heart rate and breathing rate to slow down, the blood vessels to dilate (improving blood flow), and activity to increase in many parts of the digestive tract.

peptic ulcers: A sore in the lining of the stomach or duodenum. The duodenum is the first part of the small intestine. If peptic ulcers are found in the stomach, they are called gastric ulcers. If they are found in the duodenum, they are called duodenal ulcers.

phobia: An intense fear of something that poses little or no actual danger. Some of the more common specific phobias are centered around closed-in places, heights, escalators, tunnels, highway driving, water, flying, dogs, and injuries involving blood. Such phobias aren't just extreme fear; they are irrational fear of a particular thing.

posttraumatic stress disorder (PTSD): Anxiety disorder that can occur following the experience or witnessing of a traumatic event.

progressive muscle relaxation (PMR): PMR focuses on reducing muscle tone in major muscle groups. Each of 15 major muscle groups is tensed and then relaxed in sequence.

psychiatrist: A medical doctor who specializes in the prevention, diagnosis, and treatment of mental, emotional, and behavioral disorders.

psychologist: A specialist who can talk with patients and their families about emotional and personal matters, and can help them make decisions.

psychotherapy: Psychotherapy involves talking with a trained mental health professional, such as a psychiatrist, psychologist, social worker, or counselor, to discover what caused a mental health disorder and how to deal with its symptoms.

re-experiencing symptoms: Symptoms of posttraumatic stress disorder that involve reliving the traumatic event.

serotonin: Hormone found in the brain, platelets, digestive tract, and pineal gland. It acts both as a neurotransmitter (a substance that nerves use to send messages to one another) and a vasoconstrictor (a substance that causes blood vessels to narrow). A lack of serotonin in the brain is thought to be a cause of depression. Also called 5-hydroxytryptamine.

social phobia: An anxiety disorder characterized by overwhelming anxiety and excessive self-consciousness in everyday social situations. Social phobia can be limited to only one type of situation, such as a fear of speaking in formal or informal situations, or eating or drinking in front of others, or, in its most severe form, may be so broad that a person experiences symptoms almost any time they are around other people.

stressor: A stress-causing stimulus.

sympathetic nervous system: The part of the body that helps mobilize the body for action. When a person is under stress, it produces the fight-or-flight response: the heart rate and breathing rate go up, for example, the blood vessels narrow (restricting the flow of blood), and muscles tighten.

transcendental meditation (TM): A type of meditation that originated in the Vedic tradition in India. It is a type of meditation that uses a mantra (a word, sound, or phrase repeated silently) to prevent distracting thoughts from entering the mind. The intent of TM might be described as allowing the mind to settle into a quieter state and the body into a state of deep rest. This is seen as ultimately leading to a state of relaxed alertness.

trauma: A life-threatening event such as military combat, natural disasters, terrorist incidents, serious accidents, or physical or sexual assault in adult or childhood.

valerian: A plant native to Europe and Asia; it is also found in North America. Valerian has long been used for sleep disorders and anxiety. It has also been used for other conditions, such as headaches, depression, irregular heartbeat, and trembling.

Chapter 62

Directory of Government and Private Agencies That Provide Information about Stress and Stress-Related Disorders

Government Agencies That Provide Information about Stress-Related Disorders

Centers for Disease Control and Prevention
1600 Clifton Road
Atlanta, GA 30333
Toll-Free: 800-311-3435
Phone: 404-639-3311
Website: www.cdc.gov
E-mail: cdcinfo@cdc.gov

National Institute for Occupational Safety and Health
200 Independence Avenue SW
Room 715H
Washington, DC 20201
Toll-Free: 800-356-4674
Phone: 513-533-8326
Fax: 513-533-8573
Toll-Free Fax on Demand:
888-232-3299
Website: www.cdc.gov/niosh

Federal Emergency Management Agency
500 C Street SW
Washington, DC 20472
Disaster Assistance:
800-621-FEMA (621-3362)
TTY Toll-Free: 800-462-7585
Fax: 800-827-8112
Website: www.fema.gov
E-mail:
FEMA-Correspondence-Unit
@dhs.gov

Resources in this chapter were compiled from several sources deemed reliable; all contact information was verified and updated in April 2007.

Healthfinder®
National Health Information
Center
P.O. Box 1133
Washington, DC 20013-1133
Toll-Free: 800-336-4797
Phone: 301-565-4167
Fax: 301-984-4256
Website: www.healthfinder.gov
E-mail: healthfinder@nhic.org

National Cancer Institute
Cancer Information Service
6116 Executive Boulevard
Room 3036A
Bethesda, MD 20892-8322
Toll-Free: 800-4-CANCER
(422-6237)
TTY Toll-Free: 800-332-8615
Website: www.cancer.gov
E-mail:
cancergovstaff@mail.nih.gov

National Center for Complementary and Alternative Medicine
NCCAM Clearinghouse
P.O. Box 7923
Gaithersburg, MD 20898-7923
Toll-Free: 888-644-6226
Phone: 301-519-3153
TTY: 866-464-3615
Fax: 866-464-3616
Website: nccam.nih.gov
E-mail: info@nccam.nih.gov

National Center for Health Statistics
3311 Toledo Road
Hyattsville, MD 20782
Toll-Free: 866-441-NCHS
(441-6247)
Phone: 301-458-4000
Phone: 301-458-4636
Website: www.cdc.gov/nchs
E-mail: nchsquery@cdc.gov

National Center for Post-traumatic Stress Disorder
VA Medical Center (116D)
215 N. Main Street
White River Junction, VT 05009
Phone: 802-296-6300
Phone: 802-296-5132
Fax: 802-296-5135
Website: www.ncptsd.org
E-mail: ncptsd@ncptsd.org

National Criminal Justice Reference Service (NCJRS)
P.O. Box 6000
Rockville, MD 20849-6000
Toll-Free: 800-851-3420
TTY: 877-712-9279
International: 301-519-5500
Fax: 301-519-5212
Website: www.ncjrs.gov

National Digestive Diseases Information Clearinghouse
2 Information Way
Bethesda, MD 20892-3570
Toll-Free: 800-891-5389
Fax: 703-738-4929
Website: digestive.niddk.nih.gov
E-mail:
nddic@info.niddk.nih.gov

National Heart, Lung, and Blood Institute Health Information Center
P.O. Box 30105
Bethesda, MD 20824-0105
Phone: 301-592-8573
TTY: 240-629-3255
Fax: 240-629-3246
Website: www.nhlbi.nih.gov
E-mail: nhlbiinfo@nhlbi.nih.gov

National Highway Traffic Safety Administration
400 Seventh Street, SW
Washington, DC 20590
Toll-Free: 888-327-4236
TTY Toll-Free: 800-424-9153
Website: www.nhtsa.dot.gov

National Institute of Mental Health
6001 Executive Boulevard
Room 8184, MSC 9663
Bethesda, MD 20892-9663
Toll-Free: 866-615-6464
TTY Toll-Free: 866-415-8051
TTY: 301-443-8431
Phone: 301-443-4513
Fax: 301-443-4279
Website: www.nimh.nih.gov
E-mail: nimhinfo@nih.gov

National Institute of Neurological Disorders and Stroke
NIH Neurological Institute
P.O. Box 5801
Bethesda, MD 20824
Toll-Free: 800-352-9424
Phone: 301-496-5751
TTY: 301-468-5981
Website: www.ninds.nih.gov
E-mail: braininfo@ninds.nih.gov

National Institute on Aging
Building 31C, Room 5C27
31 Center Drive, MSC 2292
Bethesda, MD 20892
Publications Toll-Free:
800-222-2225
Phone: 301-496-1752
TTY: 800-222-4225
Fax: 301-496-1072
Websites: www.nia.nih.gov
Publications Website:
www.niapublications.org
E-mail: niainfo@nia.nih.gov

National Institute on Alcohol Abuse and Alcoholism
5635 Fishers Lane, MSC 9304
Bethesda, MD 20892-9304
Phone: 301-443-3860
Website: www.niaaa.nih.gov
E-mail: niaaaweb-r@exchange
.nih.gov

National Institute on Drug Abuse
6001 Executive Boulevard,
Room 5213
Bethesda, MD 20892-9561
Phone: 301-443-1124
Website: www.nida.nih.gov
E-mail:
information@nida.nih.gov

National Institutes of Health
9000 Rockville Pike
Bethesda, MD 20892
Phone: 301-496-4000
TTY: 301-402-9612
Website: www.nih.gov
E-mail: NIHinfo@od.nih.gov

National Women's Health Information Center
8270 Willow Oaks Corporate Dr.
Fairfax, VA 22031
Toll-Free: 800-994-WOMAN
(994-9662)
TTY: 888-220-5446
Website: www.4woman.gov

President's Council on Physical Fitness and Sports
Department W
200 Independence Avenue, SW
Room 738-H
Washington, DC 20201-0004
Phone: 202-690-9000
Fax: 202-690-5211
Website: www.fitness.gov

SAMHSA National Mental Health Information Center
P.O. Box 42557
Washington, DC 20015
Toll-Free: 800-789-2647
TDD: 866-889-2647
Fax: 240-221-4295
International: 240-221-4022
Website:
mentalhealth.samhsa.gov

U.S. Department of Agriculture
1400 Independence Ave., SW
Washington, DC 20250
Phone: 202-720-4623
Fax: 202-720-5043
Website: www.usda.gov

U.S. Department of Health and Human Services
200 Independence Avenue, SW
Washington, DC 20201
Toll-Free: 877-696-6775
Phone: 202-619-0257
Website: www.hhs.gov

U.S. Food and Drug Administration
5600 Fishers Lane
HFE-50
Rockville, MD 20857-0001
Toll-Free: 888-463-6332
Phone: 301-827-4420
Fax: 301-443-9767
Website: www.fda.gov

U.S. National Library of Medicine
8600 Rockville Pike
Bethesda, MD 20894
Toll-Free: 888-346-3656
Phone: 301-594-5983
Fax: 301-402-1384
TDD: 800-735-2258
Website: www.nlm.nih.gov
E-mail: custserv@nlm.nih.gov

Weight-Control Information Network
1 WIN Way
Bethesda, MD 20892-3665
Toll-Free: 877-946-4627
Phone: 202-828-1025
Fax: 202-828-1028
Website: win.niddk.nih.gov
E-mail: win@info.niddk.nih.gov

Private Agencies That Provide Information about Stress-Related Disorders

American Academy of Allergy, Asthma, and Immunology
555 East Wells Street
Suite 1100
Milwaukee, WI 53202-3823
Patient Information and Physician Referral: 800-822-2762
Phone: 414-272-6071
Fax: 414-272-6070
Website: www.aaaai.org
E-mail: info@aaaai.org

American Academy of Child and Adolescent Psychiatry
3615 Wisconsin Avenue, NW
Washington, DC 20016-3007
Phone: 202-966-7300
Fax: 202-966-2891
Website: www.aacap.org
E-mail:
communications@aacap.org

American Academy of Dermatology
P.O. Box 4014
Schaumburg, IL 60618-4014
Toll-Free: 888-462-DERM
(462-3376)
International: 847-240-1280
Website: www.aad.org
E-mail: MRC@aad.org

American Academy of Experts in Traumatic Stress
368 Veterans Memorial Highway
Commack, NY 11725
Phone: 631-543-2217
Fax: 631-543-6977
Website: www.atsm.org
E-mail: info@aaets.org

American Academy of Family Physicians
P.O. Box 11210
Shawnee Mission, KS 66207-1210
Toll-Free: 800-274-2237
Phone: 913-906-6000
Website: www.aafp.org
E-mail: fp@aafp.org

American Association of Suicidology
5221 Wisconsin Avenue, NW
Washington, DC 20015
Phone: 202-237-2280
Fax: 202-237-2282
Website: www.suicidology.org
E-mail: info@suicidology.org

American Council for Headache Education
19 Mantua Road
Mt. Royal, NJ 08061
Phone: 856-423-0258
Fax: 856-423-0082
Website: www.achenet.org
E-mail: achehq@talley.com

American Council on Consumer Interests
415 S. Duff Avenue
Suite C
Ames, IA 50010-6600
Phone: 515-956-4666
Fax: 515-233-3101
Website:
www.consumerinterests.org
E-mail:
info@consumerinterests.org

American Dietetic Association
120 South Riverside Plaza
Suite 2000
Chicago, IL 60606-6995
Toll-Free: 800-877-1600
Website: www.eatright.org
E-mail: knowledge@eatright.org

American Federation for Aging Research
55 West 39th Street, 16th Floor
New York, NY 10018
Toll-Free: 888-582-2327
Phone: 212-703-9977
Fax: 212-997-0330
Websites: www.infoaging.org
E-mail: info@afar.org

American Foundation for Suicide Prevention
120 Wall Street, 22nd Floor
New York, NY 10005
Toll-Free: 888-333-AFSP
(333-2377)
Phone: 212-363-3500
Fax: 212-363-6237
Website: www.afsp.org
E-mail: inquiry@afsp.org

American Heart Association
7272 Greenville Avenue
Dallas, TX 75231
Toll-Free: 800-AHA-USA-1
(242-8721)
Website:
www.americanheart.org

American Institute for Cognitive Therapy
136 East 57th Street
Suite 1101
New York, NY 10022
Phone: 212-308-2440
Website:
www.cognitivetherapynyc.com
E-mail: intake
@cognitivetherapyNYC.com

American Institute of Stress
124 Park Avenue
Yonkers, NY 10703
Phone: 914-963-1200
Fax: 914-965-6267
Website: www.stress.org
E-mail: Stress125@optonline.net

American Massage Therapy Association
500 Davis Street
Suite 900
Evanston, IL 60201-4695
Toll-Free: 877-905-2700
Phone: 847-864-0123
Fax: 847-864-1178
Website: www.amtamassage.org
E-mail: info@amtamassage.org

American Medical Association/Medem
649 Mission Street, 2nd Floor
San Francisco, CA 94105
Toll-Free: 877-926-3336
Phone: 415-644-3800
Fax: 415-644-3950
Website: www.medem.com
E-mail: info@medem.com

American Psychiatric Association
1000 Wilson Boulevard
Suite 1825
Arlington, VA 22209-3901
Toll-Free: 888-357-7924
Phone: 703-907-7300
Fax: 703-907-1085
Websites: www.psych.org;
www.healthyminds.org
E-mail: apa@psych.org

American Psychiatric Nurses Association
1555 Wilson Boulevard
Suite 602
Arlington, VA 22209
Toll-Free: 866-243-2443
Fax: 703-243-3390
Website: www.apna.org
E-mail: inform@apna.org

American Psychological Association
750 First Street, NE
Washington, DC 20002-4242
Toll-Free: 800-374-2721
Phone: 202-336-5500
TDD/TTY: 202-336-6123
Website: www.apa.org

Anorexia Nervosa and Related Eating Disorders (ANRED)
Website: www.anred.com
E-mail: jarinor@rio.com

Anxiety Disorders Association of America
8730 Georgia Avenue, Suite 600
Silver Spring, MD 20910
Phone: 240-485-1001
Fax: 240-485-1035
Website: www.adaa.org
E-mail: anxdis@adaa.org

Arthritis Foundation
P.O. Box 932915
Atlanta, GA 31193-2195
Toll-Free: 800-568-4045
Phone: 404-872-7100
Website: www.arthritis.org
E-mail: help@arthritis.org

Association for Behavioral and Cognitive Therapies
305 7th Avenue, 16th Floor
New York, NY 10001-6008
Phone 212-647-1890
Fax: 212-647-1865
Website: www.abct.org
E-mail: mjeimer@abct.org

Biofeedback Certification Institute of America
10200 W. 44th Avenue
Suite 310
Wheat Ridge, CO 80033-2840
Toll-Free: 866-908-8713
Phone: 303-420-2902
Fax: 303-422-8894
Website: www.bcia.org
E-mail: bcia@resourcenter.com

British Autogenic Society
The Royal London
Homoeopathic Hospital
Great Ormond Street
London WC1N 3HR
United Kingdom
Phone: 020 7391 8908
Fax: 020 7391 8908
Website: autogenic-therapy
.org.uk

Children of Aging Parents
P.O. Box 167
Richboro, PA 18954
Toll-Free: 800-227-7294
Website:
www.caps4caregivers.org
E-mail:
info@caps4caregivers.org

Cleveland Clinic
9500 Euclid Avenue
Cleveland, OH 44195
Toll-Free: 800-223-2273
Phone: 216-444-2200
TTY: 216-444-0261
Website:
www.clevelandclinic.org

Depression and Bipolar Support Alliance (DBSA)
730 N. Franklin Street
Suite 501
Chicago, IL 60610-7224
Toll-Free: 800-826-3632
Phone: 312-642-0049
Fax: 312-642-7243
Website: www.dbsalliance.org
E-mail: info@dbsalliance.org

Family Caregiver Alliance
180 Montgomery Street
Suite 1100
San Francisco, CA 94104
Toll-Free: 800-445-8106
Phone: 415-434-3388
Fax: 415-434-3508
Website: www.caregiver.org
E-mail: info@caregiver.org

Freedom from Fear
308 Seaview Avenue
Staten Island, NY 10305
Phone: 718-351-1717
Fax: 718-980-5022
Website:
www.freedomfromfear.org
E-mail:
help@freedomfromfear.org

Gift From Within
16 Cobb Hill Road
Camden, ME 04843
Phone: 207-236-8858
Fax: 207-236-2818
Website: www.giftfromwithin.org
E-mail: JoyceB3955@aol.com

HelpGuide (Center for Healthy Aging)
2125 Arizona Avenue
Santa Monica, CA 90404
Website: www.helpguide.org

Hormone Foundation
8401 Connecticut Avenue
Suite 900
Chevy Chase, MD 20815-5817
Toll-Free: 800-HORMONE
(467-6663)
Fax: 301-941-0259
Website: www.hormone.org
E-mail: hormone@endo-society
.org

International Society for Traumatic Stress Studies
60 Revere Drive
Suite 500
Northbrook, IL 60062
Phone: 847-480-9028
Fax: 847-480-9282
Website: www.istss.org
E-mail: istss@istss.org

Iraq War Veterans Organization, Inc.
P.O. Box 571
Yucaipa, CA 92399
Website:
www.iraqwarveterans.org
E-mail:
info@iraqwarveterans.org

March of Dimes Birth Defects Foundation
1275 Mamaroneck Avenue
White Plains, NY 10605
Toll-Free English: 888-663-4637
Toll-Free Spanish: 800-925-1855
Phone: 914-997-4488
Fax: 914-997-4763
Website:
www.marchofdimes.com
E-mail:
contactus@marchofdimes.com

Mayo Foundation for Medical Education and Research
200 First Street SW
Rochester, MN 55905
Website: www.mayoclinic.com
E-mail:
comments@mayoclinic.com

National Alliance for Caregiving
4720 Montgomery Lane
5th Floor
Bethesda, MD 20814
Phone: 301-718-8444
Fax: 301-951-9067
Website: www.caregiving.org
E-mail: info@caregiving.org

National Alliance on Mental Illness (NAMI)
Colonial Place Three
2107 Wilson Boulevard
Suite 300
Arlington, VA 22201-3042
Toll-Free: 800-950-NAMI
(950-6264)
Phone: 703-524-7600
TDD: 703-516-7227
Fax: 703-524-9094
Website: www.nami.org
E-mail: info@nami.org

National Resource Center for Child Traumatic Stress
Duke University
905 W. Main Street
Suite 25-B
Durham, NC 27701
Phone: 919-682-1552 ext. 248
Fax: 919-667-9578
Website: www.nctsnet.org
E-mail: info@nctsn.org

National Center for Victims of Crime
2000 M Street NW
Suite 480
Washington, DC 20036
Phone: 202-467-8700
Fax: 202-467-8701
Website: www.ncvc.org
E-mail: gethelp@ncvc.org

National Center on Physical Activity and Disability
1640 W. Roosevelt Road
Suite 711
Chicago, IL 60608-6904
Toll-Free/TTY: 800-900-8086
Fax: 312-355-4058
Website: www.ncpad.org
E-mail: ncpad@uic.edu

National Council on Aging, Inc.
1901 L Street, NW
4th Floor
Washington, DC 20036
Phone: 202-479-1200
TDD: 202-479-6674
Fax: 202-479-0735
Website: www.ncoa.org
E-mail: info@ncoa.org

National Family Caregivers Association
10400 Connecticut Avenue
Suite 500
Kensington, MD 20895-3944
Toll-Free: 800-896-3650
Phone: 301-942-6430
Fax: 301-942-2302
Website:
www.thefamilycaregiver.org
E-mail:
info@thefamilycaregiver.org

Mental Health America
2000 N. Beauregard Street
6th Floor
Alexandria, VA 22311
Toll-Free: 800-969-6642
Phone: 703-684-7722
TTY Toll-Free: 800-433-5959
Fax: 703-684-5968
Website: www.nmha.org

National Multiple Sclerosis Society
700 Broadway
Suite 808
Denver, CO 80203
Toll-Free: 800-FIGHT-MS
(344-4867)
Website:
www.nationalmssociety.org
E-mail: general.information
@coc.mnss.org

National Organization for Victim Assistance (NOVA)
510 King Street
Suite 424
Alexandria, VA 22314
Toll-Free: 800-879-6682
Phone: 703-535-NOVA
(535-6682)
Fax: 703-535-5500
Website: www.trynova.org
E-mail: nova@try-nova.org

National Sleep Foundation
1522 K Street, NW
Suite 500
Washington, DC 20005
Phone: 202-347-3471
Fax: 202-347-3472
Website:
www.sleepfoundation.org
E-mail: nsf@sleepfoundation.org

National Women's Health Resource Center
157 Broad Street
Suite 315
Red Bank, NJ 07701
Toll-Free: 877-986-9472
Website:
www.healthywomen.org
E-mail: info@healthywomen.org

Nemours Foundation Center for Children's Health Media
1600 Rockland Road
Wilmington, DE 19803
Phone: 302-651-4000
Fax: 302-651-4055
Website: www.kidshealth.org
E-mail: info@kidshealth.org

Obsessive-Compulsive Foundation
676 State Street
New Haven, CT 06511
Phone: 203-401-2070
Fax: 203-401-2076
Website: www.ocfoundation.org
E-mail: info@ocfoundation.org

Organization of Teratology Information Specialists (OTIS)
Toll-Free: 866-626-OTIS
(626-6847)
Website: www.otispregnancy.org
E-mail: OTISPregnancy
@pharmacy.arizona.edu

Posttraumatic Stress Disorder Alliance
http://www.ptsdalliance.org

PTSDinfo.org
http://www.ptsdinfo.org

Rape, Abuse, and Incest National Network (RAINN)
2000 L Street NW
Suite 406
Washington, DC 20036
Toll-Free: 800-656-HOPE
(656-4673)
Phone: 202-544-1034
Fax: 202-544-3556
Website: www.rainn.org
E-mail: info@rainn.org

Sidran Traumatic Stress Institute
200 East Joppa Road
Suite 207
Baltimore, MD 21286-3107
Toll-Free: 888-825-8249
Phone: 410-825-8888
Fax: 410-337-0747
Website: www.sidran.org
E-mail: info@sidran.org

Suicide Prevention Advocacy Network USA
1025 Vermont Avenue, NW
Suite 1066
Washington, DC 20005
Phone: 202-449-3600
Fax: 202-449-3601
Website: www.spanusa.org
E-mail: info@spanusa.org

Transcendental Meditation Program
P.O. Box 670
Fairfield, IA 52556
Toll-Free: 888-LEARN-TM
(532-7686)
Website: www.tm.org
E-mail: tminfo@tm.org

Index

Index

Page numbers followed by 'n' indicate a footnote. Page numbers in *italics* indicate a table or illustration.

Health Reference Series
COMPLETE CATALOG
List price $87 per volume. **School and library price $78 per volume.**

Adolescent Health Sourcebook, 2nd Edition

Basic Consumer Health Information about the Physical, Mental, and Emotional Growth and Development of Adolescents, Including Medical Care, Nutritional and Physical Activity Requirements, Puberty, Sexual Activity, Acne, Tanning, Body Piercing, Common Physical Illnesses and Disorders, Eating Disorders, Attention Deficit Hyperactivity Disorder, Depression, Bullying, Hazing, and Adolescent Injuries Related to Sports, Driving, and Work

Along with Substance Abuse Information about Nicotine, Alcohol, and Drug Use, a Glossary, and Directory of Additional Resources

Edited by Joyce Brennfleck Shannon. 683 pages. 2006. 978-0-7808-0943-7.

"It is written in clear, nontechnical language aimed at general readers. . . . Recommended for public libraries, community colleges, and other agencies serving health care consumers."
—*American Reference Books Annual, 2003*

"Recommended for school and public libraries. Parents and professionals dealing with teens will appreciate the easy-to-follow format and the clearly written text. This could become a 'must have' for every high school teacher." —*E-Streams, Jan '03*

"A good starting point for information related to common medical, mental, and emotional concerns of adolescents." —*School Library Journal, Nov '02*

"This book provides accurate information in an easy to access format. It addresses topics that parents and caregivers might not be aware of and provides practical, useable information."
—*Doody's Health Sciences Book Review Journal, Sep-Oct '02*

"Recommended reference source."
—*Booklist, American Library Association, Sep '02*

■

AIDS Sourcebook, 3rd Edition

Basic Consumer Health Information about Acquired Immune Deficiency Syndrome (AIDS) and Human Immunodeficiency Virus (HIV) Infection, Including Facts about Transmission, Prevention, Diagnosis, Treatment, Opportunistic Infections, and Other Complications, with a Section for Women and Children, Including Details about Associated Gynecological Concerns, Pregnancy, and Pediatric Care

Along with Updated Statistical Information, Reports on Current Research Initiatives, a Glossary, and Directories of Internet, Hotline, and Other Resources

Edited by Dawn D. Matthews. 664 pages. 2003. 978-0-7808-0631-3.

"The 3rd edition of the *AIDS Sourcebook*, part of Omnigraphics' *Health Reference Series*, is a welcome update. . . . This resource is highly recommended for academic and public libraries."
—*American Reference Books Annual, 2004*

"Excellent sourcebook. This continues to be a highly recommended book. There is no other book that provides as much information as this book provides."
—*AIDS Book Review Journal, Dec-Jan '00*

"Recommended reference source."
—*Booklist, American Library Association, Dec '99*

■

Alcoholism Sourcebook, 2nd Edition

Basic Consumer Health Information about Alcohol Use, Abuse, and Dependence, Featuring Facts about the Physical, Mental, and Social Health Effects of Alcohol Addiction, Including Alcoholic Liver Disease, Pancreatic Disease, Cardiovascular Disease, Neurological Disorders, and the Effects of Drinking during Pregnancy

Along with Information about Alcohol Treatment, Medications, and Recovery Programs, in Addition to Tips for Reducing the Prevalence of Underage Drinking, Statistics about Alcohol Use, a Glossary of Related Terms, and Directories of Resources for More Help and Information

Edited by Amy L. Sutton. 653 pages. 2006. 978-0-7808-0942-0.

"This title is one of the few reference works on alcoholism for general readers. For some readers this will be a welcome complement to the many self-help books on the market. Recommended for collections serving general readers and consumer health collections."
—*E-Streams, Mar '01*

"This book is an excellent choice for public and academic libraries."
—*American Reference Books Annual, 2001*

"Recommended reference source."
—*Booklist, American Library Association, Dec '00*

"Presents a wealth of information on alcohol use and abuse and its effects on the body and mind, treatment, and prevention." —*SciTech Book News, Dec '00*

"Important new health guide which packs in the latest consumer information about the problems of alcoholism." —*Reviewer's Bookwatch, Nov '00*

SEE ALSO *Drug Abuse Sourcebook*

Allergies Sourcebook, 3rd Edition

Basic Consumer Health Information about Allergic Disorders, Such as Anaphylaxis, Hives, Eczema, Rhinitis, Sinusitis, and Conjunctivitis, and Their Triggers, Including Pollen, Mold, Dust Mites, Animal Dander, Insects, Chemicals, Food, Food Additives, and Medications;

Along with Advice about the Diagnosis and Treatment of Allergy Symptoms, a Glossary of Related Terms, a Directory of Resources for Help and Information, and Suggestions for Additional Reading

Edited by Amy L. Sutton. 598 pages. 2007. 978-0-7808-0950-5.

"This book brings a great deal of useful material together.... This is an excellent addition to public and consumer health library collections."
— *American Reference Books Annual, 2003*

"This second edition would be useful to laypersons with little or advanced knowledge of the subject matter. This book would also serve as a resource for nursing and other health care professions students. It would be useful in public, academic, and hospital libraries with consumer health collections." — *E-Streams, Jul '02*

■

Alternative Medicine Sourcebook

SEE Complementary & Alternative Medicine Sourcebook

■

Alzheimer's Disease Sourcebook, 3rd Edition

Basic Consumer Health Information about Alzheimer's Disease, Other Dementias, and Related Disorders, Including Multi-Infarct Dementia, AIDS Dementia Complex, Dementia with Lewy Bodies, Huntington's Disease, Wernicke-Korsakoff Syndrome (Alcohol-Related Dementia), Delirium, and Confusional States

Along with Information for People Newly Diagnosed with Alzheimer's Disease and Caregivers, Reports Detailing Current Research Efforts in Prevention, Diagnosis, and Treatment, Facts about Long-Term Care Issues, and Listings of Sources for Additional Information

Edited by Karen Bellenir. 645 pages. 2003. 978-0-7808-0666-5.

"This very informative and valuable tool will be a great addition to any library serving consumers, students and health care workers."
— *American Reference Books Annual, 2004*

"This is a valuable resource for people affected by dementias such as Alzheimer's. It is easy to navigate and includes important information and resources."
— *Doody's Review Service, Feb '04*

"Recommended reference source."
— *Booklist, American Library Association, Oct '99*

SEE ALSO *Brain Disorders Sourcebook*

Arthritis Sourcebook, 2nd Edition

Basic Consumer Health Information about Osteoarthritis, Rheumatoid Arthritis, Other Rheumatic Disorders, Infectious Forms of Arthritis, and Diseases with Symptoms Linked to Arthritis, Featuring Facts about Diagnosis, Pain Management, and Surgical Therapies

Along with Coping Strategies, Research Updates, a Glossary, and Resources for Additional Help and Information

Edited by Amy L. Sutton. 593 pages. 2004. 978-0-7808-0667-2.

"This easy-to-read volume is recommended for consumer health collections within public or academic libraries." — *E-Streams, May '05*

"As expected, this updated edition continues the excellent reputation of this series in providing sound, usable health information.... Highly recommended."
— *American Reference Books Annual, 2005*

"Excellent reference." — *The Bookwatch, Jan '05*

■

Asthma Sourcebook, 2nd Edition

Basic Consumer Health Information about the Causes, Symptoms, Diagnosis, and Treatment of Asthma in Infants, Children, Teenagers, and Adults, Including Facts about Different Types of Asthma, Common Co-Occurring Conditions, Asthma Management Plans, Triggers, Medications, and Medication Delivery Devices

Along with Asthma Statistics, Research Updates, a Glossary, a Directory of Asthma-Related Resources, and More

Edited by Karen Bellenir. 609 pages. 2006. 978-0-7808-0866-9.

"A worthwhile reference acquisition for public libraries and academic medical libraries whose readers desire a quick introduction to the wide range of asthma information." — *Choice, Association of College & Research Libraries, Jun '01*

"Recommended reference source."
— *Booklist, American Library Association, Feb '01*

"Highly recommended." — *The Bookwatch, Jan '01*

"There is much good information for patients and their families who deal with asthma daily."
— *American Medical Writers Association Journal, Winter '01*

"This informative text is recommended for consumer health collections in public, secondary school, and community college libraries and the libraries of universities with a large undergraduate population."
— *American Reference Books Annual, 2001*

■

Attention Deficit Disorder Sourcebook

Basic Consumer Health Information about Attention Deficit/Hyperactivity Disorder in Children and Adults,

Including Facts about Causes, Symptoms, Diagnostic Criteria, and Treatment Options Such as Medications, Behavior Therapy, Coaching, and Homeopathy

Along with Reports on Current Research Initiatives, Legal Issues, and Government Regulations, and Featuring a Glossary of Related Terms, Internet Resources, and a List of Additional Reading Material

Edited by Dawn D. Matthews. 470 pages. 2002. 978-0-7808-0624-5.

"Recommended reference source."
— Booklist, American Library Association, Jan '03

"This book is recommended for all school libraries and the reference or consumer health sections of public libraries." — American Reference Books Annual, 2003

Back & Neck Sourcebook, 2nd Edition

Basic Consumer Health Information about Spinal Pain, Spinal Cord Injuries, and Related Disorders, Such as Degenerative Disk Disease, Osteoarthritis, Scoliosis, Sciatica, Spina Bifida, and Spinal Stenosis, and Featuring Facts about Maintaining Spinal Health, Self-Care, Pain Management, Rehabilitative Care, Chiropractic Care, Spinal Surgeries, and Complementary Therapies

Along with Suggestions for Preventing Back and Neck Pain, a Glossary of Related Terms, and a Directory of Resources

Edited by Amy L. Sutton. 633 pages. 2004. 978-0-7808-0738-9.

"Recommended . . . an easy to use, comprehensive medical reference book." — E-Streams, Sep '05

"The strength of this work is its basic, easy-to-read format. Recommended." — Reference and User Services Quarterly, American Library Association, Winter '97

Blood & Circulatory Disorders Sourcebook, 2nd Edition

Basic Consumer Health Information about the Blood and Circulatory System and Related Disorders, Such as Anemia and Other Hemoglobin Diseases, Cancer of the Blood and Associated Bone Marrow Disorders, Clotting and Bleeding Problems, and Conditions That Affect the Veins, Blood Vessels, and Arteries, Including Facts about the Donation and Transplantation of Bone Marrow, Stem Cells, and Blood and Tips for Keeping the Blood and Circulatory System Healthy

Along with a Glossary of Related Terms and Resources for Additional Help and Information

Edited by Amy L. Sutton. 659 pages. 2005. 978-0-7808-0746-4.

"Highly recommended pick for basic consumer health reference holdings at all levels."
— The Bookwatch, Aug '05

"Recommended reference source."
— Booklist, American Library Association, Feb '99

"An important reference sourcebook written in simple language for everyday, non-technical users. "
— Reviewer's Bookwatch, Jan '99

Brain Disorders Sourcebook, 2nd Edition

Basic Consumer Health Information about Acquired and Traumatic Brain Injuries, Infections of the Brain, Epilepsy and Seizure Disorders, Cerebral Palsy, and Degenerative Neurological Disorders, Including Amyotrophic Lateral Sclerosis (ALS), Dementias, Multiple Sclerosis, and More

Along with Information on the Brain's Structure and Function, Treatment and Rehabilitation Options, Reports on Current Research Initiatives, a Glossary of Terms Related to Brain Disorders and Injuries, and a Directory of Sources for Further Help and Information

Edited by Sandra J. Judd. 625 pages. 2005. 978-0-7808-0744-0.

"Highly recommended pick for basic consumer health reference holdings at all levels."
— The Bookwatch, Aug '05

"Belongs on the shelves of any library with a consumer health collection." — E-Streams, Mar '00

"Recommended reference source."
— Booklist, American Library Association, Oct '99

SEE ALSO Alzheimer's Disease Sourcebook

Breast Cancer Sourcebook, 2nd Edition

Basic Consumer Health Information about Breast Cancer, Including Facts about Risk Factors, Prevention, Screening and Diagnostic Methods, Treatment Options, Complementary and Alternative Therapies, Post-Treatment Concerns, Clinical Trials, Special Risk Populations, and New Developments in Breast Cancer Research

Along with Breast Cancer Statistics, a Glossary of Related Terms, and a Directory of Resources for Additional Help and Information

Edited by Sandra J. Judd. 595 pages. 2004. 978-0-7808-0668-9.

"This book will be an excellent addition to public, community college, medical, and academic libraries."
— American Reference Books Annual, 2006

"It would be a useful reference book in a library or on loan to women in a support group."
— Cancer Forum, Mar '03

"Recommended reference source."
— Booklist, American Library Association, Jan '02

"This reference source is highly recommended. It is quite informative, comprehensive and detailed in nature, and yet it offers practical advice in easy-to-read language. It could be thought of as the 'bible' of breast cancer for the consumer." — *E-Streams, Jan '02*

"From the pros and cons of different screening methods and results to treatment options, *Breast Cancer Sourcebook* provides the latest information on the subject." — *Library Bookwatch, Dec '01*

"This thoroughgoing, very readable reference covers all aspects of breast health and cancer. . . . Readers will find much to consider here. Recommended for all public and patient health collections." — *Library Journal, Sep '01*

SEE ALSO *Cancer Sourcebook for Women, Women's Health Concerns Sourcebook*

Breastfeeding Sourcebook

Basic Consumer Health Information about the Benefits of Breastmilk, Preparing to Breastfeed, Breastfeeding as a Baby Grows, Nutrition, and More, Including Information on Special Situations and Concerns Such as Mastitis, Illness, Medications, Allergies, Multiple Births, Prematurity, Special Needs, and Adoption

Along with a Glossary and Resources for Additional Help and Information

Edited by Jenni Lynn Colson. 388 pages. 2002. 978-0-7808-0332-9.

"Particularly useful is the information about professional lactation services and chapters on breastfeeding when returning to work. . . . *Breastfeeding Sourcebook* will be useful for public libraries, consumer health libraries, and technical schools offering nurse assistant training, especially in areas where Internet access is problematic." — *American Reference Books Annual, 2003*

SEE ALSO *Pregnancy & Birth Sourcebook*

Burns Sourcebook

Basic Consumer Health Information about Various Types of Burns and Scalds, Including Flame, Heat, Cold, Electrical, Chemical, and Sun Burns

Along with Information on Short-Term and Long-Term Treatments, Tissue Reconstruction, Plastic Surgery, Prevention Suggestions, and First Aid

Edited by Allan R. Cook. 604 pages. 1999. 978-0-7808-0204-9.

"This is an exceptional addition to the series and is highly recommended for all consumer health collections, hospital libraries, and academic medical centers." — *E-Streams, Mar '00*

"This key reference guide is an invaluable addition to all health care and public libraries in confronting this ongoing health issue." — *American Reference Books Annual, 2000*

"Recommended reference source." — *Booklist, American Library Association, Dec '99*

SEE ALSO *Dermatological Disorders Sourcebook*

Cancer Sourcebook, 5th Edition

Basic Consumer Health Information about Major Forms and Stages of Cancer, Featuring Facts about Head and Neck Cancers, Lung Cancers, Gastrointestinal Cancers, Genitourinary Cancers, Lymphomas, Blood Cell Cancers, Endocrine Cancers, Skin Cancers, Bone Cancers, Metastatic Cancers, and More

Along with Facts about Cancer Treatments, Cancer Risks and Prevention, a Glossary of Related Terms, Statistical Data, and a Directory of Resources for Additional Information

Edited by Karen Bellenir. 1,133 pages. 2007. 978-0-7808-0947-5.

"With cancer being the second leading cause of death for Americans, a prodigious work such as this one, which locates centrally so much cancer-related information, is clearly an asset to this nation's citizens and others." — *Journal of the National Medical Association, 2004*

"This title is recommended for health sciences and public libraries with consumer health collections." — *E-Streams, Feb '01*

". . . can be effectively used by cancer patients and their families who are looking for answers in a language they can understand. Public and hospital libraries should have it on their shelves." — *American Reference Books Annual, 2001*

"Recommended reference source." — *Booklist, American Library Association, Dec '00*

SEE ALSO *Breast Cancer Sourcebook, Cancer Sourcebook for Women, Pediatric Cancer Sourcebook, Prostate Cancer Sourcebook*

Cancer Sourcebook for Women, 3rd Edition

Basic Consumer Health Information about Leading Causes of Cancer in Women, Featuring Facts about Gynecologic Cancers and Related Concerns, Such as Breast Cancer, Cervical Cancer, Endometrial Cancer, Uterine Sarcoma, Vaginal Cancer, Vulvar Cancer, and Common Non-Cancerous Gynecologic Conditions, in Addition to Facts about Lung Cancer, Colorectal Cancer, and Thyroid Cancer in Women

Along with Information about Cancer Risk Factors, Screening and Prevention, Treatment Options, and Tips on Coping with Life after Cancer Treatment, a Glossary of Cancer Terms, and a Directory of Resources for Additional Help and Information

Edited by Amy L. Sutton. 715 pages. 2006. 978-0-7808-0867-6.

"An excellent addition to collections in public, consumer health, and women's health libraries." — *American Reference Books Annual, 2003*

"Overall, the information is excellent, and complex topics are clearly explained. As a reference book for the consumer it is a valuable resource to assist them to make informed decisions about cancer and its treatments." — *Cancer Forum, Nov '02*

"Highly recommended for academic and medical reference collections." — *Library Bookwatch, Sep '02*

"This is a highly recommended book for any public or consumer library, being reader friendly and containing accurate and helpful information."
— *E-Streams, Aug '02*

"Recommended reference source."
—*Booklist, American Library Association, Jul '02*

SEE ALSO *Breast Cancer Sourcebook, Women's Health Concerns Sourcebook*

■

Cancer Survivorship Sourcebook

Basic Consumer Health Information about the Physical, Educational, Emotional, Social, and Financial Needs of Cancer Patients from Diagnosis, through Cancer Treatment, and Beyond, Including Facts about Researching Specific Types of Cancer and Learning about Clinical Trials and Treatment Options, and Featuring Tips for Coping with the Side Effects of Cancer Treatments and Adjusting to Life after Cancer Treatment Concludes

Along with Suggestions for Caregivers, Friends, and Family Members of Cancer Patients, a Glossary of Cancer Care Terms, and Directories of Related Resources

Edited by Karen Bellenir. 6561 pages. 2007. 978-0-7808-0985-7.

■

Cardiovascular Diseases & Disorders Sourcebook, 3rd Edition

Basic Consumer Health Information about Heart and Vascular Diseases and Disorders, Such as Angina, Heart Attacks, Arrhythmias, Cardiomyopathy, Valve Disease, Atherosclerosis, and Aneurysms, with Information about Managing Cardiovascular Risk Factors and Maintaining Heart Health, Medications and Procedures Used to Treat Cardiovascular Disorders, and Concerns of Special Significance to Women

Along with Reports on Current Research Initiatives, a Glossary of Related Medical Terms, and a Directory of Sources for Further Help and Information

Edited by Sandra J. Judd. 713 pages. 2005. 978-0-7808-0739-6.

"This updated sourcebook is still the best first stop for comprehensive introductory information on cardiovascular diseases."
— *American Reference Books Annual, 2006*

"Recommended for public libraries and libraries supporting health care professionals."
— *E-Streams, Sep '05*

"This should be a standard health library reference."
—*The Bookwatch, Jun '05*

"Recommended reference source."
—*Booklist, American Library Association, Dec '00*

". . . comprehensive format provides an extensive overview on this subject."
— *Choice, Association of College & Research Libraries*

■

Caregiving Sourcebook

Basic Consumer Health Information for Caregivers, Including a Profile of Caregivers, Caregiving Responsibilities and Concerns, Tips for Specific Conditions, Care Environments, and the Effects of Caregiving

Along with Facts about Legal Issues, Financial Information, and Future Planning, a Glossary, and a Listing of Additional Resources

Edited by Joyce Brennfleck Shannon. 600 pages. 2001. 978-0-7808-0331-2.

"Essential for most collections."
—*Library Journal, Apr 1, 2002*

"An ideal addition to the reference collection of any public library. Health sciences information professionals may also want to acquire the *Caregiving Sourcebook* for their hospital or academic library for use as a ready reference tool by health care workers interested in aging and caregiving." —*E-Streams, Jan '02*

"Recommended reference source."
—*Booklist, American Library Association, Oct '01*

■

Child Abuse Sourcebook

Basic Consumer Health Information about the Physical, Sexual, and Emotional Abuse of Children, with Additional Facts about Neglect, Munchausen Syndrome by Proxy (MSBP), Shaken Baby Syndrome, and Controversial Issues Related to Child Abuse, Such as Withholding Medical Care, Corporal Punishment, and Child Maltreatment in Youth Sports, and Featuring Facts about Child Protective Services, Foster Care, Adoption, Parenting Challenges, and Other Abuse Prevention Efforts

Along with a Glossary of Related Terms and Resources for Additional Help and Information

Edited by Dawn D. Matthews. 620 pages. 2004. 978-0-7808-0705-1.

"A valuable and highly recommended resource for school, academic and public libraries whether used on its own or as a starting point for more in-depth research." — *E-Streams, Apr '05*

"Every week the news brings cases of child abuse or neglect, so it is useful to have a source that supplies so much helpful information. . . . Recommended. Public and academic libraries, and child welfare offices."
— *Choice, Association of College & Research Libraries, Mar '05*

"Packed with insights on all kinds of issues, from foster care and adoption to parenting and abuse prevention."
—*The Bookwatch, Nov '04*

SEE ALSO: *Domestic Violence Sourcebook*

Childhood Diseases & Disorders Sourcebook

Basic Consumer Health Information about Medical Problems Often Encountered in Pre-Adolescent Children, Including Respiratory Tract Ailments, Ear Infections, Sore Throats, Disorders of the Skin and Scalp, Digestive and Genitourinary Diseases, Infectious Diseases, Inflammatory Disorders, Chronic Physical and Developmental Disorders, Allergies, and More

Along with Information about Diagnostic Tests, Common Childhood Surgeries, and Frequently Used Medications, with a Glossary of Important Terms and Resource Directory

Edited by Chad T. Kimball. 662 pages. 2003. 978-0-7808-0458-6.

"This is an excellent book for new parents and should be included in all health care and public libraries."
— *American Reference Books Annual, 2004*

SEE ALSO: *Healthy Children Sourcebook*

■

Colds, Flu & Other Common Ailments Sourcebook

Basic Consumer Health Information about Common Ailments and Injuries, Including Colds, Coughs, the Flu, Sinus Problems, Headaches, Fever, Nausea and Vomiting, Menstrual Cramps, Diarrhea, Constipation, Hemorrhoids, Back Pain, Dandruff, Dry and Itchy Skin, Cuts, Scrapes, Sprains, Bruises, and More

Along with Information about Prevention, Self-Care, Choosing a Doctor, Over-the-Counter Medications, Folk Remedies, and Alternative Therapies, and Including a Glossary of Important Terms and a Directory of Resources for Further Help and Information

Edited by Chad T. Kimball. 638 pages. 2001. 978-0-7808-0435-7.

"A good starting point for research on common illnesses. It will be a useful addition to public and consumer health library collections."
— *American Reference Books Annual, 2002*

"Will prove valuable to any library seeking to maintain a current, comprehensive reference collection of health resources. . . . Excellent reference."
— *The Bookwatch, Aug '01*

"Recommended reference source."
— *Booklist, American Library Association, Jul '01*

■

Communication Disorders Sourcebook

Basic Information about Deafness and Hearing Loss, Speech and Language Disorders, Voice Disorders, Balance and Vestibular Disorders, and Disorders of Smell, Taste, and Touch

Edited by Linda M. Ross. 533 pages. 1996. 978-0-7808-0077-9.

"This is skillfully edited and is a welcome resource for the layperson. It should be found in every public and medical library." — *Booklist Health Sciences Supplement, American Library Association, Oct '97*

■

Complementary & Alternative Medicine Sourcebook, 3rd Edition

Basic Consumer Health Information about Complementary and Alternative Medical Therapies, Including Acupuncture, Ayurveda, Traditional Chinese Medicine, Herbal Medicine, Homeopathy, Naturopathy, Biofeedback, Hypnotherapy, Yoga, Art Therapy, Aromatherapy, Clinical Nutrition, Vitamin and Mineral Supplements, Chiropractic, Massage, Reflexology, Crystal Therapy, Therapeutic Touch, and More

Along with Facts about Alternative and Complementary Treatments for Specific Conditions Such as Cancer, Diabetes, Osteoarthritis, Chronic Pain, Menopause, Gastrointestinal Disorders, Headaches, and Mental Illness, a Glossary, and a Resource List for Additional Help and Information

Edited by Sandra J. Judd. 657 pages. 2006. 978-0-7808-0864-5.

"Recommended for public, high school, and academic libraries that have consumer health collections. Hospital libraries that also serve the public will find this to be a useful resource." — *E-Streams, Feb '03*

"Recommended reference source."
— *Booklist, American Library Association, Jan '03*

"An important alternate health reference."
— *MBR Bookwatch, Oct '02*

"A great addition to the reference collection of every type of library." — *American Reference Books Annual, 2000*

■

Congenital Disorders Sourcebook, 2nd Edition

Basic Consumer Health Information about Nonhereditary Birth Defects and Disorders Related to Prematurity, Gestational Injuries, Congenital Infections, and Birth Complications, Including Heart Defects, Hydrocephalus, Spina Bifida, Cleft Lip and Palate, Cerebral Palsy, and More

Along with Facts about the Prevention of Birth Defects, Fetal Surgery and Other Treatment Options, Research Initiatives, a Glossary of Related Terms, and Resources for Additional Information and Support

Edited by Sandra J. Judd. 647 pages. 2006. 978-0-7808-0945-1.

"Recommended reference source."
— *Booklist, American Library Association, Oct '97*

SEE ALSO *Pregnancy & Birth Sourcebook*

■

Contagious Diseases Sourcebook

Basic Consumer Health Information about Infectious Diseases Spread by Person-to-Person Contact through

Direct Touch, Airborne Transmission, Sexual Contact, or Contact with Blood or Other Body Fluids, Including Hepatitis, Herpes, Influenza, Lice, Measles, Mumps, Pinworm, Ringworm, Severe Acute Respiratory Syndrome (SARS), Streptococcal Infections, Tuberculosis, and Others

Along with Facts about Disease Transmission, Antimicrobial Resistance, and Vaccines, with a Glossary and Directories of Resources for More Information

Edited by Karen Bellenir. 643 pages. 2004. 978-0-7808-0736-5.

"This easy-to-read volume is recommended for consumer health collections within public or academic libraries." — E-Streams, May '05

"This informative book is highly recommended for public libraries, consumer health collections, and secondary schools and undergraduate libraries." — American Reference Books Annual, 2005

"Excellent reference." — The Bookwatch, Jan '05

■

Death & Dying Sourcebook, 2nd Edition

Basic Consumer Health Information about End-of-Life Care and Related Perspectives and Ethical Issues, Including End-of-Life Symptoms and Treatments, Pain Management, Quality-of-Life Concerns, the Use of Life Support, Patients' Rights and Privacy Issues, Advance Directives, Physician-Assisted Suicide, Caregiving, Organ and Tissue Donation, Autopsies, Funeral Arrangements, and Grief

Along with Statistical Data, Information about the Leading Causes of Death, a Glossary, and Directories of Support Groups and Other Resources

Edited by Joyce Brennfleck Shannon. 653 pages. 2006. 978-0-7808-0871-3.

"Public libraries, medical libraries, and academic libraries will all find this sourcebook a useful addition to their collections." — American Reference Books Annual, 2001

"An extremely useful resource for those concerned with death and dying in the United States." — Respiratory Care, Nov '00

"Recommended reference source." — Booklist, American Library Association, Aug '00

"This book is a definite must for all those involved in end-of-life care." — Doody's Review Service, 2000

■

Dental Care & Oral Health Sourcebook, 2nd Edition

Basic Consumer Health Information about Dental Care, Including Oral Hygiene, Dental Visits, Pain Management, Cavities, Crowns, Bridges, Dental Implants, and Fillings, and Other Oral Health Concerns, Such as Gum Disease, Bad Breath, Dry Mouth, Genetic and Developmental Abnormalities, Oral Cancers, Orthodontics, and Temporomandibular Disorders

Along with Updates on Current Research in Oral Health, a Glossary, a Directory of Dental and Oral Health Organizations, and Resources for People with Dental and Oral Health Disorders

Edited by Amy L. Sutton. 609 pages. 2003. 978-0-7808-0634-4.

"This book could serve as a turning point in the battle to educate consumers in issues concerning oral health." — American Reference Books Annual, 2004

"Unique source which will fill a gap in dental sources for patients and the lay public. A valuable reference tool even in a library with thousands of books on dentistry. Comprehensive, clear, inexpensive, and easy to read and use. It fills an enormous gap in the health care literature." — Reference & User Services Quarterly, American Library Association, Summer '98

"Recommended reference source." — Booklist, American Library Association, Dec '97

■

Depression Sourcebook

Basic Consumer Health Information about Unipolar Depression, Bipolar Disorder, Postpartum Depression, Seasonal Affective Disorder, and Other Types of Depression in Children, Adolescents, Women, Men, the Elderly, and Other Selected Populations

Along with Facts about Causes, Risk Factors, Diagnostic Criteria, Treatment Options, Coping Strategies, Suicide Prevention, a Glossary, and a Directory of Sources for Additional Help and Information

Edited by Karen Bellenir. 602 pages. 2002. 978-0-7808-0611-5.

"Depression Sourcebook is of a very high standard. Its purpose, which is to serve as a reference source to the lay reader, is very well served." — Journal of the National Medical Association, 2004

"Invaluable reference for public and school library collections alike." — Library Bookwatch, Apr '03

"Recommended for purchase." — American Reference Books Annual, 2003

■

Dermatological Disorders Sourcebook, 2nd Edition

Basic Consumer Health Information about Conditions and Disorders Affecting the Skin, Hair, and Nails, Such as Acne, Rosacea, Rashes, Dermatitis, Pigmentation Disorders, Birthmarks, Skin Cancer, Skin Injuries, Psoriasis, Scleroderma, and Hair Loss, Including Facts about Medications and Treatments for Dermatological Disorders and Tips for Maintaining Healthy Skin, Hair, and Nails

Along with Information about How Aging Affects the Skin, a Glossary of Related Terms, and a Directory of Resources for Additional Help and Information

Edited by Amy L. Sutton. 645 pages. 2005. 978-0-7808-0795-2.

"... comprehensive, easily read reference book."
—*Doody's Health Sciences Book Reviews, Oct '97*

SEE ALSO *Burns Sourcebook*

▪

Diabetes Sourcebook, 3rd Edition

Basic Consumer Health Information about Type 1 Diabetes (Insulin-Dependent or Juvenile-Onset Diabetes), Type 2 Diabetes (Noninsulin-Dependent or Adult-Onset Diabetes), Gestational Diabetes, Impaired Glucose Tolerance (IGT), and Related Complications, Such as Amputation, Eye Disease, Gum Disease, Nerve Damage, and End-Stage Renal Disease, Including Facts about Insulin, Oral Diabetes Medications, Blood Sugar Testing, and the Role of Exercise and Nutrition in the Control of Diabetes

Along with a Glossary and Resources for Further Help and Information

Edited by Dawn D. Matthews. 622 pages. 2003. 978-0-7808-0629-0.

"This edition is even more helpful than earlier versions. . . . It is a truly valuable tool for anyone seeking readable and authoritative information on diabetes."
— *American Reference Books Annual, 2004*

"An invaluable reference." — *Library Journal, May '00*

Selected as one of the 250 "Best Health Sciences Books of 1999." — *Doody's Rating Service, Mar-Apr '00*

"Provides useful information for the general public."
— *Healthlines, University of Michigan Health Management Research Center, Sep/Oct '99*

". . . provides reliable mainstream medical information . . . belongs on the shelves of any library with a consumer health collection." — *E-Streams, Sep '99*

"Recommended reference source."
— *Booklist, American Library Association, Feb '99*

▪

Diet & Nutrition Sourcebook, 3rd Edition

Basic Consumer Health Information about Dietary Guidelines and the Food Guidance System, Recommended Daily Nutrient Intakes, Serving Proportions, Weight Control, Vitamins and Supplements, Nutrition Issues for Different Life Stages and Lifestyles, and the Needs of People with Specific Medical Concerns, Including Cancer, Celiac Disease, Diabetes, Eating Disorders, Food Allergies, and Cardiovascular Disease

Along with Facts about Federal Nutrition Support Programs, a Glossary of Nutrition and Dietary Terms, and Directories of Additional Resources for More Information about Nutrition

Edited by Joyce Brennfleck Shannon. 633 pages. 2006. 978-0-7808-0800-3.

"This book is an excellent source of basic diet and nutrition information." — *Booklist Health Sciences Supplement, American Library Association, Dec '00*

"This reference document should be in any public library, but it would be a very good guide for beginning students in the health sciences. If the other books in this publisher's series are as good as this, they should all be in the health sciences collections."
— *American Reference Books Annual, 2000*

"This book is an excellent general nutrition reference for consumers who desire to take an active role in their health care for prevention. Consumers of all ages who select this book can feel confident they are receiving current and accurate information." — *Journal of Nutrition for the Elderly, Vol. 19, No. 4, 2000*

SEE ALSO *Digestive Diseases & Disorders Sourcebook, Eating Disorders Sourcebook, Gastrointestinal Diseases & Disorders Sourcebook, Vegetarian Sourcebook*

▪

Digestive Diseases & Disorders Sourcebook

Basic Consumer Health Information about Diseases and Disorders that Impact the Upper and Lower Digestive System, Including Celiac Disease, Constipation, Crohn's Disease, Cyclic Vomiting Syndrome, Diarrhea, Diverticulosis and Diverticulitis, Gallstones, Heartburn, Hemorrhoids, Hernias, Indigestion (Dyspepsia), Irritable Bowel Syndrome, Lactose Intolerance, Ulcers, and More

Along with Information about Medications and Other Treatments, Tips for Maintaining a Healthy Digestive Tract, a Glossary, and Directory of Digestive Diseases Organizations

Edited by Karen Bellenir. 335 pages. 2000. 978-0-7808-0327-5.

"This title would be an excellent addition to all public or patient-research libraries."
— *American Reference Books Annual, 2001*

"This title is recommended for public, hospital, and health sciences libraries with consumer health collections." — *E-Streams, Jul-Aug '00*

"Recommended reference source."
— *Booklist, American Library Association, May '00*

SEE ALSO *Eating Disorders Sourcebook, Gastrointestinal Diseases & Disorders Sourcebook*

▪

Disabilities Sourcebook

Basic Consumer Health Information about Physical and Psychiatric Disabilities, Including Descriptions of Major Causes of Disability, Assistive and Adaptive Aids, Workplace Issues, and Accessibility Concerns

Along with Information about the Americans with Disabilities Act, a Glossary, and Resources for Additional Help and Information

Edited by Dawn D. Matthews. 616 pages. 2000. 978-0-7808-0389-3.

"It is a must for libraries with a consumer health section." — *American Reference Books Annual, 2002*

"A much needed addition to the Omnigraphics *Health Reference Series*. A current reference work to provide people with disabilities, their families, caregivers or those who work with them, a broad range of information in one volume, has not been available until now. . . . It is recommended for all public and academic library reference collections." —*E-Streams, May '01*

"An excellent source book in easy-to-read format covering many current topics; highly recommended for all libraries." —*Choice, Association of College & Research Libraries, Jan '01*

"Recommended reference source."
—*Booklist, American Library Association, Jul '00*

Domestic Violence Sourcebook, 2nd Edition

Basic Consumer Health Information about the Causes and Consequences of Abusive Relationships, Including Physical Violence, Sexual Assault, Battery, Stalking, and Emotional Abuse, and Facts about the Effects of Violence on Women, Men, Young Adults, and the Elderly, with Reports about Domestic Violence in Selected Populations, and Featuring Facts about Medical Care, Victim Assistance and Protection, Prevention Strategies, Mental Health Services, and Legal Issues

Along with a Glossary of Related Terms and Resources for Additional Help and Information

Edited by Dawn D. Matthews. 628 pages. 2004. 978-0-7808-0669-6.

"Educators, clergy, medical professionals, police, and victims and their families will benefit from this realistic and easy-to-understand resource."
—*American Reference Books Annual, 2005*

"Recommended for all collections supporting consumer health information. It should also be considered for any collection needing general, readable information on domestic violence." —*E-Streams, Jan '05*

"This sourcebook complements other books in its field, providing a one-stop resource . . . Recommended."
—*Choice, Association of College & Research Libraries, Jan '05*

"Interested lay persons should find the book extremely beneficial. . . . A copy of *Domestic Violence and Child Abuse Sourcebook* should be in every public library in the United States."
—*Social Science & Medicine, No. 56, 2003*

"This is important information. The Web has many resources but this sourcebook fills an important societal need. I am not aware of any other resources of this type." —*Doody's Review Service, Sep '01*

"Recommended reference source."
—*Booklist, American Library Association, Apr '01*

"Important pick for college-level health reference libraries." —*The Bookwatch, Mar '01*

"Because this problem is so widespread and because this book includes a lot of issues within one volume, this work is recommended for all public libraries."
—*American Reference Books Annual, 2001*

SEE ALSO *Child Abuse Sourcebook*

Drug Abuse Sourcebook, 2nd Edition

Basic Consumer Health Information about Illicit Substances of Abuse and the Misuse of Prescription and Over-the-Counter Medications, Including Depressants, Hallucinogens, Inhalants, Marijuana, Stimulants, and Anabolic Steroids

Along with Facts about Related Health Risks, Treatment Programs, Prevention Programs, a Glossary of Abuse and Addiction Terms, a Glossary of Drug-Related Street Terms, and a Directory of Resources for More Information

Edited by Catherine Ginther. 607 pages. 2004. 978-0-7808-0740-2.

"Commendable for organizing useful, normally scattered government and association-produced data into a logical sequence."
—*American Reference Books Annual, 2006*

"This easy-to-read volume is recommended for consumer health collections within public or academic libraries." —*E-Streams, Sep '05*

"An excellent library reference."
—*The Bookwatch, May '05*

"Containing a wealth of information, this book will be useful to the college student just beginning to explore the topic of substance abuse. This resource belongs in libraries that serve a lower-division undergraduate or community college clientele as well as the general public." —*Choice, Association of College & Research Libraries, Jun '01*

"Recommended reference source."
—*Booklist, American Library Association, Feb '01*

SEE ALSO *Alcoholism Sourcebook*

Ear, Nose & Throat Disorders Sourcebook, 2nd Edition

Basic Consumer Health Information about Disorders of the Ears, Hearing Loss, Vestibular Disorders, Nasal and Sinus Problems, Throat and Vocal Cord Disorders, and Otolaryngologic Cancers, Including Facts about Ear Infections and Injuries, Genetic and Congenital Deafness, Sensorineural Hearing Disorders, Tinnitus, Vertigo, Ménière Disease, Rhinitis, Sinusitis, Snoring, Sore Throats, Hoarseness, and More

Along with Reports on Current Research Initiatives, a Glossary of Related Medical Terms, and a Directory of Sources for Further Help and Information

Edited by Sandra J. Judd. 659 pages. 2006. 978-0-7808-0872-0.

"Overall, this sourcebook is helpful for the consumer seeking information on ENT issues. It is recommended for public libraries."
— *American Reference Books Annual, 1999*

"Recommended reference source."
— *Booklist, American Library Association, Dec '98*

Eating Disorders Sourcebook, 2nd Edition

Basic Consumer Health Information about Anorexia Nervosa, Bulimia Nervosa, Binge Eating, Compulsive Exercise, Female Athlete Triad, and Other Eating Disorders, Including Facts about Body Image and Other Cultural and Age-Related Risk Factors, Prevention Efforts, Adverse Health Effects, Treatment Options, and the Recovery Process

Along with Guidelines for Healthy Weight Control, a Glossary, and Directories of Additional Resources

Edited by Joyce Brennfleck Shannon. 585 pages. 2007. 978-0-7808-0948-2.

"Recommended for health science libraries that are open to the public, as well as hospital libraries. This book is a good resource for the consumer who is concerned about eating disorders." — *E-Streams, Mar '02*

"This volume is another convenient collection of excerpted articles. Recommended for school and public library patrons; lower-division undergraduates; and two-year technical program students."
— *Choice, Association of College & Research Libraries, Jan '02*

"Recommended reference source."
— *Booklist, American Library Association, Oct '01*

SEE ALSO *Diet & Nutrition Sourcebook, Digestive Diseases & Disorders Sourcebook, Gastrointestinal Diseases & Disorders Sourcebook*

Emergency Medical Services Sourcebook

Basic Consumer Health Information about Preventing, Preparing for, and Managing Emergency Situations, When and Who to Call for Help, What to Expect in the Emergency Room, the Emergency Medical Team, Patient Issues, and Current Topics in Emergency Medicine

Along with Statistical Data, a Glossary, and Sources of Additional Help and Information

Edited by Jenni Lynn Colson. 494 pages. 2002. 978-0-7808-0420-3.

"Handy and convenient for home, public, school, and college libraries. Recommended."
— *Choice, Association of College & Research Libraries, Apr '03*

"This reference can provide the consumer with answers to most questions about emergency care in the United States, or it will direct them to a resource where the answer can be found."
— *American Reference Books Annual, 2003*

"Recommended reference source."
— *Booklist, American Library Association, Feb '03*

Endocrine & Metabolic Disorders Sourcebook

Basic Information for the Layperson about Pancreatic and Insulin-Related Disorders Such as Pancreatitis, Diabetes, and Hypoglycemia; Adrenal Gland Disorders Such as Cushing's Syndrome, Addison's Disease, and Congenital Adrenal Hyperplasia; Pituitary Gland Disorders Such as Growth Hormone Deficiency, Acromegaly, and Pituitary Tumors; Thyroid Disorders Such as Hypothyroidism, Graves' Disease, Hashimoto's Disease, and Goiter; Hyperparathyroidism; and Other Diseases and Syndromes of Hormone Imbalance or Metabolic Dysfunction

Along with Reports on Current Research Initiatives

Edited by Linda M. Shin. 574 pages. 1998. 978-0-7808-0207-0.

"Omnigraphics has produced another needed resource for health information consumers."
— *American Reference Books Annual, 2000*

"Recommended reference source."
— *Booklist, American Library Association, Dec '98*

Environmental Health Sourcebook, 2nd Edition

Basic Consumer Health Information about the Environment and Its Effect on Human Health, Including the Effects of Air Pollution, Water Pollution, Hazardous Chemicals, Food Hazards, Radiation Hazards, Biological Agents, Household Hazards, Such as Radon, Asbestos, Carbon Monoxide, and Mold, and Information about Associated Diseases and Disorders, Including Cancer, Allergies, Respiratory Problems, and Skin Disorders

Along with Information about Environmental Concerns for Specific Populations, a Glossary of Related Terms, and Resources for Further Help and Information

Edited by Dawn D. Matthews. 673 pages. 2003. 978-0-7808-0632-0.

"This recently updated edition continues the level of quality and the reputation of the numerous other volumes in Omnigraphics' *Health Reference Series*."
— *American Reference Books Annual, 2004*

"An excellent updated edition."
— *The Bookwatch, Oct '03*

"Recommended reference source."
— *Booklist, American Library Association, Sep '98*

"This book will be a useful addition to anyone's library." — *Choice Health Sciences Supplement, Association of College & Research Libraries, May '98*

". . . a good survey of numerous environmentally induced physical disorders . . . a useful addition to anyone's library."
— *Doody's Health Sciences Book Reviews, Jan '98*

Ethnic Diseases Sourcebook

Basic Consumer Health Information for Ethnic and Racial Minority Groups in the United States, Including General Health Indicators and Behaviors, Ethnic Diseases, Genetic Testing, the Impact of Chronic Diseases, Women's Health, Mental Health Issues, and Preventive Health Care Services

Along with a Glossary and a Listing of Additional Resources

Edited by Joyce Brennfleck Shannon. 664 pages. 2001. 978-0-7808-0336-7.

"Recommended for health sciences libraries where public health programs are a priority."
— E-Streams, Jan '02

"Not many books have been written on this topic to date, and the *Ethnic Diseases Sourcebook* is a strong addition to the list. It will be an important introductory resource for health consumers, students, health care personnel, and social scientists. It is recommended for public, academic, and large hospital libraries."
— American Reference Books Annual, 2002

"Recommended reference source."
— Booklist, American Library Association, Oct '01

"Will prove valuable to any library seeking to maintain a current, comprehensive reference collection of health resources. . . . An excellent source of health information about genetic disorders which affect particular ethnic and racial minorities in the U.S."
— The Bookwatch, Aug '01

Eye Care Sourcebook, 2nd Edition

Basic Consumer Health Information about Eye Care and Eye Disorders, Including Facts about the Diagnosis, Prevention, and Treatment of Common Refractive Problems Such as Myopia, Hyperopia, Astigmatism, and Presbyopia, and Eye Diseases, Including Glaucoma, Cataract, Age-Related Macular Degeneration, and Diabetic Retinopathy

Along with a Section on Vision Correction and Refractive Surgeries, Including LASIK and LASEK, a Glossary, and Directories of Resources for Additional Help and Information

Edited by Amy L. Sutton. 543 pages. 2003. 978-0-7808-0635-1.

". . . a solid reference tool for eye care and a valuable addition to a collection."
— American Reference Books Annual, 2004

Family Planning Sourcebook

Basic Consumer Health Information about Planning for Pregnancy and Contraception, Including Traditional Methods, Barrier Methods, Hormonal Methods, Permanent Methods, Future Methods, Emergency Contraception, and Birth Control Choices for Women at Each Stage of Life

Along with Statistics, a Glossary, and Sources of Additional Information

Edited by Amy Marcaccio Keyzer. 520 pages. 2001. 978-0-7808-0379-4.

"Recommended for public, health, and undergraduate libraries as part of the circulating collection."
— E-Streams, Mar '02

"Information is presented in an unbiased, readable manner, and the sourcebook will certainly be a necessary addition to those public and high school libraries where Internet access is restricted or otherwise problematic." *— American Reference Books Annual, 2002*

"Recommended reference source."
— Booklist, American Library Association, Oct '01

"Will prove valuable to any library seeking to maintain a current, comprehensive reference collection of health resources. . . . Excellent reference."
— The Bookwatch, Aug '01

SEE ALSO Pregnancy & Birth Sourcebook

Fitness & Exercise Sourcebook, 3rd Edition

Basic Consumer Health Information about the Physical and Mental Benefits of Fitness, Including Cardiorespiratory Endurance, Muscular Strength, Muscular Endurance, and Flexibility, with Facts about Sports Nutrition and Exercise-Related Injuries and Tips about Physical Activity and Exercises for People of All Ages and for People with Health Concerns

Along with Advice on Selecting and Using Exercise Equipment, Maintaining Exercise Motivation, a Glossary of Related Terms, and a Directory of Resources for More Help and Information

Edited by Amy L. Sutton. 663 pages. 2007. 978-0-7808-0946-8.

"This work is recommended for all general reference collections."
— American Reference Books Annual, 2002

"Highly recommended for public, consumer, and school grades fourth through college." *— E-Streams, Nov '01*

"Recommended reference source."
— Booklist, American Library Association, Oct '01

"The information appears quite comprehensive and is considered reliable. . . . This second edition is a welcomed addition to the series."
— Doody's Review Service, Sep '01

Food Safety Sourcebook

Basic Consumer Health Information about the Safe Handling of Meat, Poultry, Seafood, Eggs, Fruit Juices, and Other Food Items, and Facts about Pesticides, Drinking Water, Food Safety Overseas, and the Onset, Duration, and Symptoms of Foodborne Illnesses, Including Types of Pathogenic Bacteria, Parasitic Protozoa, Worms, Viruses, and Natural Toxins

Along with the Role of the Consumer, the Food Handler, and the Government in Food Safety; a Glossary, and Resources for Additional Help and Information

Edited by Dawn D. Matthews. 339 pages. 1999. 978-0-7808-0326-8.

"This book is recommended for public libraries and universities with home economic and food science programs."
— E-Streams, Nov '00

"Recommended reference source."
— Booklist, American Library Association, May '00

"This book takes the complex issues of food safety and foodborne pathogens and presents them in an easily understood manner. [It does] an excellent job of covering a large and often confusing topic."
— American Reference Books Annual, 2000

Forensic Medicine Sourcebook

Basic Consumer Information for the Layperson about Forensic Medicine, Including Crime Scene Investigation, Evidence Collection and Analysis, Expert Testimony, Computer-Aided Criminal Identification, Digital Imaging in the Courtroom, DNA Profiling, Accident Reconstruction, Autopsies, Ballistics, Drugs and Explosives Detection, Latent Fingerprints, Product Tampering, and Questioned Document Examination

Along with Statistical Data, a Glossary of Forensics Terminology, and Listings of Sources for Further Help and Information

Edited by Annemarie S. Muth. 574 pages. 1999. 978-0-7808-0232-2.

"Given the expected widespread interest in its content and its easy to read style, this book is recommended for most public and all college and university libraries."
— E-Streams, Feb '01

"Recommended for public libraries."
— Reference & User Services Quarterly, American Library Association, Spring 2000

"Recommended reference source."
— Booklist, American Library Association, Feb '00

"A wealth of information, useful statistics, references are up-to-date and extremely complete. This wonderful collection of data will help students who are interested in a career in any type of forensic field. It is a great resource for attorneys who need information about types of expert witnesses needed in a particular case. It also offers useful information for fiction and nonfiction writers whose work involves a crime. A fascinating compilation. All levels."
— Choice, Association of College & Research Libraries, Jan '00

"There are several items that make this book attractive to consumers who are seeking certain forensic data. . . . This is a useful current source for those seeking general forensic medical answers."
— American Reference Books Annual, 2000

Gastrointestinal Diseases & Disorders Sourcebook, 2nd Edition

Basic Consumer Health Information about the Upper and Lower Gastrointestinal (GI) Tract, Including the Esophagus, Stomach, Intestines, Rectum, Liver, and Pancreas, with Facts about Gastroesophageal Reflux Disease, Gastritis, Hernias, Ulcers, Celiac Disease, Diverticulitis, Irritable Bowel Syndrome, Hemorrhoids, Gastrointestinal Cancers, and Other Diseases and Disorders Related to the Digestive Process

Along with Information about Commonly Used Diagnostic and Surgical Procedures, Statistics, Reports on Current Research Initiatives and Clinical Trials, a Glossary, and Resources for Additional Help and Information

Edited by Sandra J. Judd. 681 pages. 2006. 978-0-7808-0798-3.

". . . very readable form. The successful editorial work that brought this material together into a useful and understandable reference makes accessible to all readers information that can help them more effectively understand and obtain help for digestive tract problems."
— Choice, Association of College & Research Libraries, Feb '97

SEE ALSO Diet & Nutrition Sourcebook, Digestive Diseases & Disorders Sourcebook, Eating Disorders Sourcebook

Genetic Disorders Sourcebook, 3rd Edition

Basic Consumer Health Information about Hereditary Diseases and Disorders, Including Facts about the Human Genome, Genetic Inheritance Patterns, Disorders Associated with Specific Genes, Such as Sickle Cell Disease, Hemophilia, and Cystic Fibrosis, Chromosome Disorders, Such as Down Syndrome, Fragile X Syndrome, and Turner Syndrome, and Complex Diseases and Disorders Resulting from the Interaction of Environmental and Genetic Factors, Such as Allergies, Cancer, and Obesity

Along with Facts about Genetic Testing, Suggestions for Parents of Children with Special Needs, Reports on Current Research Initiatives, a Glossary of Genetic Terminology, and Resources for Additional Help and Information

Edited by Karen Bellenir. 777 pages. 2004. 978-0-7808-0742-6.

"This text is recommended for any library with an interest in providing consumer health resources."
— E-Streams, Aug '05

"This is a valuable resource for anyone wishing to have an understandable description of any of the topics or disorders included. The editor succeeds in making complex genetic issues understandable."
— Doody's Book Review Service, May '05

"A good acquisition for public libraries."
— American Reference Books Annual, 2005

620

"Excellent reference." — *The Bookwatch, Jan '05*

"Recommended reference source."
— *Booklist, American Library Association, Apr '01*

"Important pick for college-level health reference libraries." — *The Bookwatch, Mar '01*

Head Trauma Sourcebook

Basic Information for the Layperson about Open-Head and Closed-Head Injuries, Treatment Advances, Recovery, and Rehabilitation

Along with Reports on Current Research Initiatives

Edited by Karen Bellenir. 414 pages. 1997. 978-0-7808-0208-7.

Headache Sourcebook

Basic Consumer Health Information about Migraine, Tension, Cluster, Rebound and Other Types of Headaches, with Facts about the Cause and Prevention of Headaches, the Effects of Stress and the Environment, Headaches during Pregnancy and Menopause, and Childhood Headaches

Along with a Glossary and Other Resources for Additional Help and Information

Edited by Dawn D. Matthews. 362 pages. 2002. 978-0-7808-0337-4.

"Highly recommended for academic and medical reference collections." — *Library Bookwatch, Sep '02*

Healthy Aging Sourcebook

Basic Consumer Health Information about Maintaining Health through the Aging Process, Including Advice on Nutrition, Exercise, and Sleep, Help in Making Decisions about Midlife Issues and Retirement, and Guidance Concerning Practical and Informed Choices in Health Consumerism

Along with Data Concerning the Theories of Aging, Different Experiences in Aging by Minority Groups, and Facts about Aging Now and Aging in the Future; and Featuring a Glossary, a Guide to Consumer Help, Additional Suggested Reading, and Practical Resource Directory

Edited by Jenifer Swanson. 536 pages. 1999. 978-0-7808-0390-9.

"Recommended reference source."
— *Booklist, American Library Association, Feb '00*

SEE ALSO *Physical & Mental Issues in Aging Sourcebook*

Healthy Children Sourcebook

Basic Consumer Health Information about the Physical and Mental Development of Children between the Ages of 3 and 12, Including Routine Health Care, Preventative Health Services, Safety and First Aid,

Healthy Sleep, Dental Care, Nutrition, and Fitness, and Featuring Parenting Tips on Such Topics as Bedwetting, Choosing Day Care, Monitoring TV and Other Media, and Establishing a Foundation for Substance Abuse Prevention

Along with a Glossary of Commonly Used Pediatric Terms and Resources for Additional Help and Information.

Edited by Chad T. Kimball. 647 pages. 2003. 978-0-7808-0247-6.

"It is hard to imagine that any other single resource exists that would provide such a comprehensive guide of timely information on health promotion and disease prevention for children aged 3 to 12."
— *American Reference Books Annual, 2004*

"The strengths of this book are many. It is clearly written, presented and structured."
— *Journal of the National Medical Association, 2004*

SEE ALSO *Childhood Diseases & Disorders Sourcebook*

Healthy Heart Sourcebook for Women

Basic Consumer Health Information about Cardiac Issues Specific to Women, Including Facts about Major Risk Factors and Prevention, Treatment and Control Strategies, and Important Dietary Issues

Along with a Special Section Regarding the Pros and Cons of Hormone Replacement Therapy and Its Impact on Heart Health, and Additional Help, Including Recipes, a Glossary, and a Directory of Resources

Edited by Dawn D. Matthews. 336 pages. 2000. 978-0-7808-0329-9.

"A good reference source and recommended for all public, academic, medical, and hospital libraries."
— *Medical Reference Services Quarterly, Summer '01*

"Because of the lack of information specific to women on this topic, this book is recommended for public libraries and consumer libraries."
— *American Reference Books Annual, 2001*

"Contains very important information about coronary artery disease that all women should know. The information is current and presented in an easy-to-read format. The book will make a good addition to any library." — *American Medical Writers Association Journal, Summer '00*

"Important, basic reference."
— *Reviewer's Bookwatch, Jul '00*

SEE ALSO *Cardiovascular Diseases & Disorders Sourcebook, Women's Health Concerns Sourcebook*

Hepatitis Sourcebook

Basic Consumer Health Information about Hepatitis A, Hepatitis B, Hepatitis C, and Other Forms of Hepatitis, Including Autoimmune Hepatitis, Alcoholic Hepatitis, Nonalcoholic Steatohepatitis, and Toxic Hepatitis, with

Facts about Risk Factors, Screening Methods, Diagnostic Tests, and Treatment Options

Along with Information on Liver Health, Tips for People Living with Chronic Hepatitis, Reports on Current Research Initiatives, a Glossary of Terms Related to Hepatitis, and a Directory of Sources for Further Help and Information

Edited by Sandra J. Judd. 597 pages. 2005. 978-0-7808-0749-5.

"Highly recommended."
— *American Reference Books Annual, 2006*

∎

Household Safety Sourcebook

Basic Consumer Health Information about Household Safety, Including Information about Poisons, Chemicals, Fire, and Water Hazards in the Home

Along with Advice about the Safe Use of Home Maintenance Equipment, Choosing Toys and Nursery Furniture, Holiday and Recreation Safety, a Glossary, and Resources for Further Help and Information

Edited by Dawn D. Matthews. 606 pages. 2002. 978-0-7808-0338-1.

"This work will be useful in public libraries with large consumer health and wellness departments."
— *American Reference Books Annual, 2003*

"As a sourcebook on household safety this book meets its mark. It is encyclopedic in scope and covers a wide range of safety issues that are commonly seen in the home." — *E-Streams, Jul '02*

∎

Hypertension Sourcebook

Basic Consumer Health Information about the Causes, Diagnosis, and Treatment of High Blood Pressure, with Facts about Consequences, Complications, and Co-Occurring Disorders, Such as Coronary Heart Disease, Diabetes, Stroke, Kidney Disease, and Hypertensive Retinopathy, and Issues in Blood Pressure Control, Including Dietary Choices, Stress Management, and Medications

Along with Reports on Current Research Initiatives and Clinical Trials, a Glossary, and Resources for Additional Help and Information

Edited by Dawn D. Matthews and Karen Bellenir. 613 pages. 2004. 978-0-7808-0674-0.

"Academic, public, and medical libraries will want to add the *Hypertension Sourcebook* to their collections."
— *E-Streams, Aug '05*

"The strength of this source is the wide range of information given about hypertension."
— *American Reference Books Annual, 2005*

∎

Immune System Disorders Sourcebook, 2nd Edition

Basic Consumer Health Information about Disorders of the Immune System, Including Immune System Function and Response, Diagnosis of Immune Disorders, Information about Inherited Immune Disease, Acquired Immune Disease, and Autoimmune Diseases, Including Primary Immune Deficiency, Acquired Immunodeficiency Syndrome (AIDS), Lupus, Multiple Sclerosis, Type 1 Diabetes, Rheumatoid Arthritis, and Graves' Disease

Along with Treatments, Tips for Coping with Immune Disorders, a Glossary, and a Directory of Additional Resources.

Edited by Joyce Brennfleck Shannon. 671 pages. 2005. 978-0-7808-0748-8.

"Highly recommended for academic and public libraries." — *American Reference Books Annual, 2006*

"The updated second edition is a 'must' for any consumer health library seeking a solid resource covering the treatments, symptoms, and options for immune disorder sufferers. . . . An excellent guide."
— *MBR Bookwatch, Jan '06*

∎

Infant & Toddler Health Sourcebook

Basic Consumer Health Information about the Physical and Mental Development of Newborns, Infants, and Toddlers, Including Neonatal Concerns, Nutrition Recommendations, Immunization Schedules, Common Pediatric Disorders, Assessments and Milestones, Safety Tips, and Advice for Parents and Other Caregivers

Along with a Glossary of Terms and Resource Listings for Additional Help

Edited by Jenifer Swanson. 585 pages. 2000. 978-0-7808-0246-9.

"As a reference for the general public, this would be useful in any library." — *E-Streams, May '01*

"Recommended reference source."
— *Booklist, American Library Association, Feb '01*

"This is a good source for general use."
— *American Reference Books Annual, 2001*

∎

Infectious Diseases Sourcebook

Basic Consumer Health Information about Non-Contagious Bacterial, Viral, Prion, Fungal, and Parasitic Diseases Spread by Food and Water, Insects and Animals, or Environmental Contact, Including Botulism, E. Coli, Encephalitis, Legionnaires' Disease, Lyme Disease, Malaria, Plague, Rabies, Salmonella, Tetanus, and Others, and Facts about Newly Emerging Diseases, Such as Hantavirus, Mad Cow Disease, Monkeypox, and West Nile Virus

Along with Information about Preventing Disease Transmission, the Threat of Bioterrorism, and Current Research Initiatives, with a Glossary and Directory of Resources for More Information

Edited by Karen Bellenir. 634 pages. 2004. 978-0-7808-0675-7.

"This reference continues the excellent tradition of the *Health Reference Series* in consolidating a wealth of information on a selected topic into a format that is easy to use and accessible to the general public."
— *American Reference Books Annual, 2005*

"Recommended for public and academic libraries."
— *E-Streams, Jan '05*

███

Injury & Trauma Sourcebook

Basic Consumer Health Information about the Impact of Injury, the Diagnosis and Treatment of Common and Traumatic Injuries, Emergency Care, and Specific Injuries Related to Home, Community, Workplace, Transportation, and Recreation

Along with Guidelines for Injury Prevention, a Glossary, and a Directory of Additional Resources

Edited by Joyce Brennfleck Shannon. 696 pages. 2002. 978-0-7808-0421-0.

"This publication is the most comprehensive work of its kind about injury and trauma."
— *American Reference Books Annual, 2003*

"This sourcebook provides concise, easily readable, basic health information about injuries. . . . This book is well organized and an easy to use reference resource suitable for hospital, health sciences and public libraries with consumer health collections."
— *E-Streams, Nov '02*

"Practitioners should be aware of guides such as this in order to facilitate their use by patients and their families."
— *Doody's Health Sciences Book Review Journal, Sep-Oct '02*

"Recommended reference source."
— *Booklist, American Library Association, Sep '02*

"Highly recommended for academic and medical reference collections."
— *Library Bookwatch, Sep '02*

███

Kidney & Urinary Tract Diseases & Disorders Sourcebook

SEE Urinary Tract & Kidney Diseases & Disorders Sourcebook

███

Learning Disabilities Sourcebook, 2nd Edition

Basic Consumer Health Information about Learning Disabilities, Including Dyslexia, Developmental Speech and Language Disabilities, Non-Verbal Learning Disorders, Developmental Arithmetic Disorder, Developmental Writing Disorder, and Other Conditions That Impede Learning Such as Attention Deficit/Hyperactivity Disorder, Brain Injury, Hearing Impairment, Klinefelter Syndrome, Dyspraxia, and Tourette's Syndrome

Along with Facts about Educational Issues and Assistive Technology, Coping Strategies, a Glossary of Related Terms, and Resources for Further Help and Information

Edited by Dawn D. Matthews. 621 pages. 2003. 978-0-7808-0626-9.

"The second edition of Learning Disabilities Sourcebook far surpasses the earlier edition in that it is more focused on information that will be useful as a consumer health resource."
— *American Reference Books Annual, 2004*

"Teachers as well as consumers will find this an essential guide to understanding various syndromes and their latest treatments. [An] invaluable reference for public and school library collections alike."
— *Library Bookwatch, Apr '03*

Named "Outstanding Reference Book of 1999."
— *New York Public Library, Feb '00*

"An excellent candidate for inclusion in a public library reference section. It's a great source of information. Teachers will also find the book useful. Definitely worth reading."
— *Journal of Adolescent & Adult Literacy, Feb 2000*

"Readable . . . provides a solid base of information regarding successful techniques used with individuals who have learning disabilities, as well as practical suggestions for educators and family members. Clear language, concise descriptions, and pertinent information for contacting multiple resources add to the strength of this book as a useful tool."
— *Choice, Association of College & Research Libraries, Feb '99*

"Recommended reference source."
— *Booklist, American Library Association, Sep '98*

"A useful resource for libraries and for those who don't have the time to identify and locate the individual publications."
— *Disability Resources Monthly, Sep '98*

███

Leukemia Sourcebook

Basic Consumer Health Information about Adult and Childhood Leukemias, Including Acute Lymphocytic Leukemia (ALL), Chronic Lymphocytic Leukemia (CLL), Acute Myelogenous Leukemia (AML), Chronic Myelogenous Leukemia (CML), and Hairy Cell Leukemia, and Treatments Such as Chemotherapy, Radiation Therapy, Peripheral Blood Stem Cell and Marrow Transplantation, and Immunotherapy

Along with Tips for Life During and After Treatment, a Glossary, and Directories of Additional Resources

Edited by Joyce Brennfleck Shannon. 587 pages. 2003. 978-0-7808-0627-6.

"Unlike other medical books for the layperson, . . . the language does not talk down to the reader. . . . This volume is highly recommended for all libraries."
— *American Reference Books Annual, 2004*

". . . a fine title which ranges from diagnosis to alternative treatments, staging, and tips for life during and after diagnosis."
— *The Bookwatch, Dec '03*

Liver Disorders Sourcebook

Basic Consumer Health Information about the Liver and How It Works; Liver Diseases, Including Cancer, Cirrhosis, Hepatitis, and Toxic and Drug Related Diseases; Tips for Maintaining a Healthy Liver; Laboratory Tests, Radiology Tests, and Facts about Liver Transplantation

Along with a Section on Support Groups, a Glossary, and Resource Listings

Edited by Joyce Brennfleck Shannon. 591 pages. 2000. 978-0-7808-0383-1.

"A valuable resource."
—*American Reference Books Annual, 2001*

"This title is recommended for health sciences and public libraries with consumer health collections."
—*E-Streams, Oct '00*

"Recommended reference source."
—*Booklist, American Library Association, Jun '00*

Lung Disorders Sourcebook

Basic Consumer Health Information about Emphysema, Pneumonia, Tuberculosis, Asthma, Cystic Fibrosis, and Other Lung Disorders, Including Facts about Diagnostic Procedures, Treatment Strategies, Disease Prevention Efforts, and Such Risk Factors as Smoking, Air Pollution, and Exposure to Asbestos, Radon, and Other Agents

Along with a Glossary and Resources for Additional Help and Information

Edited by Dawn D. Matthews. 678 pages. 2002. 978-0-7808-0339-8.

"This title is a great addition for public and school libraries because it provides concise health information on the lungs."
—*American Reference Books Annual, 2003*

"Highly recommended for academic and medical reference collections."
—*Library Bookwatch, Sep '02*

SEE ALSO *Respiratory Diseases & Disorders Sourcebook*

Medical Tests Sourcebook, 2nd Edition

Basic Consumer Health Information about Medical Tests, Including Age-Specific Health Tests, Important Health Screenings and Exams, Home-Use Tests, Blood and Specimen Tests, Electrical Tests, Scope Tests, Genetic Testing, and Imaging Tests, Such as X-Rays, Ultrasound, Computed Tomography, Magnetic Resonance Imaging, Angiography, and Nuclear Medicine

Along with a Glossary and Directory of Additional Resources

Edited by Joyce Brennfleck Shannon. 654 pages. 2004. 978-0-7808-0670-2.

"Recommended for hospital and health sciences libraries with consumer health collections."
—*E-Streams, Mar '00*

"This is an overall excellent reference with a wealth of general knowledge that may aid those who are reluctant to get vital tests performed."
—*Today's Librarian, Jan '00*

"A valuable reference guide."
—*American Reference Books Annual, 2000*

Men's Health Concerns Sourcebook, 2nd Edition

Basic Consumer Health Information about the Medical and Mental Concerns of Men, Including Theories about the Shorter Male Lifespan, the Leading Causes of Death and Disability, Physical Concerns of Special Significance to Men, Reproductive and Sexual Concerns, Sexually Transmitted Diseases, Men's Mental and Emotional Health, and Lifestyle Choices That Affect Wellness, Such as Nutrition, Fitness, and Substance Use

Along with a Glossary of Related Terms and a Directory of Organizational Resources in Men's Health

Edited by Robert Aquinas McNally. 644 pages. 2004. 978-0-7808-0671-9.

"A very accessible reference for non-specialist general readers and consumers." —*The Bookwatch, Jun '04*

"This comprehensive resource and the series are highly recommended."
—*American Reference Books Annual, 2000*

"Recommended reference source."
—*Booklist, American Library Association, Dec '98*

Mental Health Disorders Sourcebook, 3rd Edition

Basic Consumer Health Information about Mental and Emotional Health and Mental Illness, Including Facts about Depression, Bipolar Disorder, and Other Mood Disorders, Phobias, Post-Traumatic Stress Disorder (PTSD), Obsessive-Compulsive Disorder, and Other Anxiety Disorders, Impulse Control Disorders, Eating Disorders, Personality Disorders, and Psychotic Disorders, Including Schizophrenia and Dissociative Disorders

Along with Statistical Information, a Special Section Concerning Mental Health Issues in Children and Adolescents, a Glossary, and Directories of Resources for Additional Help and Information

Edited by Karen Bellenir. 661 pages. 2005. 978-0-7808-0747-1.

"Recommended for public libraries and academic libraries with an undergraduate program in psychology."
—*American Reference Books Annual, 2006*

"Recommended reference source."
—*Booklist, American Library Association, Jun '00*

Mental Retardation Sourcebook

Basic Consumer Health Information about Mental Retardation and Its Causes, Including Down Syndrome, Fetal Alcohol Syndrome, Fragile X Syndrome, Genetic Conditions, Injury, and Environmental Sources

Along with Preventive Strategies, Parenting Issues, Educational Implications, Health Care Needs, Employment and Economic Matters, Legal Issues, a Glossary, and a Resource Listing for Additional Help and Information

Edited by Joyce Brennfleck Shannon. 642 pages. 2000. 978-0-7808-0377-0.

"Public libraries will find the book useful for reference and as a beginning research point for students, parents, and caregivers."
— *American Reference Books Annual, 2001*

"The strength of this work is that it compiles many basic fact sheets and addresses for further information in one volume. It is intended and suitable for the general public. This sourcebook is relevant to any collection providing health information to the general public."
— *E-Streams, Nov '00*

"From preventing retardation to parenting and family challenges, this covers health, social and legal issues and will prove an invaluable overview."
— *Reviewer's Bookwatch, Jul '00*

Movement Disorders Sourcebook

Basic Consumer Health Information about Neurological Movement Disorders, Including Essential Tremor, Parkinson's Disease, Dystonia, Cerebral Palsy, Huntington's Disease, Myasthenia Gravis, Multiple Sclerosis, and Other Early-Onset and Adult-Onset Movement Disorders, Their Symptoms and Causes, Diagnostic Tests, and Treatments

Along with Mobility and Assistive Technology Information, a Glossary, and a Directory of Additional Resources

Edited by Joyce Brennfleck Shannon. 655 pages. 2003. 978-0-7808-0628-3.

". . . a good resource for consumers and recommended for public, community college and undergraduate libraries." — *American Reference Books Annual, 2004*

Muscular Dystrophy Sourcebook

Basic Consumer Health Information about Congenital, Childhood-Onset, and Adult-Onset Forms of Muscular Dystrophy, Such as Duchenne, Becker, Emery-Dreifuss, Distal, Limb-Girdle, Facioscapulohumeral (FSHD), Myotonic, and Ophthalmoplegic Muscular Dystrophies, Including Facts about Diagnostic Tests, Medical and Physical Therapies, Management of Co-Occurring Conditions, and Parenting Guidelines

Along with Practical Tips for Home Care, a Glossary, and Directories of Additional Resources

Edited by Joyce Brennfleck Shannon. 577 pages. 2004. 978-0-7808-0676-4.

"This book is highly recommended for public and academic libraries as well as health care offices that support the information needs of patients and their families."
— *E-Streams, Apr '05*

"Excellent reference." — *The Bookwatch, Jan '05*

Obesity Sourcebook

Basic Consumer Health Information about Diseases and Other Problems Associated with Obesity, and Including Facts about Risk Factors, Prevention Issues, and Management Approaches

Along with Statistical and Demographic Data, Information about Special Populations, Research Updates, a Glossary, and Source Listings for Further Help and Information

Edited by Wilma Caldwell and Chad T. Kimball. 376 pages. 2001. 978-0-7808-0333-6.

"The book synthesizes the reliable medical literature on obesity into one easy-to-read and useful resource for the general public."
— *American Reference Books Annual, 2002*

"This is a very useful resource book for the lay public."
— *Doody's Review Service, Nov '01*

"Well suited for the health reference collection of a public library or an academic health science library that serves the general population." — *E-Streams, Sep '01*

"Recommended reference source."
— *Booklist, American Library Association, Apr '01*

"Recommended pick both for specialty health library collections and any general consumer health reference collection." — *The Bookwatch, Apr '01*

Oral Health Sourcebook

SEE Dental Care & Oral Health Sourcebook

Osteoporosis Sourcebook

Basic Consumer Health Information about Primary and Secondary Osteoporosis and Juvenile Osteoporosis and Related Conditions, Including Fibrous Dysplasia, Gaucher Disease, Hyperthyroidism, Hypophosphatasia, Myeloma, Osteopetrosis, Osteogenesis Imperfecta, and Paget's Disease

Along with Information about Risk Factors, Treatments, Traditional and Non-Traditional Pain Management, a Glossary of Related Terms, and a Directory of Resources

Edited by Allan R. Cook. 584 pages. 2001. 978-0-7808-0239-1.

"This would be a book to be kept in a staff or patient library. The targeted audience is the layperson, but the therapist who needs a quick bit of information on a particular topic will also find the book useful."
— *Physical Therapy, Jan '02*

"This resource is recommended as a great reference source for public, health, and academic libraries, and is another triumph for the editors of Omnigraphics."
— *American Reference Books Annual, 2002*

"Recommended for all public libraries and general health collections, especially those supporting patient education or consumer health programs."
— *E-Streams, Nov '01*

"Will prove valuable to any library seeking to maintain a current, comprehensive reference collection of health resources. . . . From prevention to treatment and associated conditions, this provides an excellent survey."
— *The Bookwatch, Aug '01*

"Recommended reference source."
— *Booklist, American Library Association, Jul '01*

SEE ALSO *Healthy Aging Sourcebook, Physical & Mental Issues in Aging Sourcebook, Women's Health Concerns Sourcebook*

■

Pain Sourcebook, 2nd Edition

Basic Consumer Health Information about Specific Forms of Acute and Chronic Pain, Including Muscle and Skeletal Pain, Nerve Pain, Cancer Pain, and Disorders Characterized by Pain, Such as Fibromyalgia, Shingles, Angina, Arthritis, and Headaches

Along with Information about Pain Medications and Management Techniques, Complementary and Alternative Pain Relief Options, Tips for People Living with Chronic Pain, a Glossary, and a Directory of Sources for Further Information

Edited by Karen Bellenir. 670 pages. 2002. 978-0-7808-0612-2.

"A source of valuable information. . . . This book offers help to nonmedical people who need information about pain and pain management. It is also an excellent reference for those who participate in patient education."
— *Doody's Review Service, Sep '02*

"Highly recommended for academic and medical reference collections." — *Library Bookwatch, Sep '02*

"The text is readable, easily understood, and well indexed. This excellent volume belongs in all patient education libraries, consumer health sections of public libraries, and many personal collections."
— *American Reference Books Annual, 1999*

"The information is basic in terms of scholarship and is appropriate for general readers. Written in journalistic style . . . intended for non-professionals. Quite thorough in its coverage of different pain conditions and summarizes the latest clinical information regarding pain treatment." — *Choice, Association of College and Research Libraries, Jun '98*

"Recommended reference source."
— *Booklist, American Library Association, Mar '98*

■

Pediatric Cancer Sourcebook

Basic Consumer Health Information about Leukemias, Brain Tumors, Sarcomas, Lymphomas, and Other Cancers in Infants, Children, and Adolescents, Including Descriptions of Cancers, Treatments, and Coping Strategies

Along with Suggestions for Parents, Caregivers, and Concerned Relatives, a Glossary of Cancer Terms, and Resource Listings

Edited by Edward J. Prucha. 587 pages. 1999. 978-0-7808-0245-2.

"An excellent source of information. Recommended for public, hospital, and health science libraries with consumer health collections." — *E-Streams, Jun '00*

"Recommended reference source."
— *Booklist, American Library Association, Feb '00*

"A valuable addition to all libraries specializing in health services and many public libraries."
— *American Reference Books Annual, 2000*

SEE ALSO *Childhood Diseases & Disorders Sourcebook, Healthy Children Sourcebook*

■

Physical & Mental Issues in Aging Sourcebook

Basic Consumer Health Information on Physical and Mental Disorders Associated with the Aging Process, Including Concerns about Cardiovascular Disease, Pulmonary Disease, Oral Health, Digestive Disorders, Musculoskeletal and Skin Disorders, Metabolic Changes, Sexual and Reproductive Issues, and Changes in Vision, Hearing, and Other Senses

Along with Data about Longevity and Causes of Death, Information on Acute and Chronic Pain, Descriptions of Mental Concerns, a Glossary of Terms, and Resource Listings for Additional Help

Edited by Jenifer Swanson. 660 pages. 1999. 978-0-7808-0233-9.

"This is a treasure of health information for the layperson." — *Choice Health Sciences Supplement, Association of College & Research Libraries, May '00*

"Recommended for public libraries."
— *American Reference Books Annual, 2000*

"Recommended reference source."
— *Booklist, American Library Association, Oct '99*

SEE ALSO *Healthy Aging Sourcebook*

■

Podiatry Sourcebook, 2nd Edition

Basic Consumer Health Information about Disorders, Diseases, Deformities, and Injuries that Affect the Foot and Ankle, Including Sprains, Corns, Calluses, Bunions, Plantar Warts, Plantar Fasciitis, Neuromas, Clubfoot, Flat Feet, Achilles Tendonitis, and Much More

Along with Information about Selecting a Foot Care Specialist, Foot Fitness, Shoes and Socks, Diagnostic Tests and Corrective Procedures, Financial Assistance for Corrective Devices, a Glossary of Related Terms, and a Directory of Resources for Additional Help and Information

Edited by Ivy L. Alexander. 543 pages. 2007. 978-0-7808-0944-4.

"Recommended reference source."
— Booklist, American Library Association, Feb '02

"There is a lot of information presented here on a topic that is usually only covered sparingly in most larger comprehensive medical encyclopedias."
— American Reference Books Annual, 2002

■

Pregnancy & Birth Sourcebook, 2nd Edition

Basic Consumer Health Information about Conception and Pregnancy, Including Facts about Fertility, Infertility, Pregnancy Symptoms and Complications, Fetal Growth and Development, Labor, Delivery, and the Postpartum Period, as Well as Information about Maintaining Health and Wellness during Pregnancy and Caring for a Newborn

Along with Information about Public Health Assistance for Low-Income Pregnant Women, a Glossary, and Directories of Agencies and Organizations Providing Help and Support

Edited by Amy L. Sutton. 626 pages. 2004. 978-0-7808-0672-6.

"Will appeal to public and school reference collections strong in medicine and women's health. . . . Deserves a spot on any medical reference shelf."
— The Bookwatch, Jul '04

"A well-organized handbook. Recommended."
— Choice, Association of College & Research Libraries, Apr '98

"Recommended reference source."
— Booklist, American Library Association, Mar '98

"Recommended for public libraries."
— American Reference Books Annual, 1998

SEE ALSO Breastfeeding Sourcebook, Congenital Disorders Sourcebook, Family Planning Sourcebook

■

Prostate & Urological Disorders Sourcebook

Basic Consumer Health Information about Urogenital and Sexual Disorders in Men, Including Prostate and Other Andrological Cancers, Prostatitis, Benign Prostatic Hyperplasia, Testicular and Penile Trauma, Cryptorchidism, Peyronie Disease, Erectile Dysfunction, and Male Factor Infertility, and Facts about Commonly Used Tests and Procedures, Such as Prostatectomy, Vasectomy, Vasectomy Reversal, Penile Implants, and Semen Analysis

Along with a Glossary of Andrological Terms and a Directory of Resources for Additional Information

Edited by Karen Bellenir. 631 pages. 2005. 978-0-7808-0797-6.

Prostate Cancer Sourcebook

Basic Consumer Health Information about Prostate Cancer, Including Information about the Associated Risk Factors, Detection, Diagnosis, and Treatment of Prostate Cancer

Along with Information on Non-Malignant Prostate Conditions, and Featuring a Section Listing Support and Treatment Centers and a Glossary of Related Terms

Edited by Dawn D. Matthews. 358 pages. 2001. 978-0-7808-0324-4.

"Recommended reference source."
— Booklist, American Library Association, Jan '02

"A valuable resource for health care consumers seeking information on the subject. . . . All text is written in a clear, easy-to-understand language that avoids technical jargon. Any library that collects consumer health resources would strengthen their collection with the addition of the Prostate Cancer Sourcebook."
— American Reference Books Annual, 2002

SEE ALSO Men's Health Concerns Sourcebook

■

Reconstructive & Cosmetic Surgery Sourcebook

Basic Consumer Health Information on Cosmetic and Reconstructive Plastic Surgery, Including Statistical Information about Different Surgical Procedures, Things to Consider Prior to Surgery, Plastic Surgery Techniques and Tools, Emotional and Psychological Considerations, and Procedure-Specific Information

Along with a Glossary of Terms and a Listing of Resources for Additional Help and Information

Edited by M. Lisa Weatherford. 374 pages. 2001. 978-0-7808-0214-8.

"An excellent reference that addresses cosmetic and medically necessary reconstructive surgeries. . . . The style of the prose is calm and reassuring, discussing the many positive outcomes now available due to advances in surgical techniques."
— American Reference Books Annual, 2002

"Recommended for health science libraries that are open to the public, as well as hospital libraries that are open to the patients. This book is a good resource for the consumer interested in plastic surgery."
— E-Streams, Dec '01

"Recommended reference source."
— Booklist, American Library Association, Jul '01

■

Rehabilitation Sourcebook

Basic Consumer Health Information about Rehabilitation for People Recovering from Heart Surgery, Spinal Cord Injury, Stroke, Orthopedic Impairments, Amputation, Pulmonary Impairments, Traumatic Injury, and More, Including Physical Therapy, Occupational Therapy, Speech/Language Therapy, Massage Therapy, Dance Therapy, Art Therapy, and Recreational Therapy

Along with Information on Assistive and Adaptive Devices, a Glossary, and Resources for Additional Help and Information

Edited by Dawn D. Matthews. 531 pages. 1999. 978-0-7808-0236-0.

"This is an excellent resource for public library reference and health collections."
— American Reference Books Annual, 2001

"Recommended reference source."
— Booklist, American Library Association, May '00

Respiratory Diseases & Disorders Sourcebook

Basic Information about Respiratory Diseases and Disorders, Including Asthma, Cystic Fibrosis, Pneumonia, the Common Cold, Influenza, and Others, Featuring Facts about the Respiratory System, Statistical and Demographic Data, Treatments, Self-Help Management Suggestions, and Current Research Initiatives

Edited by Allan R. Cook and Peter D. Dresser. 771 pages. 1995. 978-0-7808-0037-3.

"Designed for the layperson and for patients and their families coping with respiratory illness. . . . an extensive array of information on diagnosis, treatment, management, and prevention of respiratory illnesses for the general reader." — Choice, Association of College & Research Libraries, Jun '96

"A highly recommended text for all collections. It is a comforting reminder of the power of knowledge that good books carry between their covers."
— Academic Library Book Review, Spring '96

"A comprehensive collection of authoritative information presented in a nontechnical, humanitarian style for patients, families, and caregivers."
—Association of Operating Room Nurses, Sep/Oct '95

SEE ALSO Lung Disorders Sourcebook

Sexually Transmitted Diseases Sourcebook, 3rd Edition

Basic Consumer Health Information about Chlamydial Infections, Gonorrhea, Hepatitis, Herpes, HIV/AIDS, Human Papillomavirus, Pubic Lice, Scabies, Syphilis, Trichomoniasis, Vaginal Infections, and Other Sexually Transmitted Diseases, Including Facts about Risk Factors, Symptoms, Diagnosis, Treatment, and the Prevention of Sexually Transmitted Infections

Along with Updates on Current Research Initiatives, a Glossary of Related Terms, and Resources for Additional Help and Information

Edited by Amy L. Sutton. 629 pages. 2006. 978-0-7808-0824-9.

"Recommended for consumer health collections in public libraries, and secondary school and community college libraries."
— American Reference Books Annual, 2002

"Every school and public library should have a copy of this comprehensive and user-friendly reference book."
— Choice, Association of College & Research Libraries, Sep '01

"This is a highly recommended book. This is an especially important book for all school and public libraries."
— AIDS Book Review Journal, Jul-Aug '01

"Recommended reference source."
— Booklist, American Library Association, Apr '01

Sleep Disorders Sourcebook, 2nd Edition

Basic Consumer Health Information about Sleep and Sleep Disorders, Including Insomnia, Sleep Apnea, Restless Legs Syndrome, Narcolepsy, Parasomnias, and Other Health Problems That Affect Sleep, Plus Facts about Diagnostic Procedures, Treatment Strategies, Sleep Medications, and Tips for Improving Sleep Quality

Along with a Glossary of Related Terms and Resources for Additional Help and Information

Edited by Amy L. Sutton. 567 pages. 2005. 978-0-7808-0743-3.

"This book will be useful for just about everybody, especially the 40 million Americans with sleep disorders."
— American Reference Books Annual, 2006

"Recommended for public libraries and libraries supporting health care professionals." — E-Streams, Sep '05

". . . key medical library acquisition."
— The Bookwatch, Jun '05

Smoking Concerns Sourcebook

Basic Consumer Health Information about Nicotine Addiction and Smoking Cessation, Featuring Facts about the Health Effects of Tobacco Use, Including Lung and Other Cancers, Heart Disease, Stroke, and Respiratory Disorders, Such as Emphysema and Chronic Bronchitis

Along with Information about Smoking Prevention Programs, Suggestions for Achieving and Maintaining a Smoke-Free Lifestyle, Statistics about Tobacco Use, Reports on Current Research Initiatives, a Glossary of Related Terms, and Directories of Resources for Additional Help and Information

Edited by Karen Bellenir. 621 pages. 2004. 978-0-7808-0323-7.

"Provides everything needed for the student or general reader seeking practical details on the effects of tobacco use." — The Bookwatch, Mar '05

"Public libraries and consumer health care libraries will find this work useful."
— American Reference Books Annual, 2005

Sports Injuries Sourcebook, 3rd Edition

Basic Consumer Health Information about Sprains and Strains, Fractures, Growth Plate Injuries, Overtraining Injuries, and Injuries to the Head, Face, Shoulders, Elbows, Hands, Spinal Column, Knees, Ankles, and Feet, and with Facts about Heat-Related Illness, Steroids and Sport Supplements, Protective Equipment, Diagnostic Procedures, Treatment Options, and Rehabilitation

Along with a Glossary of Related Terms and a Directory of Resources for Additional Help and Information

Edited by Sandra J. Judd. 651 pages. 2007. 978-0-7808-0949-9.

"This is an excellent reference for consumers and it is recommended for public, community college, and undergraduate libraries."
— *American Reference Books Annual, 2003*

"Recommended reference source."
— *Booklist, American Library Association, Feb '03*

Stress-Related Disorders Sourcebook

Basic Consumer Health Information about Stress and Stress-Related Disorders, Including Stress Origins and Signals, Environmental Stress at Work and Home, Mental and Emotional Stress Associated with Depression, Post-Traumatic Stress Disorder, Panic Disorder, Suicide, and the Physical Effects of Stress on the Cardiovascular, Immune, and Nervous Systems

Along with Stress Management Techniques, a Glossary, and a Listing of Additional Resources

Edited by Joyce Brennfleck Shannon. 610 pages. 2002. 978-0-7808-0560-6.

"Well written for a general readership, the *Stress-Related Disorders Sourcebook* is a useful addition to the health reference literature."
— *American Reference Books Annual, 2003*

"I am impressed by the amount of information. It offers a thorough overview of the causes and consequences of stress for the layperson. . . . A well-done and thorough reference guide for professionals and nonprofessionals alike."
— *Doody's Review Service, Dec '02*

Stroke Sourcebook

Basic Consumer Health Information about Stroke, Including Ischemic, Hemorrhagic, Transient Ischemic Attack (TIA), and Pediatric Stroke, Stroke Triggers and Risks, Diagnostic Tests, Treatments, and Rehabilitation Information

Along with Stroke Prevention Guidelines, Legal and Financial Information, a Glossary, and a Directory of Additional Resources

Edited by Joyce Brennfleck Shannon. 606 pages. 2003. 978-0-7808-0630-6.

"This volume is highly recommended and should be in every medical, hospital, and public library."
— *American Reference Books Annual, 2004*

"Highly recommended for the amount and variety of topics and information covered." — *Choice, Nov '03*

Surgery Sourcebook

Basic Consumer Health Information about Inpatient and Outpatient Surgeries, Including Cardiac, Vascular, Orthopedic, Ocular, Reconstructive, Cosmetic, Gynecologic, and Ear, Nose, and Throat Procedures and More

Along with Information about Operating Room Policies and Instruments, Laser Surgery Techniques, Hospital Errors, Statistical Data, a Glossary, and Listings of Sources for Further Help and Information

Edited by Annemarie S. Muth and Karen Bellenir. 596 pages. 2002. 978-0-7808-0380-0.

"Large public libraries and medical libraries would benefit from this material in their reference collections."
— *American Reference Books Annual, 2004*

"Invaluable reference for public and school library collections alike." — *Library Bookwatch, Apr '03*

Thyroid Disorders Sourcebook

Basic Consumer Health Information about Disorders of the Thyroid and Parathyroid Glands, Including Hypothyroidism, Hyperthyroidism, Graves Disease, Hashimoto Thyroiditis, Thyroid Cancer, and Parathyroid Disorders, Featuring Facts about Symptoms, Risk Factors, Tests, and Treatments

Along with Information about the Effects of Thyroid Imbalance on Other Body Systems, Environmental Factors That Affect the Thyroid Gland, a Glossary, and a Directory of Additional Resources

Edited by Joyce Brennfleck Shannon. 599 pages. 2005. 978-0-7808-0745-7.

"Recommended for consumer health collections."
— *American Reference Books Annual, 2006*

"Highly recommended pick for basic consumer health reference holdings at all levels."
— *The Bookwatch, Aug '05*

Transplantation Sourcebook

Basic Consumer Health Information about Organ and Tissue Transplantation, Including Physical and Financial Preparations, Procedures and Issues Relating to Specific Solid Organ and Tissue Transplants, Rehabilitation, Pediatric Transplant Information, the Future of Transplantation, and Organ and Tissue Donation

Along with a Glossary and Listings of Additional Resources

Edited by Joyce Brennfleck Shannon. 628 pages. 2002. 978-0-7808-0322-0.

"Along with these advances [in transplantation technology] have come a number of daunting questions for potential transplant patients, their families, and their health care providers. This reference text is the best single tool to address many of these questions. . . . It will be a much-needed addition to the reference collections in health care, academic, and large public libraries."
— *American Reference Books Annual, 2003*

"Recommended for libraries with an interest in offering consumer health information." — *E-Streams, Jul '02*

"This is a unique and valuable resource for patients facing transplantation and their families."
— *Doody's Review Service, Jun '02*

■

Traveler's Health Sourcebook

Basic Consumer Health Information for Travelers, Including Physical and Medical Preparations, Transportation Health and Safety, Essential Information about Food and Water, Sun Exposure, Insect and Snake Bites, Camping and Wilderness Medicine, and Travel with Physical or Medical Disabilities

Along with International Travel Tips, Vaccination Recommendations, Geographical Health Issues, Disease Risks, a Glossary, and a Listing of Additional Resources

Edited by Joyce Brennfleck Shannon. 613 pages. 2000. 978-0-7808-0384-8.

"Recommended reference source."
— *Booklist, American Library Association, Feb '01*

"This book is recommended for any public library, any travel collection, and especially any collection for the physically disabled."
— *American Reference Books Annual, 2001*

SEE ALSO *Worldwide Health Sourcebook*

■

Urinary Tract & Kidney Diseases & Disorders Sourcebook, 2nd Edition

Basic Consumer Health Information about the Urinary System, Including the Bladder, Urethra, Ureters, and Kidneys, with Facts about Urinary Tract Infections, Incontinence, Congenital Disorders, Kidney Stones, Cancers of the Urinary Tract and Kidneys, Kidney Failure, Dialysis, and Kidney Transplantation

Along with Statistical and Demographic Information, Reports on Current Research in Kidney and Urologic Health, a Summary of Commonly Used Diagnostic Tests, a Glossary of Related Terms, and a Directory of Resources for Additional Help and Information

Edited by Ivy L. Alexander. 649 pages. 2005. 978-0-7808-0750-1.

"A good choice for a consumer health information library or for a medical library needing information to refer to their patients."
— *American Reference Books Annual, 2006*

Vegetarian Sourcebook

Basic Consumer Health Information about Vegetarian Diets, Lifestyle, and Philosophy, Including Definitions of Vegetarianism and Veganism, Tips about Adopting Vegetarianism, Creating a Vegetarian Pantry, and Meeting Nutritional Needs of Vegetarians, with Facts Regarding Vegetarianism's Effect on Pregnant and Lactating Women, Children, Athletes, and Senior Citizens

Along with a Glossary of Commonly Used Vegetarian Terms and Resources for Additional Help and Information

Edited by Chad T. Kimball. 360 pages. 2002. 978-0-7808-0439-5.

"Organizes into one concise volume the answers to the most common questions concerning vegetarian diets and lifestyles. This title is recommended for public and secondary school libraries." — *E-Streams, Apr '03*

"Invaluable reference for public and school library collections alike." — *Library Bookwatch, Apr '03*

"The articles in this volume are easy to read and come from authoritative sources. The book does not necessarily support the vegetarian diet but instead provides the pros and cons of this important decision. The Vegetarian Sourcebook is recommended for public libraries and consumer health libraries."
— *American Reference Books Annual, 2003*

SEE ALSO *Diet & Nutrition Sourcebook*

■

Women's Health Concerns Sourcebook, 2nd Edition

Basic Consumer Health Information about the Medical and Mental Concerns of Women, Including Maintaining Health and Wellness, Gynecological Concerns, Breast Health, Sexuality and Reproductive Issues, Menopause, Cancer in Women, Leading Causes of Death and Disability among Women, Physical Concerns of Special Significance to Women, and Women's Mental and Emotional Health

Along with a Glossary of Related Terms and Directories of Resources for Additional Help and Information

Edited by Amy L. Sutton. 746 pages. 2004. 978-0-7808-0673-3.

"This is a useful reference book, which makes the reader knowledgeable about several issues that concern women's health. It is recommended for public libraries and home library collections." — *E-Streams, May '05*

"A useful addition to public and consumer health library collections."
— *American Reference Books Annual, 2005*

"A highly recommended title."
— *The Bookwatch, May '04*

"Handy compilation. There is an impressive range of diseases, devices, disorders, procedures, and other physical and emotional issues covered . . . well organized, illustrated, and indexed." — *Choice, Association of College & Research Libraries, Jan '98*

SEE ALSO *Breast Cancer Sourcebook, Cancer Sourcebook for Women, Healthy Heart Sourcebook for Women, Osteoporosis Sourcebook*

Workplace Health & Safety Sourcebook

Basic Consumer Health Information about Workplace Health and Safety, Including the Effect of Workplace Hazards on the Lungs, Heart, Ears, Eyes, Brain, Reproductive Organs, Musculoskeletal System, and Other Organs and Body Parts

Along with Information about Occupational Cancer, Personal Protective Equipment, Toxic and Hazardous Chemicals, Child Labor, Stress, and Workplace Violence

Edited by Chad T. Kimball. 626 pages. 2000. 978-0-7808-0231-5.

"As a reference for the general public, this would be useful in any library."   —*E-Streams, Jun '01*

"Provides helpful information for primary care physicians and other caregivers interested in occupational medicine. . . . General readers; professionals."
       —*Choice, Association of College & Research Libraries, May '01*

"Recommended reference source."
       —*Booklist, American Library Association, Feb '01*

"Highly recommended."   —*The Bookwatch, Jan '01*

Worldwide Health Sourcebook

Basic Information about Global Health Issues, Including Malnutrition, Reproductive Health, Disease Dispersion and Prevention, Emerging Diseases, Risky Health Behaviors, and the Leading Causes of Death

Along with Global Health Concerns for Children, Women, and the Elderly, Mental Health Issues, Research and Technology Advancements, and Economic, Environmental, and Political Health Implications, a Glossary, and a Resource Listing for Additional Help and Information

Edited by Joyce Brennfleck Shannon. 614 pages. 2001. 978-0-7808-0330-5.

"Named an Outstanding Academic Title."
       —*Choice, Association of College & Research Libraries, Jan '02*

"Yet another handy but also unique compilation in the extensive *Health Reference Series,* this is a useful work because many of the international publications reprinted or excerpted are not readily available. Highly recommended."   —*Choice, Association of College & Research Libraries, Nov '01*

"Recommended reference source."
       —*Booklist, American Library Association, Oct '01*

SEE ALSO *Traveler's Health Sourcebook*

Teen Health Series
Helping Young Adults Understand, Manage, and Avoid Serious Illness

List price $65 per volume. **School and library price $58 per volume.**

Alcohol Information for Teens
Health Tips about Alcohol and Alcoholism
Including Facts about Underage Drinking, Preventing Teen Alcohol Use, Alcohol's Effects on the Brain and the Body, Alcohol Abuse Treatment, Help for Children of Alcoholics, and More

Edited by Joyce Brennfleck Shannon. 370 pages. 2005. 978-0-7808-0741-9.

"Boxed facts and tips add visual interest to the well-researched and clearly written text."
— *Curriculum Connection, Apr '06*

Allergy Information for Teens
Health Tips about Allergic Reactions Such as Anaphylaxis, Respiratory Problems, and Rashes
Including Facts about Identifying and Managing Allergies to Food, Pollen, Mold, Animals, Chemicals, Drugs, and Other Substances

Edited by Karen Bellenir. 410 pages. 2006. 978-0-7808-0799-0.

Asthma Information for Teens
Health Tips about Managing Asthma and Related Concerns
Including Facts about Asthma Causes, Triggers, Symptoms, Diagnosis, and Treatment

Edited by Karen Bellenir. 386 pages. 2005. 978-0-7808-0770-9.

"Highly recommended for medical libraries, public school libraries, and public libraries."
— *American Reference Books Annual, 2006*

"It is so clearly written and well organized that even hesitant readers will be able to find the facts they need, whether for reports or personal information. . . . A succinct but complete resource."
— *School Library Journal, Sep '05*

Body Information for Teens
Health Tips about Maintaining Well-Being for a Lifetime
Including Facts about the Development and Functioning of the Body's Systems, Organs, and Structures and the Health Impact of Lifestyle Choices

Edited by Sandra Augustyn Lawton. 458 pages. 2007. 978-0-7808-0443-2.

Cancer Information for Teens
Health Tips about Cancer Awareness, Prevention, Diagnosis, and Treatment
Including Facts about Frequently Occurring Cancers, Cancer Risk Factors, and Coping Strategies for Teens Fighting Cancer or Dealing with Cancer in Friends or Family Members

Edited by Wilma R. Caldwell. 428 pages. 2004. 978-0-7808-0678-8.

"Recommended for school libraries, or consumer libraries that see a lot of use by teens."
— *E-Streams, May '05*

"A valuable educational tool."
— *American Reference Books Annual, 2005*

"Young adults and their parents alike will find this new addition to the *Teen Health Series* an important reference to cancer in teens."
— *Children's Bookwatch, Feb '05*

Complementary and Alternative Medicine Information for Teens
Health Tips about Non-Traditional and Non-Western Medical Practices
Including Information about Acupuncture, Chiropractic Medicine, Dietary and Herbal Supplements, Hypnosis, Massage Therapy, Prayer and Spirituality, Reflexology, Yoga, and More

Edited by Sandra Augustyn Lawton. 405 pages. 2006. 978-0-7808-0966-6.

Diabetes Information for Teens
Health Tips about Managing Diabetes and Preventing Related Complications
Including Information about Insulin, Glucose Control, Healthy Eating, Physical Activity, and Learning to Live with Diabetes

Edited by Sandra Augustyn Lawton. 410 pages. 2006. 978-0-7808-0811-9.

Diet Information for Teens, 2nd Edition

Health Tips about Diet and Nutrition

Including Facts about Dietary Guidelines, Food Groups, Nutrients, Healthy Meals, Snacks, Weight Control, Medical Concerns Related to Diet, and More

Edited by Karen Bellenir. 432 pages. 2006. 978-0-7808-0820-1.

"Full of helpful insights and facts throughout the book. . . . An excellent resource to be placed in public libraries or even in personal collections."
— *American Reference Books Annual, 2002*

"Recommended for middle and high school libraries and media centers as well as academic libraries that educate future teachers of teenagers. It is also a suitable addition to health science libraries that serve patrons who are interested in teen health promotion and education."
— *E-Streams, Oct '01*

"This comprehensive book would be beneficial to collections that need information about nutrition, dietary guidelines, meal planning, and weight control. . . . This reference is so easy to use that its purchase is recommended."
— *The Book Report, Sep-Oct '01*

"This book is written in an easy to understand format describing issues that many teens face every day, and then provides thoughtful explanations so that teens can make informed decisions. This is an interesting book that provides important facts and information for today's teens."
— *Doody's Health Sciences Book Review Journal, Jul-Aug '01*

"A comprehensive compendium of diet and nutrition. The information is presented in a straightforward, plain-spoken manner. This title will be useful to those working on reports on a variety of topics, as well as to general readers concerned about their dietary health."
— *School Library Journal, Jun '01*

Drug Information for Teens, 2nd Edition

Health Tips about the Physical and Mental Effects of Substance Abuse

Including Information about Marijuana, Inhalants, Club Drugs, Stimulants, Hallucinogens, Opiates, Prescription and Over-the-Counter Drugs, Herbal Products, Tobacco, Alcohol, and More

Edited by Sandra Augustyn Lawton. 468 pages. 2006. 978-0-7808-0862-1.

"A clearly written resource for general readers and researchers alike."
— *School Library Journal*

"This book is well-balanced. . . . a must for public and school libraries."
— *VOYA: Voice of Youth Advocates, Dec '03*

"The chapters are quick to make a connection to their teenage reading audience. The prose is straightforward and the book lends itself to spot reading. It should be useful both for practical information and for research, and it is suitable for public and school libraries."
— *American Reference Books Annual, 2003*

"Recommended reference source."
— *Booklist, American Library Association, Feb '03*

"This is an excellent resource for teens and their parents. Education about drugs and substances is key to discouraging teen drug abuse and this book provides this much needed information in a way that is interesting and factual."
— *Doody's Review Service, Dec '02*

Eating Disorders Information for Teens

Health Tips about Anorexia, Bulimia, Binge Eating, and Other Eating Disorders

Including Information on the Causes, Prevention, and Treatment of Eating Disorders, and Such Other Issues as Maintaining Healthy Eating and Exercise Habits

Edited by Sandra Augustyn Lawton. 337 pages. 2005. 978-0-7808-0783-9.

"An excellent resource for teens and those who work with them."
— *VOYA: Voice of Youth Advocates, Apr '06*

"A welcome addition to high school and undergraduate libraries." — *American Reference Books Annual, 2006*

"This book covers the topic in a lucid manner but delves deeper into every aspect of an eating disorder. A solid addition for any nonfiction or reference collection."
— *School Library Journal, Dec '05*

Fitness Information for Teens

Health Tips about Exercise, Physical Well-Being, and Health Maintenance

Including Facts about Aerobic and Anaerobic Conditioning, Stretching, Body Shape and Body Image, Sports Training, Nutrition, and Activities for Non-Athletes

Edited by Karen Bellenir. 425 pages. 2004. 978-0-7808-0679-5.

"Another excellent offering from Omnigraphics in their *Teen Health Series*. . . . This book will be a great addition to any public, junior high, senior high, or secondary school library."
— *American Reference Books Annual, 2005*

Learning Disabilities Information for Teens

Health Tips about Academic Skills Disorders and Other Disabilities That Affect Learning

Including Information about Common Signs of Learning Disabilities, School Issues, Learning to Live with a Learning Disability, and Other Related Issues

Edited by Sandra Augustyn Lawton. 337 pages. 2005. 978-0-7808-0796-9.

"This book provides a wealth of information for any reader interested in the signs, causes, and consequences

of learning disabilities, as well as related legal rights and educational interventions. . . . Public and academic libraries should want this title for both students and general readers."
— *American Reference Books Annual, 2006*

Mental Health Information for Teens, 2nd Edition

Health Tips about Mental Wellness and Mental Illness

Including Facts about Mental and Emotional Health, Depression and Other Mood Disorders, Anxiety Disorders, Behavior Disorders, Self-Injury, Psychosis, Schizophrenia, and More

Edited by Karen Bellenir. 400 pages. 2006. 978-0-7808-0863-8.

"In both language and approach, this user-friendly entry in the *Teen Health Series* is on target for teens needing information on mental health concerns."
— *Booklist, American Library Association, Jan '02*

"Readers will find the material accessible and informative, with the shaded notes, facts, and embedded glossary insets adding appropriately to the already interesting and succinct presentation."
— *School Library Journal, Jan '02*

"This title is highly recommended for any library that serves adolescents and parents/caregivers of adolescents."
— *E-Streams, Jan '02*

"Recommended for high school libraries and young adult collections in public libraries. Both health professionals and teenagers will find this book useful."
— *American Reference Books Annual, 2002*

"This is a nice book written to enlighten the society, primarily teenagers, about common teen mental health issues. It is highly recommended to teachers and parents as well as adolescents."
— *Doody's Review Service, Dec '01*

Sexual Health Information for Teens

Health Tips about Sexual Development, Human Reproduction, and Sexually Transmitted Diseases

Including Facts about Puberty, Reproductive Health, Chlamydia, Human Papillomavirus, Pelvic Inflammatory Disease, Herpes, AIDS, Contraception, Pregnancy, and More

Edited by Deborah A. Stanley. 391 pages. 2003. 978-0-7808-0445-6.

"This work should be included in all high school libraries and many larger public libraries. . . . highly recommended."
— *American Reference Books Annual, 2004*

"*Sexual Health* approaches its subject with appropriate seriousness and offers easily accessible advice and information."
— *School Library Journal, Feb '04*

Skin Health Information for Teens

Health Tips about Dermatological Concerns and Skin Cancer Risks

Including Facts about Acne, Warts, Hives, and Other Conditions and Lifestyle Choices, Such as Tanning, Tattooing, and Piercing, That Affect the Skin, Nails, Scalp, and Hair

Edited by Robert Aquinas McNally. 429 pages. 2003. 978-0-7808-0446-3.

"This volume, as with others in the series, will be a useful addition to school and public library collections." — *American Reference Books Annual, 2004*

"There is no doubt that this reference tool is valuable."
— *VOYA: Voice of Youth Advocates, Feb '04*

"This volume serves as a one-stop source and should be a necessity for any health collection."
— *Library Media Connection*

Sports Injuries Information for Teens

Health Tips about Sports Injuries and Injury Protection

Including Facts about Specific Injuries, Emergency Treatment, Rehabilitation, Sports Safety, Competition Stress, Fitness, Sports Nutrition, Steroid Risks, and More

Edited by Joyce Brennfleck Shannon. 405 pages. 2003. 978-0-7808-0447-0.

"This work will be useful in the young adult collections of public libraries as well as high school libraries."
— *American Reference Books Annual, 2004*

Suicide Information for Teens

Health Tips about Suicide Causes and Prevention

Including Facts about Depression, Risk Factors, Getting Help, Survivor Support, and More

Edited by Joyce Brennfleck Shannon. 368 pages. 2005. 978-0-7808-0737-2.

Tobacco Information for Teens

Health Tips about the Hazards of Using Cigarettes, Smokeless Tobacco, and Other Nicotine Products

Including Facts about Nicotine Addiction, Immediate and Long-Term Health Effects of Tobacco Use, Related Cancers, Smoking Cessation, Tobacco Use Prevention, and Tobacco Use Statistics

Edited by Karen Bellenir. 440 pages. 2007. 978-0-7808-0976-5.

Health Reference Series